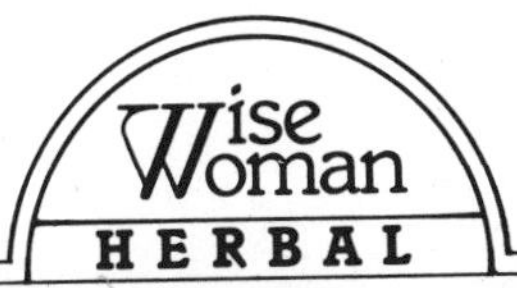

HEALING WISE

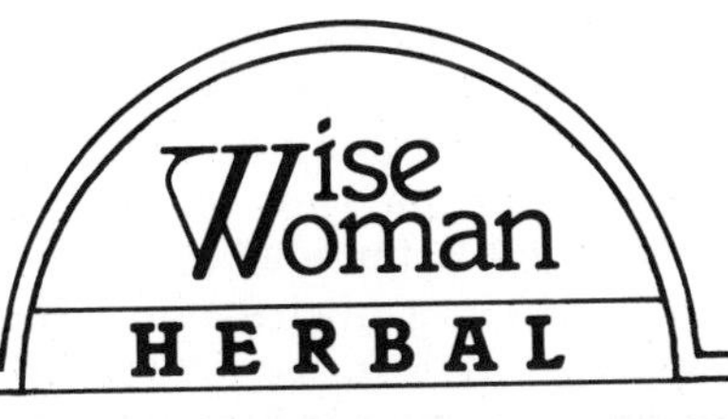

HEALING WISE

Susun S. Weed

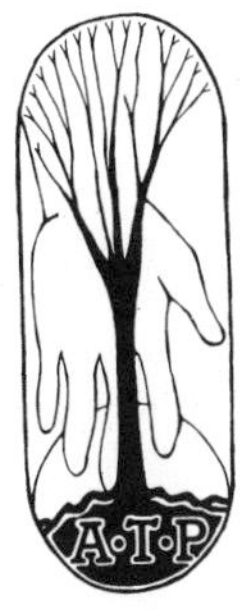

Ash Tree Publishing
Woodstock, New York

All information in the *Wise Woman Herbal* is based on the experiences and research of the author and other professional healers. This information is shared with the understanding that you accept complete responsibility for your own health and well-being. You have a unique body and the action of each herbal medicine is unique and health care is full of variables. The result of any treatment suggested herein cannot always be anticipated and never guaranteed. The author and publisher are not responsible for any adverse effects or consequences resulting from the use of any remedies, procedures, or preparations included in this *Wise Woman Herbal*. Consult your inner guidance, knowledgeable friends, and trained healers in addition to the words written here.

Ash Tree Publishing, PO Box 64, Woodstock, NY 12498.

Illustrations on pages xii-xiii, 1, 4, 6, 7, 10, 11, 14, 16, 23, 28-29, 30, 42-46, 60, 61, 70, 82-83, 88, 112, 120, 130, 141, 149, 164, 180, 192, 212, 213, 236, 239, 254-255, 274-278 by Toni Bernhard.

All other illustrations, and fairies throughout, by Susun Weed.

Green Ally titles, pages 86, 111, 129, 163, 191, 211, and 235:
design: Toni Bernhard
calligraphy: Alan McKnight
fairies & additions: Susun Weed.

Cover design by Janet Woodman.

Cover art by Alan McKnight.

Library of Congress Catalog Card Number: 89-084619

ISBN 0-9614620-2-7

May the seven directions empower this medicine work.
May it be pleasing to my grandmothers, the ancient ones.
And may it be of benefit to all beings.

So mote it be.

Acknowledgements

My heart overflows with gratitude for the joy, care, and energy that so many people gave to this project.

My nostalgic thanks to Peter Blum, Maria Dolores Hajosy, Cyndi Heath, Jane Poehler, Haleya Priest, and Janet Woodman for their help in the early stages.

My consistent and punctual thanks to Cynthia Werthamer and Betsy Grace Sandlin for vigilant editing, and to Kent Babcock for compassionate typesetting.

My graphic thanks to Toni Bernhard for her magical interior illustrations, to Alan McKnight for his glorious cover watercolor and exquisite calligraphic plant names, and to Mark Poole for his attentive camera work.

My spiralic thanks to the Wise Woman herbalists who reviewed the Green Allies: Robin Bennett, Jane Bothwell, Ryan Drum, Jane LaForce, Rosemary Gladstar, Cascade Anderson-Geller, Ellen Greenlaw, Mara Levin, Deborah Maia, Brigitte Mars, Pam Montgomery, Carol Petherbridge, Pela Sander, Deb Soule, Sher Willis, and Wren; and to Laura O'Banion, MD, for reviewing the entire manuscript.

My mythic thanks to Jean Houston, mentor, guide, and Athena to my Artemis.

My orderly thanks to Peg Goddard for paste-up and to Barry Koffler for indexing.

My bucolic thanks to those special friends and loves who tended to me while I devoted myself to "Healing Wise": Veronica Daggett, Kim Gormley, Estherelke Kaplan, Chuck Orenic, Justine Swede, and Ellen Weaver.

My ecstatic thanks to my consort, Michael Dattorre, who helped me nourish this child of love.

And my thanks, as well, to the trees, who have given their substance that you might hold this book.

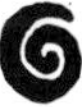

Contents

Introduction viii

Foreword x

The Image xii

Notes on My Way xiv

PART I: **Traditions of Healing** 1

WISE WOMAN *ways nourish spiraling transformations* 5

HEROIC *ways cleanse the spirit's dirty temple* 47

SCIENTIFIC *ways fix the measurable machine/body* 61

SPIRALS OF TRANSFORMATION *put it all in perspective* 74

Chart of the Healing Traditions 2–3

Medicine Wheel of the Wise Woman Tradition 81

PART II: **Green Allies and Deep Roots** 83

BURDOCK: *"Get down!"* 86

CHICKWEED: *The Little Star Lady* 111

DANDELION: *"Doctor Dent-de-leon, s'il vous plaît"* 129

NETTLE: *"Pay attention"* 163

OATSTRAW: *Secret Sexy Goddess Reveals All* 191

SEAWEEDS: *The Salt of Life* 211

VIOLET: *Sweet (Shy) Aunt Vi* 235

Herbal Pharmacy 255

Glossary 279

Index 285

Recipe Index 295

Introduction

A wise woman of my acquaintance, a tiny and intense Italian *strega,* peers into the murkiness of the immediate future and announces with operatic bravado that we humans have, at most, fifteen years to create the big turnaround of healing and wholing ourselves and our planet. That's the time frame, she swears, and unless we make the massive changes of mind and body, brain and spirit, to enact the required transitions from disaster and devastation to nurturing and balance, this beautiful planet, her human children and perhaps all living things as we know them, will be lost. And physicist Max Bjorn's painful assessment will have proven true: that Nature's attempt to evolve a thinking creature on this earth has failed.

On a more positive note, however, possibilities, plans, and hopes for making the necessary changes in person and in our personal relationships to our earth are vigorously alive. In fact, the planet herself feels more and more alive, molding us into skillful partners of her processes, willing us to relearn her ancient mysteries and share them through the gracing of those whom she claims most deeply as her daughters and sons.

One such Earth Daughter, perhaps the most vivid and original of my acquaintance, is Susun Weed. The secrets she is willing to share, through her role as keeper of the Wise Woman tradition, are among those which can reawaken us to a new understanding of health and earth/body wisdom.

Susun frankly and provocatively offers the Wise Woman way of life as a healing alternative to the body-alienating, body-objectifying methods she describes as the Scientific and Heroic traditions.

Inviting us to nestle into her sense of union with the earth, Susun engages us in learning to perceive health and wholeness as the essence of any condition and teaches the questions of "how" and "what" instead of "why" as the real issues to ponder when we seek healing wisdom.

She gives us a renewed sense of the power of true enabling, working, as she says the wise woman does, from the center of the void, which she feels is the place of female energy. In fact, her entire description of the Way of the Wise Woman is refreshing, courageous, and clear. One feels after reading it that one has raced through tall meadow grasses to the top of a high hill and been wrestled to the ground by three happy Airedales.

But Susun saves her wildest whimsy and most extensive explorations—dare I say her most scientific understanding?—for her detailed discussions of the Mother's gifts, in the form of the plants with which she works. The plants talk to us, sing to us, tell us stories. We are treated to rich descriptions of the powers each plant embodies, if we are thoughtful and caring enough to harvest and work with them appropriately.

Susun offers us her understanding that the way to learn a plant fully and deeply is to live with it for a year, in all weathers, in all variations of daylight and starlight. Working with her book in the same manner will also grant you the Yeargiftings of Nature's Way.

Jean Houston, PhD
March 1989

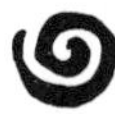

Foreword

Healing Wise nourishes. Healing Wise springs from love. Healing Wise flows through compassion. Healing Wise is as natural as birth, as certain as death. Healing Wise is the joy of the individual and the strength of the community.

If you think the only health care options are the established, scientific way, and alternative methods, it is because the third—an intuitive, individualized way, the unique Wise Woman way—is invisible.

Healing Wise is done with the eyes. Healing Wise is done by hand. Healing Wise is charged with meaning. Healing Wise is in tune with the seasons. Healing Wise is wholing and holy. Healing Wise is letting go. Healing Wise is timing.

Most of the health caring done world-wide, and most of the health care in your own life, is part of this third, invisible tradition.

Healing Wise the ancient ones know. Healing Wise speaks the truth. Healing Wise walks in beauty. Healing Wise says **you** are the beloved child of the universe. Healing Wise is a deep-rooted oak tree. Healing Wise is a waterfall. Healing Wise is full of smells. Healing Wise is an awe-full mess. Healing Wise is often earthy. Healing Wise is real.

Why do I give words to this invisible, this hard-to-know Wise Woman way? It is time now to see with clarity and wisdom, as crones have always seen.

Healing Wise is green, gold, glancing, rainbows sparkling dancing.

The Wise Woman way heals the planet as well as the people. It is time now for us all to remember how this can be. Time for us to be fully conscious of our choices for ourselves and for our Earth.

Healing Wise is right at your doorstep. Healing Wise is your granny's memories. Healing Wise requires effort. Healing Wise knows change. Healing Wise honors transformation. Healing Wise allows perfection.

The Wise Woman tradition of health care focuses on prevention and on remedies which are accessible, inexpensive, effective, and safe. It is time now for us to recognize and support the wise old woman in ourselves, our communities, and the global village.

Healing Wise lives inside you. Healing Wise is fun. Healing Wise is a clear course through turbulent waters. Healing Wise: the way of the wise one. Healing Wise: the Wise Woman ways.

The Wise Woman tradition of healing is the thread out of our current medical/legal maze and into heartfelt, wise use of our life resources, with respect for all life and all people. It is time now for us to trust this thread, to name it and claim it. *Healing Wise* does this.

Healing Wise, the second in my Wise Woman Herbal series, is about the Wise Woman tradition: a way to help us all name, claim, know, acknowledge, recognize, support, and nourish the wise woman within, wherever we see her.

Healing Wise identifies and explains the three traditions of healing: Wise Woman (spiralic), Heroic (cyclical), and Scientific (linear). Understanding the nature of each tradition will help you choose the health care helpers most supportive of your own motivations and health goals. Understanding the viewpoint of each tradition will help you make sense out of conflicting claims about the validity of specific healing substances and procedures.

Healing Wise introduces you to green allies, so you can choose a friend or two to help you through. Each herb talks to you, tells you tales, reveals her uses, and gives you remedies and recipes. Before you know it, the green leaves of chickweed, dandelion, violet, nettle, oats, and seaweeds will be your daily supporters. And, with a bit of effort, you'll have the deep roots of dandelion and burdock to lend a hand when times are hard. It's such a pleasure to share some of my most beloved friends with you.

Here then is *Healing Wise*, my thanks to the midwives, clowns, artists, storytellers, cooks, mothers, musicians, farmers, herbalists, healers, doctors, and lovers who have shared their lives and wisdoms with me. Here then is *Healing Wise,* my give-away to the health/wholeness/holiness of our planet and every being on it.

(The first book in this series, *Wise Woman Herbal for the Childbearing Year,* is available for $11.95 postpaid from Ash Tree Publishing, PO Box 64, Woodstock, NY 12498. It is also available in German through Orlanda Frauenverlag.)

SSW
April '89

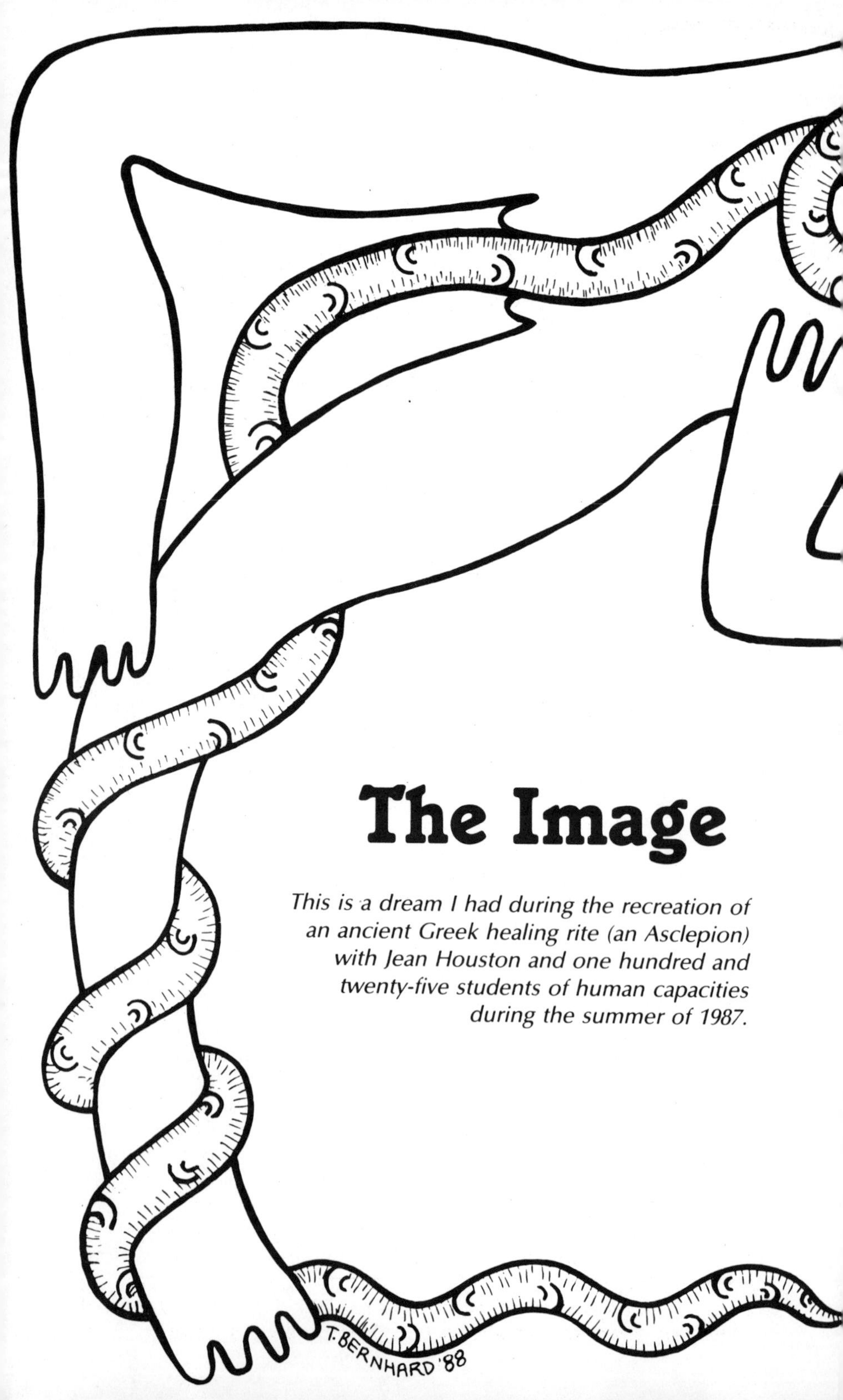

The Image

This is a dream I had during the recreation of an ancient Greek healing rite (an Asclepion) with Jean Houston and one hundred and twenty-five students of human capacities during the summer of 1987.

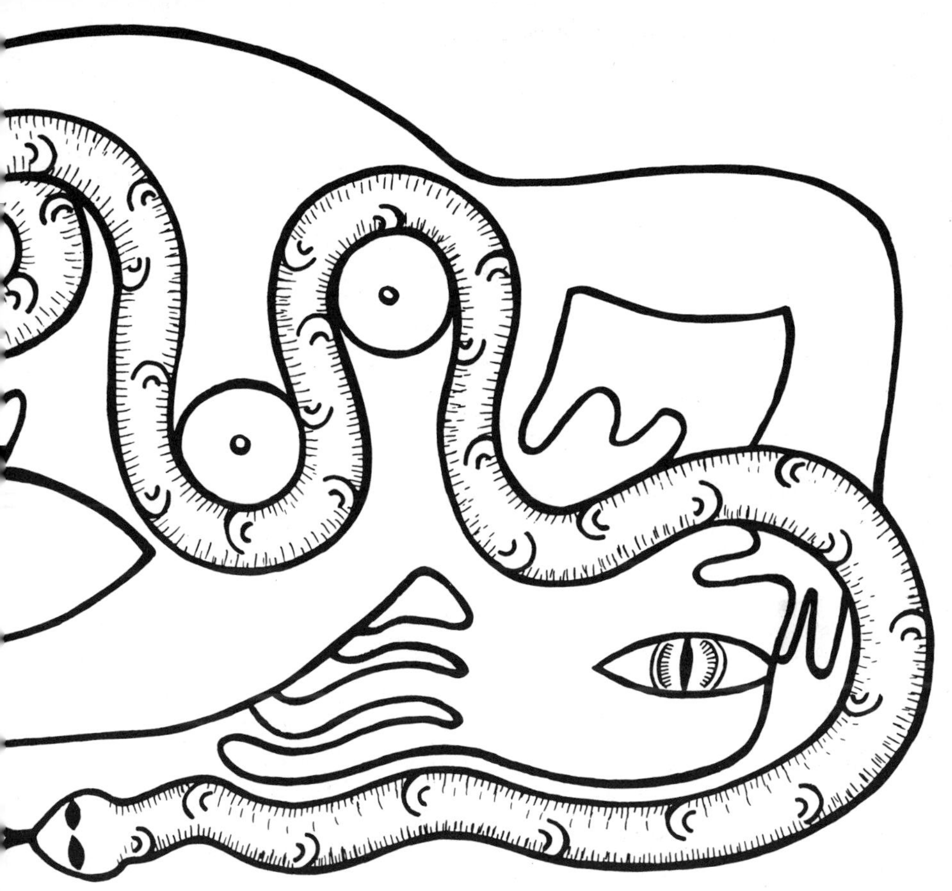

In a time very long ago, very far in the future, there were many temples and shrines of healing, so many that there seemed to be none at all. Every home was a sacred healing space; the whole earth a shrine, an altar. The healers were priestesses and priests, queens and kings. The healers were all ordinary people. Their robes and costumes were the ordinary clothes of their time: beautiful and colorful, plainly and exquisitely stitched garb. Their names were ordinary names: evocative, wonderful names such as goddesses and gods everywhere are called. Though they could heal, there was no disease. There was no disease they could heal; there was no disease they could not heal. There was no disease in the land, no need for healing. All were whole. All holy. All were healed. All healers. Miracles were the ordinary play of all. All miracles were to be played in an ordinary way, a common way, a vulgar way. Vulgar miracles always evoking the healing laughter. Everyday laughter healing the whole. Holy jokes. Wholly funny. The game of healing . . . joyous amusement. Amusing the muses, a muse filled with light. Trying out the game of disease to learn the fun of healing. Healers make disease so they can play miraculous games. We are all healers. We play to heal. We call to you from the future, from the past: "Come healing playing laughing with us miraculous ones. Tickle us. Touch us. Heal us. Hold us dear. We are always you. We are always here."

Notes on My Way to the Wise Woman Tradition

I was confused about health as a child. My parents had to ask a stranger if I was healthy. I was confused about health because the stranger said I was healthy and then gave me an injection. No one ever asked *me* if I felt healthy.

I was confused about health as a young adult. There were so many ways to stop pain, feel good, look my best, and enjoy life, and sometimes I did and sometimes I didn't, and how could I tell what really helped anyhow? I was confused about health because some of the ways others tried to be healthy seemed to harm me and some ways of staying healthy I tried seem to contradict or undo the benefits of other ways. I was also confused about the validity of claims and studies and folklore and my own experiences of being sick and staying healthy. What could I trust?

On my own as a grown-up, I attempted to clear my confusion. I was confused by the damage I saw from drugs and surgery, so I rejected modern medicine and its doctors. I was confused by the damage technology did to people and the earth, so I left the city and went to live in the country, where I built, by hand, a cabin—no plumbing, no electricity, no phone—in a meadow in the Catskills. I ate what I grew and what I and others accidentally killed on the road. I became a goatherd and cheese maker. I practiced yoga. I meditated. I cut down trees to dry and burn for winter warmth. I made love. I went for long walks. But none of this exempted me from illness and injury.

I continued to be confused. Sometimes I had my health, and sometimes I lost it. Sometimes I had accidents, and sometimes avoided them. Sometimes I overextended myself, overate, and overworked, yet I often remembered to relax and to reward myself sensuously and well. If I did all the "right" things, would I be healthy, happy and free from trouble and pain? If living simply in the country and avoiding chemicals wasn't enough, what was?

I studied alternative health. I read Jethro Kloss, Bernard Jensen, Arnold Ehret, Ann Wigmore, Adele Davis, Dr. Walker, and Euell Gibbons. I worked in several health food stores as resident herbalist. I was still confused about my health.

Like the customers of the health food stores, I thought of health care as being either traditional or alternative. Traditional medicine was M.D.s and the AMA. I was victim: powerless, drugged, and cut open. We would have none of that. Alternative medicine was enemas and wheatgrass juice and vitamin pills and personal power; and we were all doing it. But I became confused when I saw the loss of vitality in people on severely restricted diets such as strictly vegetarian, only raw foods, or extended and frequent fasting regimes. And I was really confused when I saw that everything and anything helped some of the people, some of the time.

In a seemingly unrelated part of my life, I fell in love with women, the Goddess, and myself. And I pursued my love completely, committedly, devotedly. I turned my vision to see the Goddess in all. And as I looked for the Goddess everywhere, in everything, and especially in all women, I realized that "traditional" and "alternative" healing were not so different. Just as suddenly, I knew there was another way, an invisible way, a woman's way, the way of the Great Mother, the Wise Woman way, and at last my confusion cleared. I began to walk the beauty way, the unique, spiral maze of the wise woman. I walk there still. Come join me.

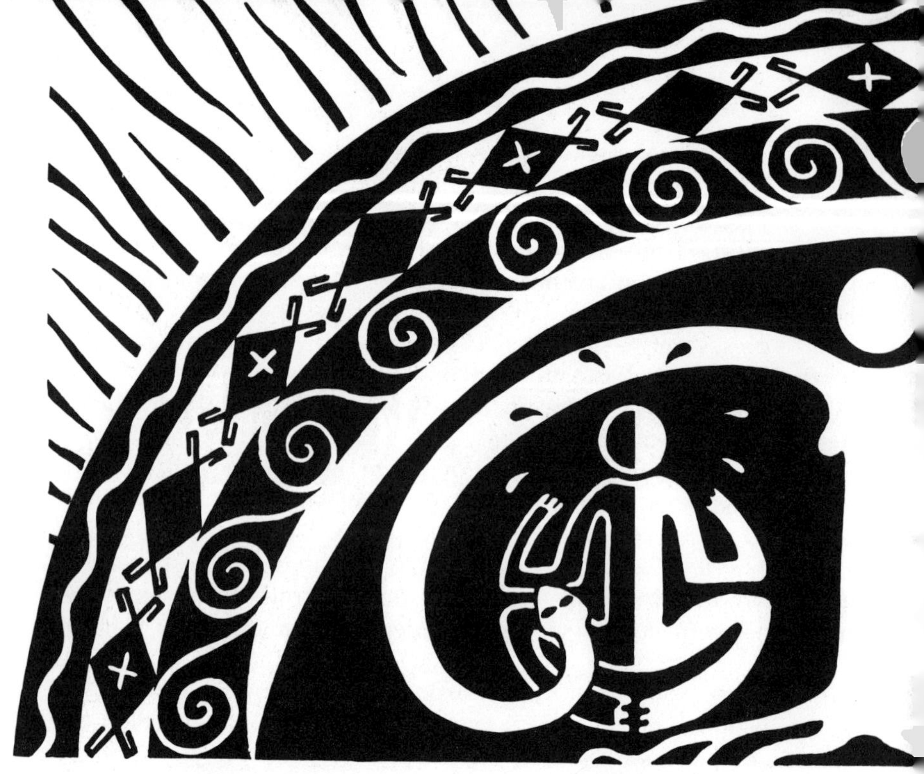

Three Traditions

There is more than the choice between modern Western medicine and alternatives. There are three traditions of healing.

The Wise Woman tradition, focusing on integration and nourishment, and insisting on attention to uniqueness and holographic interconnectedness, is another choice: a new way that is also the most ancient healing way known. A way that follows a spiral path, a give-away dance of nourishment, change, and self love. "Trust yourself."

Alternative health care practitioners usually think in the Heroic tradition: the way of the savior, a circular path of rules, punishment, and purification. "Trust me."

AMA-approved, legal, covered-by-insurance health care practitioners are trained to think in the Scientific tradition: walking the knife edge of keen intellect, the straight line of analytical thought, measuring and repeating, measuring and repeating. Excellent for fixing broken things. "Trust my machine."

The Scientific, Heroic, and Wise Woman traditions are ways of thinking, not ways of acting. Any practice, any technique, any substance can be used by a practitioner/helper in any of the three traditions. There are, for instance, herbalists, and midwives, and MDs in each tradition.

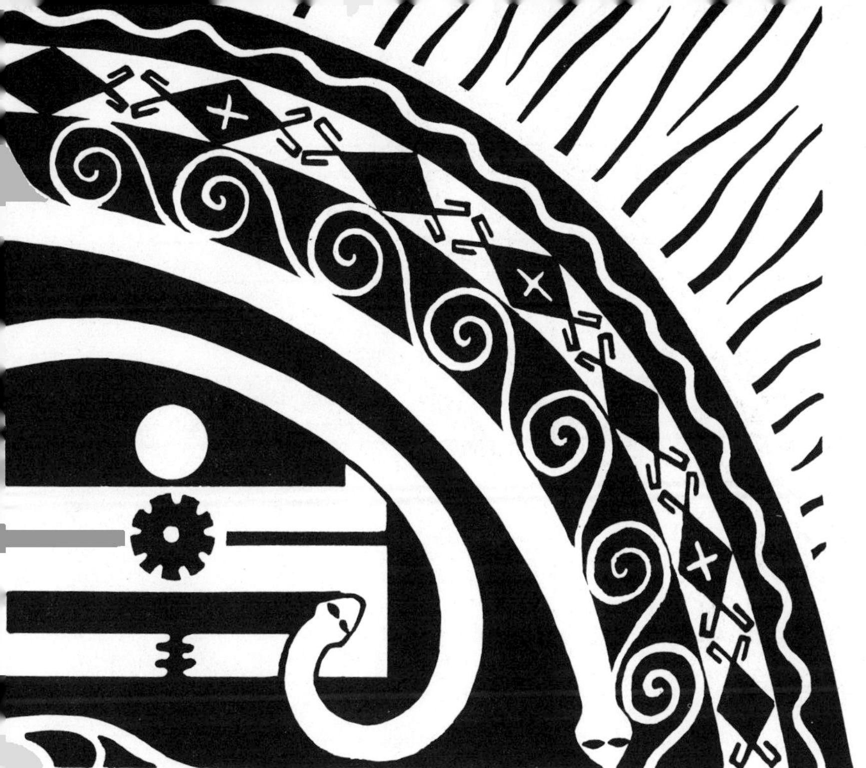

# of Healing

The practitioner and the practice are different. The same techniques, the same herbs are seen and used differently by a person thinking in Scientific, Heroic, or Wise Woman ways.

Thinking these ways does lead to a preference for certain cures. The Wise Woman helper frequently nourishes with herbs and words. The Heroic savior lays down the law to clean up your act fast. The Scientific technician is most at ease with laboratory tests and repeatable, predictable, reliable drugs. But still, the practices do not conclusively identify the practitioner as being in a particular tradition.

The intent, the thought behind the technique points to the tradition: scientific fixing, heroic elimination, or wise womanly digestion and integration.

You contain some aspects of each tradition. And the three traditions are not limited to the realm of healing. The Scientific, Heroic, and Wise Woman ways of thinking are found in politics, legal systems, religions, psychologies, teaching styles, economics. As the Wise Woman way becomes more clearly identified, it opens the way to an integrated, whole, sacred, peaceful global village, interactive with Gaia, mother, earth. As each discipline spins anew its wise woman thread, we reweave the web of interconnectedness with all beings.

THREE TRADITIONS

		SCIENTIFIC TRADITION
	Symbol	line/monolith
	Time span	1500 AD to now
	Overall vision	homeostatic
	Disease/death	the enemy
	Cure	fix/fight
	Body view	machine
	Healer as	mechanic
	Troubled one says	"It's beyond me. I want the expert to do it."
	Healer says	"Trust the test results."
	Preferred treatments	drugs, surgery
	Health/life	young, fully-functioning white male
	Health care	elite
	Characteristic	visible
	Assumes	measurable repetition
	World view	atomic
	Lineage	Newton, Descartes
	Overview	The whole is the same as its parts
	Place of power	machine/tests/drugs
VISIONS OF:	**Women/womb**	unstable
	Snakes	caduceus
	Moon/blood	inconsequential
	The void	avoid it
	Birth	impossible
HERBAL MEDICINE:	**Favorite plants**	tobacco, coffee, drugs
	Sought-after plant parts	alkaloids, active ingredients
	Ideal remedy	precise, odorless, tasteless

OF HEALING

HEROIC TRADITION	WISE WOMAN TRADITION
circle	spiral
1000 BC to now	50,000 BC to now
dualistic	holographic
result of toxins	natural allies for transformation
clean/punish	nourish
(dirty) temple of the spirit	perfect manifestation of complete being
savior/ruler	compassionate, self-loving one
"I've been bad and need someone to punish me."	"I seek support so I can let go to my depths."
"I'll save you."	"I'll play with you in the sacred garden."
stimulants, purges, enemas	unconditional love and nourishment
fully-functioning white people	unimagined transformations
popular	common
alternative	invisible
endless cycles	unique variations
good/bad	interconnected web
St. Paul, Hippocrates, Galen	crone, midwife
The whole is the sum of its parts	The whole is more than the sum of its parts
healer	self
unclean	central
Ouroboros	snake and egg (void)
dangerous	fertile
will get you	source of all being
trauma	empowerment
lobelia, cayenne, goldenseal	common local weeds
medicinal ones, strong ones	vitamins, minerals, chlorophyll
complex, difficult, scarce	familiar, simple, messy, fun

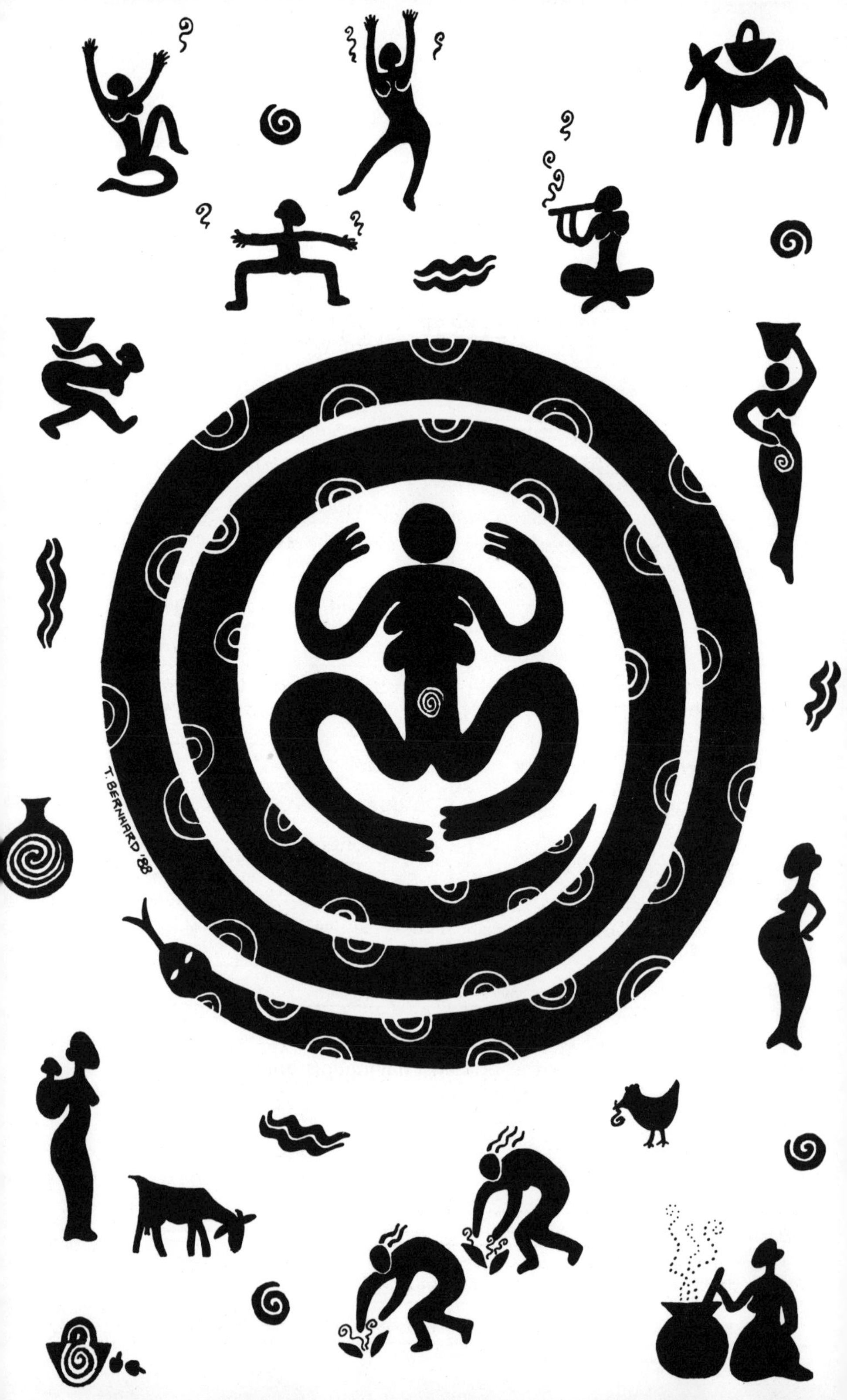
T. BERNHARD '88

Wise Woman Tradition

The Wise Woman tradition is the oldest tradition of healing known on our planet, yet one that is rarely identified, rarely written or talked about. A woman-centered tradition of self love, respectful of the earth and all her creatures, the Wise Woman tradition tells us that compassion, simple ritual, and common herbs heal the whole person and maintain health/wholeness/holiness.

In the Wise Woman tradition good health is flexibility, openness to change, availability to transformation, and groundedness. The spiral is the symbol of the Wise Woman tradition.

The special powers and sensibilities of women (especially menstrual powers) are central to the Wise Woman tradition. Men in the Wise Woman tradition find the wise woman within themselves and become her.

In the Wise Woman tradition we nourish. We do not fix or cure or balance. We nourish health/wholeness/holiness in each individual, ever aware of each individual as holographically related to family/community/universe, in spiraling, ever-changing completeness. Problems become doorways of transformation.

Substance, thought, feeling, and spirit are inseparable in the Wise Woman tradition. Wholism, holographic imagery, and unified field physics are parts of the holy wisdom of the Wise Woman way: a choiceless "both/and" wisdom. Everyone wins. Each one is the best.

In the spiralic and amazing Wise Woman tradition, our self-healing options are as diverse as the human imagination and as complex as the human psyche. The Wise Woman tradition has no rules, no texts, no rites; it is constantly changing, constantly being re-invented.

The wise woman and the Wise Woman tradition have been invisible for thousands of years of our recent past. Now the time has come for us to recognize this invisible thread woven into our lives, this common thread that runs from our earliest foremothers to us, this thread of love and nurturance which can lead us out of the maze of planetary destruction, war, and self-hatred.

I see the wise woman.

She carries a blanket of compassion. She wears a robe of wisdom. Around her throat flutters a veil of shifting shapes. From her shoulders, a mantle of power flows. A story band encircles her forehead. She stitches a quilt; she spins fibers into yarn; she knits; she sews; she weaves. She ties the threads of our lives together. She forms a web of spiraling threads.

I see the wise woman. She is at her loom: a loom warped with days and nights. White threads, black threads receive her flying shuttle, a shuttle filled with threads of many colors. Threads the colors of the earth, the common ground; threads the colors of the people of the earth. Some threads short; some threads long; each thread different, each perfect. These threads are alive with sound and color. These threads are mutable; they change at a touch. These threads are crystal antennae; they respond at a thought.

And intertwined with each thread is a thread blood red: a thread of such sensitivity, it cannot be seen, yet a thread of such vitality, it can never be hidden. As our blood flows over and under the days and nights of our lives and binds each moment to the whole, so the red thread of the wise woman binds us in the tapestried, cosmic web.

I see the wise woman.

And she sees me.

The Wise Woman Tradition

Who Is This Crippled Old Black Woman?

I see the wise woman. She is old and black and walks with the aid of a beautifully carved stick. She's the ancient grandmother of us all and she represents health/wholeness/holiness in the Wise Woman tradition.

She's the one who brought me here. She brought me to the Wise Woman tradition, and she has guided me in the writing of this book. I have been following her traces for years, finding here and there a thread from her cloak.

I find many of her threads, vibrant threads, when I visit with and read about aboriginal women. The aboriginal woman, the original woman, the earth-based woman, the woman of earth colors, the woman of the mother cultures speaks to me. She speaks in a gesture, in a color, in a glance. She speaks in a smile, in a song, in a dance. She speaks to me of Wise Woman ways.

The crippled old black woman winks at me and spreads her arms.

"These are the ways of our ancient grandmothers, the ancient ones who still live. These wise women are one with all life as they tread the ever-changing spiral. Every pain, every plant, every stone, every feeling, every problem is cherished as teacher: not teacher who grades, but teacher who guides. Night is loved for darkness and the stars. Day is loved for light and the sun. Uniqueness is our treasure, not normalcy. Our universe includes all; it is 'both/and,' not 'either/or.' This is the Wise Woman way the world 'round.

"These are the ways of our ancient grandmothers, the ancient ones who still live. These wise women receive nourishment from and give nourishment to the great mother of all. They receive her abundance with compassion, knowing they themselves will be food for others. They know that dying is the portal to the existence of death as birth is the portal to the existence of life. They celebrate all comings and goings. This is the Wise Woman way the world 'round.

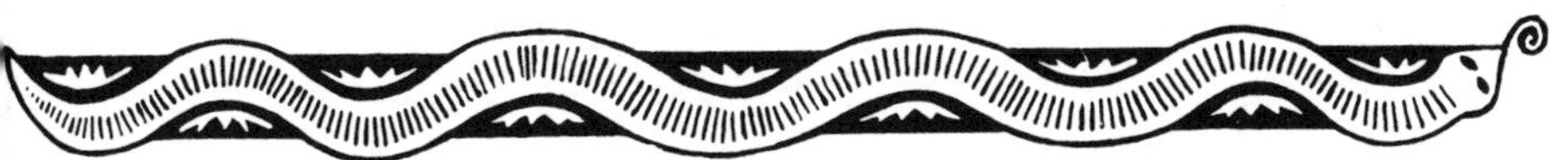

"These are the ways of our ancient grandmothers, the ancient ones who still live. These wise women spin the invisible web which weaves us all together. They invite you to weave the threads of your own life back into the cloak of the ancient one, the holy blanket of the wise woman. They thank you for reweaving, wherever you can, the sacred threads of planetary, animal, plant, and personal kinship.

"These are the ways of our ancient grandmothers, the ancient ones who still live. The joy of life is the give-away. They give you a gift of a robe, a robe woven of unconditional self love: luminous, resonant, shimmering.

"Here, put it on. Ah! Do you feel it?

"As you emerge through the neckhole you become the center of the universe. All revolves around you, the world's axis, life's matrix, the still point in the ever-moving. The designs of the universe itself radiate down your sleeves and bodice. It is an ancient design. Lift your arms. You are the tree of life, the goddess, unique and whole.

"And as you trace the invisible way of the Wise Woman, wearing your robe, know that the ancient ones offer you safe journey. They offer you safe journey and the possibility of finding yourself healthy/whole/holy. This is the Wise Woman way the world 'round."

The Wise Woman Tradition is Invisible

The Wise Woman tradition is the oldest tradition of healing known on our planet, yet one that is rarely identified, rarely written or talked about. It is an invisible tradition.

Flexible and common, claiming no healers, having no universities, no institutions, the Wise Woman tradition is hard to see. I feel it as an invisible thread humming with wholeness, ancient and vibrant, stitched through my life, stitched through the lives of all who went before and all who come after me. An invisible, tenacious thread.

The reasons for the invisibility of the Wise Woman tradition are manifold:

• Nourishing is an invisible process.

The Wise Woman tradition is based on nourishment, a basic process generally taken for granted, not considered worthy of much note. Nourishment through giving suck and gathering and preparing food is presented as background by anthropologists who are fascinated by the occasional dramatic hunt. Wise women nourish in invisible ways, helping others to empower themselves without saying, "Hey, look at me healing you. Look at me teaching you!"

• Mothers are invisible.

Virtually all health care given worldwide (99% say some experts) is provided by mothers who care for their families' health, and most of this is done in the Wise Woman tradition. But this is not measured nor paid for, and anyway, isn't that what mothers do?

• Women, especially women of color, are invisible to white men and white male society.

The Wise Woman tradition is a woman-centered tradition. For hundreds of years, the news of the world has been given to us by white men who hardly see women at all, let alone black women. And they do not see women as powerful even when they do perceive women's existence. Women healers, midwives, and herbalists are frequently written out of accounts, omitted when lists are recopied, or known only by a husband's name. And the lineage of the European Wise Woman tradition has gone up in flames so often that tracing that thread is difficult indeed.

• A woman making dinner is invisible.

To claim that she is engaged in healing her family and community and keeping her universe in balance is a lot to claim for dinner. This is the Wise Woman way.

• Spoken words are invisible.

The Wise Woman tradition is an oral tradition, and we have grown accustomed to believing things only if they are written down, in books, like this one. The Wise Woman tradition flows from experience rather than faith in books; from creativity rather than dogma; from many unique individuals creating new ways to heal/whole, creating new/old wise ways, rather than a monolithic tradition. It is nonrepeatable, nonreplicable, ever changing.

• There's no visible structure in the Wise Woman tradition.

There is no hierarchy in the Wise Woman tradition: no difference between above and below, no order of authority, no sense of "man" as better than all other forms of life. There's no president, no guru, no chairman of the board. There are no rules to follow. You can't get a degree or certificate in the Wise Woman tradition. You can't be tested on it, because there are no right and wrong answers.

• Uniqueness is invisible.

Each healing/wholing ritual encounter in the Wise Woman tradition is unique. Repetition is neither sought nor valued. In the Scientific world view, a single instance of anything is virtually invisible. The more repeatable something is, the more visible it is.

• Commonness is invisible.

It's just too familiar. When the European came upon native cultures he could not see that there were medicine women, because all women were medicine women. The few medicine men (often dressed up as women) were visible to him. And so European cultural biases perpetrated the myth of the medicine man, and the medicine woman remained invisible.

• Prevention is invisible.

If I drink nettle infusion while pregnant and don't hemorrhage, I haven't done anything visible or noticeable. We have become so used to invasive preventive medicine (as with mammograms) that nourishing as prevention is invisible to us. With Wise Woman ways we resonate in health/wholeness/holiness throughout our lives, so there are fewer emergencies and fewer heroic measures needed.

• One of the powers of the wise woman is invisibility.

A Wise Woman tradition midwife tells me that when she is profusely thanked (right at the birth), she reconsiders what she did, looking for ways to be more invisible.

"I'm there to help her remember *her* power, not to display mine. I'm there to support *her* to deliver the baby; I don't deliver. I'm only there if I'm needed. The more invisible I am, the more I can really help."

Because it's invisible, the Wise Woman tradition is difficult to discover and easy to ignore. At the same time, because the Wise Woman tradition is the oldest tradition of health care among humans, its ways are deeply embedded in our collective consciousness, in our morphogenetic fields, in our ancient brain parts. We can try to ignore the Wise Woman tradition, but it won't leave us alone.

The wisdom of the Wise Woman way exists within each of us; it exists within you and it can come to life through you. The Wise Woman tradition lives in the woman-self memory of each person. How do I know? The most frequent comment (and my favorite compliment) after a talk on the Wise Woman tradition: "I already knew everything you had to say, I just needed you to remind me."

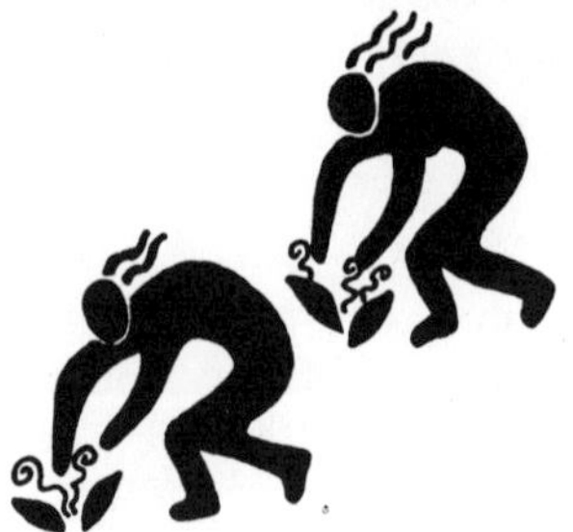

The Wise Woman Tradition is a Spiral

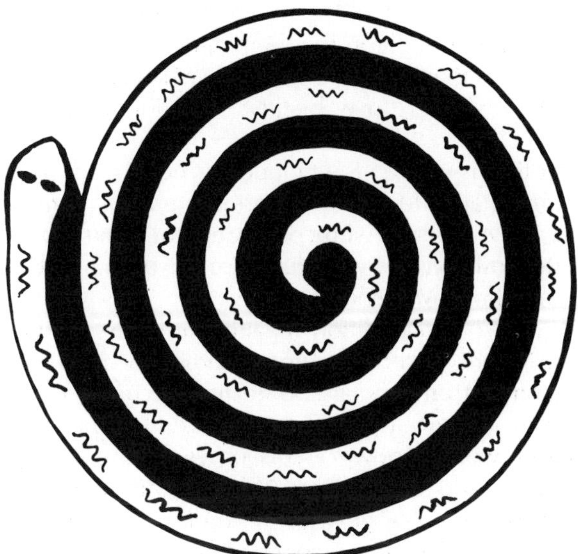

The symbol of the Wise Woman tradition is a spiral. A spiral is a cycle as it moves through time. A spiral is movement around and beyond a circle, always returning to itself, but never at exactly the same place. Spirals never repeat themselves. Spirals remind us that life is movement, that each moment is unique, and that form is the essence of transformation.

The symbol of the Wise Woman tradition is the spiral. The spiral is the bubbling cauldron, the curl of the wave, the lift of the wind, the whirlpool of water, the umbilical cord, the great serpent, the path of the earth, the twist of the helix, the spin of our galaxy. The spiral is the soft guts. The spiral is the labyrinth. The spiral is the womb-moon-tide möbius pull. The spiral is your individual life. The spiral is the passage between worlds: birth passing into death, death passing into birth. The path of enlightenment is the spiral dance of bliss.

The symbol of the Wise Woman tradition is a spiral. Spirals never repeat. Walk a circle and you can stay in balance, know the cycles, trust your every step. Walk a spiral, you will inevitably come to the unique next step, the unknown, the thirteenth step, the opportunity for change, the window of transformation.

The thirteenth step creates the spiral. Twelve is the number of established order. Twelve is easily divided and ordered into halves and quarters and thirds, easily categorized and labeled and defined. One step beyond the mutable twelve is thirteen, the wild card, the unique number, the indivisible prime. Thirteen, the number of change.

The Wise Woman Tradition is Woman-Centered

The Wise Woman tradition is a woman-centered tradition. Everything is perceived as manifesting from the female center: life, nourishment, song, story, shelter, love, beauty, sacredness, healing, wholeness.

Earth is mother is woman is wholeness is health. So, whether they are men or women, all self-healing helpers in the Wise Woman tradition are perceived as women. (In some cultures, the men act this out by wearing female clothing, or by cutting themselves, so that they bleed like women [see **Blood Mysteries**].)

In the Wise Woman tradition, health/wholeness/holiness comes through nourishment, and nourishment comes through the mother; nourishment comes from woman. So healing occurs in the ground of woman power, in the ground of heart-centered compassion.

What is this woman power? This power of nourishment? This power of creation and destruction? What is this female energy? It certainly is not the opposite of what we think of as male energy. It is not "the passive" or even "the receptive." It is the void.

Female energy is the void of all being: the all-consuming void, the all-birthing void.

The Power of the Void

In the Wise Woman tradition, all health, all coming to wholeness, begins with a return to the void. To heal, to become whole, we turn again around the spiral of our life. We turn again around the spiral and enter the void, the great unknown, knowing only that our form is reformed, that our form is transformed, that rebirth inevitably follows death.

When we resist our death, our return to the void, we call it "our problem."

The problem is I am in pain. The problem is I am out of control. The problem is I am falling, without chance of stopping, falling into the void of all beginnings, into the void of all ends.

The Wise Woman tradition asks us to let go and fall. Fall into the void. Fall into the open arms of the mother. Add on to yourself by letting go of everything. Become whole and healthy by turning on the spiral, by returning to the void.

Where does the spiral end? Where begin? In the void. Place of female power. Place we are taught to avoid. Nothing. Chaos. The spiral emerges from and ends in invisibility, the great nothing dark womb of the goddess, endlessly empty, endlessly full, doorway of life, window of transformation, entry to death.

Death is part of successful healing in the Wise Woman tradition. Death the invisible, unique void. The void is woman power: simultaneously dynamic and relaxed; empty yet completely full; satiated yet always consuming; creative, abundant, insatiable, unfillable, unquenchable, wild, having nothing to receive, knowing everything is already present, completely calm.

Here in the void lives the Crone. Here we encounter the Crone in her power: Hecate chants words of power at the crossing. Kali, bedecked with musical, runic skulls, dances on the corpses. Cerridwen, the sacred sow, cosmic pig, feeds eternally. Hel, full of passion, guards the sacred fire. The unknowable goddess flutters her veil. The void contains all and consumes all.

From the void comes the Virgin who gives birth: Mary sits spinning the red thread of life. Persephone weaves the tapestry of the universe. Ishtar performs the sacred belly dance for her sisters. All life arises from the creative void.

Where is the void? Is it heaven? Is it hell? Up the mountain in my town, at the Tibetan monastery, the day begins with an invocation to the goddess Tara, life giver. An invocation to Mahakala (Kali), the goddess of death, closes each day. All things begin from woman. All things return to woman. In sickness, in death, we are the food, the nourishment of the void, the great goddess. Now I eat you. In life, in birth, she gives to us, nourishes us abundantly, cares for us compassionately. Now you eat me.

The Wise Woman Tradition Heals with Nourishment

In the Wise Woman tradition, health/wholeness/holiness comes through adding on to, that is, through nourishment. Problems, pains, diseases, and illnesses are not fixed, or cured, or even brought into balance, in the Wise Woman tradition, but honored, supported, respected for their truth, nourished, and added on to the truth of the whole being. Nourishment helps us incorporate ("to intimately blend, to make into a body") all of our experiences. Each problem is acknowledged as a potential thirteenth step to transformation and growth.

Nourishment encourages expansion and growth. Nourishment includes. Nourishment supports each being as unique, holy, individual. Nourishing our problems encourages love for all parts of ourselves.

We become whole, and genuinely who we are, rather than the fixed, cured, balanced person we suppose we are supposed to be.

The Wise Woman tradition sees everything as nourishment. Nourishment insures life. Nourishment is the great grounding root and green leaf of the Wise Woman tradition. All health occurs through nourishment. (The immune system nourishes itself on viruses.) All is nourishment. Now you eat me. Now I eat you.

Cell by cell, you replace yourself. Thought by thought, you create yourself. Dream by dream, you envision the universe. You create a million new cells every second: impressionable, vulnerable cells. From what do you create them? With what do you imprint them?

Nourish yourself optimally, with health/wholeness/holiness, to create healthy/whole/holy cells. Imprint them with vibrations of wholeness, resonate holographically, and you create health and flexibility in the Wise Woman way. *Not* "good health" as in the absence of pain and problems. *Not* immunity to all germs, viruses, hoaxes, disappointments, heartbreaks, setbacks, and sheer galactic perversity, but the stamina and grace to find the thirteenth step of every problem, to find pain's gift.

With optimum nourishment, says the Wise Woman tradition, we find ourselves walking an ever-increasing spiral of health/wholeness/holiness.

What of cleaning? What of toxins? How can you be healthy, holy, and happy if you're full of crap? Don't you have to clean the liver? Don't you have to clean the blood?

Nourish the new cells, optimally, says the Wise Woman tradition, and the old cells and other waste will be cleared away easily. The liver is replaced, every cell of it, in six weeks. Nourish each new liver cell optimally, and the liver will clean the blood. The kidneys are replaced, every cell, in a month. Nourish each new cell optimally, let the kidneys clean the blood. The blood volume itself is replaced, every cell, in three weeks. What cleaner blood than new and optimally nourished cells?

Partake of optimum nourishment, as understood by wise women through the ages, and soon every cell of your body is healthy/whole/holy: the nervous system functions more smoothly, the hormonal system fluctuates more evenly, the liver and kidneys are more effective, the immune system is better organized, and the digestive system makes better use of all available nourishment.

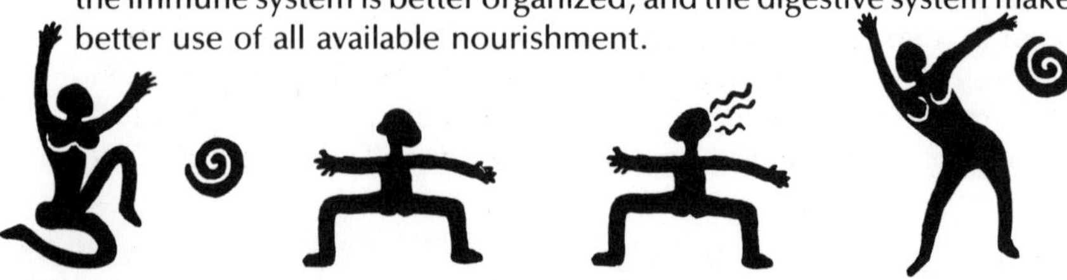

Blood Mysteries

In the beginning, according to the Wise Woman tradition, everything began, as everything does, at birth. The Great Mother of All gave birth and the earth appeared out of the void. Then the Great Mother of All gave birth again, and again, and again, and people, and animals, and plants appeared on the earth. They were all very hungry. "What shall we eat?" they asked the Great Mother. "Now you eat me," she said, smiling. Soon there were a very great many lives, but the Great Mother of All was enjoying creating and giving birth so much that she didn't want to stop. "Ah," she said smiling, "now I eat you." And so she still does.

We all come from the same mother. She is the wise woman. We all return to her embrace, her bloody-rich womb place, when we die. Every woman is a whole/holy form of her, able to be whole/holy mother of all life, able to be whole/holy destroyer of life. Her power is her blood that flows and flows, her blood which is life and gives life. Every woman's menstrual blood and birth-time blood is a holy mystery.

What are the blood mysteries? Why are they central to the understanding of the Wise Woman tradition?

Blood mysteries teach that menstrual blood and birthing blood are holy blood, power blood, healing blood. The blood mysteries teach us to remember that life and healing come from and return to woman, to the wise woman, to the woman who bleeds and bleeds. And does not die.

Blood mysteries reveal that menstrual (moontime) blood and birth blood are so holy, so full of potential, so full of the void, that they are to be used only to heal, to heal by nourishing. Holy woman-blood is nourishing blood, blood of love, blood of abundance, blood that heals the earth.

Blood mysteries recall the immense power of the bleeding woman. Power enough to share in great nourishing give-aways. Give-away from woman womb to earth womb, give-away from mother to matrix, give-away of nourisher to nourisher. When we bleed into the ground (in reality or in fantasy) our power regrounds as our blood flows through the personal root chakra and into the earth.

Bleeding into the ground, bleeding freely, we know ourselves as women, as nourishers of life, as givers of nourishment to the plants, givers of holy nourishment: our moontime blood.

I am woman giving away nourishment to ensure this planet's life. With my moontime power, my blood, with my birthing power, my blood, I feed the earth who feeds us all. Every month I remember: I am woman. I am earth. I am life. I am nourishment. I am change.

I am woman, blatantly and repeatedly confronted with my changes: hormonal harmonics stirring moon time visions, ovulatory oracles, pre-menstrual crazies, orgasmic knowings, birth ecstasies, breast-feeding bliss, menopausal moods.

I am wholeness. I am woman of wisdom. I know life, death, pain, and health in my marrow, in my womb. I know the bloody places: the narrow bloody space between life and death, the bloody place of birth, the bloody mess of nourishing life, the bloody flow of letting life go. I am woman. My blood is power. Peaceful power. Peaceful blood.

My blood is holy nourishment. My blood nourishes the growing fetus. My blood becomes milk to nourish the young child. My blood flows into the ground as holy nourishment for the Great Mother, Gaia, Mother Earth.

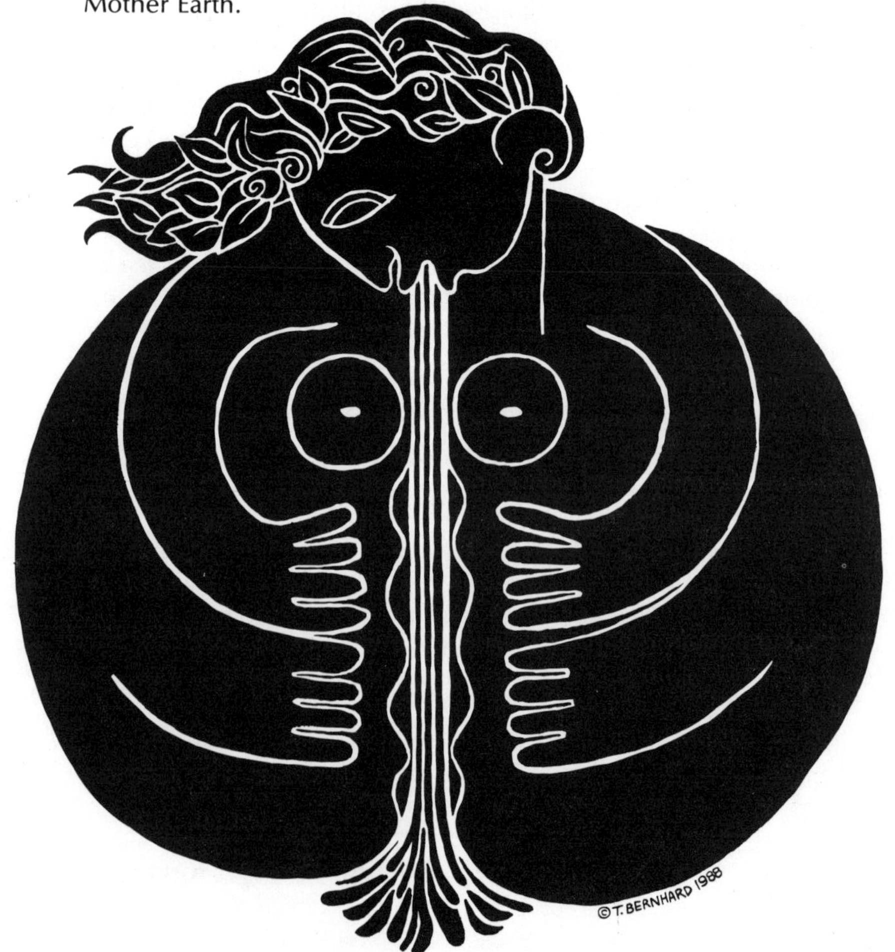

Gaia, whose ways are bloody. Woman, whose ways are bloody. Blood of nourishment. But bloody. Bloody menstrual blood, bloody birth blood. Blood of peace, nourishing blood. Blood of health/wholeness/holiness, not of sacrifice. The Wise Woman tradition is a bloody-handed woman, a bloody-thighed woman, a woman who gives birth, a woman who sees to the other side of things.

Health/wholeness/holiness is always changing. Life is mysterious, moving in spirals of change. Spirals moving to, through, from the void. Change making the hole so we can see the holy healthy gift of our wholeness.

"Sit, sister, here on the soft green moss, and give your sacred moon blood to the earth, back again to the spiral of life. Let flow your womb's blood red to the green and brown of earth. Sit here. Relax and close your eyes and let the visions come. Rest now and give your moon blood to nourish the mother who nourishes us. Relax and let the visions come."

The time of menstrual bleeding, according to the Wise Woman tradition, is a time of visions. Any woman who pays attention to these visions will find the powers of shamans, witch doctors, medicine wo/men.

"Add a bit of red leaf to your herbal mixtures, any red leaf except poison ivy. That will make the medicine strong," says a friend, apprentice to a Native American shaman. And the wise woman inside me whispers: "They do this to evoke the power of menstrual blood."

These are the natural powers of menstruating, menopausal, and post-menopausal women:

- Oneness with the earth as a responsive nurturing presence
- Communication with plants, animals, rocks
- Weather making
- Shape shifting
- Invisibility
- Communication with fairies, devas, elves, dragons, unicorns
- Foreknowledge
- Acutely sensitive senses of smell, taste, hearing, sight, touch
- Healing

The Wise Woman tradition understands healing/wholing as blood mysteries. The blood of birth and death, and the blood of nourishment, these are the natural knowledge of women, these are the things that make us wise.

Holographic Understanding is a Wise Woman Way

The whole is more than the sum of its parts in the Wise Woman tradition. And every part is seen *as* the whole in the Wise Woman tradition. The part is as whole as the whole is. These are holographic understandings. They follow the way of the hologram.

Hologram is derived from the Greek words *holo,* meaning *whole,* and *gram,* meaning *to write.* Thus the hologram writes the whole.

A hologram is formed by splitting a laser beam into two parts: one travels directly to a photographic plate, one is bounced off an object and onto the plate. The resulting interference pattern at the intersection of the beams, which is recorded on the photographic plate, is not only extremely complex, but usually invisible to the unaided eye. When the photographic plate is illuminated with laser light, the original object is seen three-dimensionally, with luminous depth and great detail, from many viewpoints. If only a small part of the plate is illuminated, the entire object is still visible, though somewhat less sharply, with less definition and detail, and from fewer viewpoints.

The individual cell in the body is one small, whole picture of the entire being. The person is composed of millions of cells, millions of pictures, collected together and becoming more than the sum of the parts. In this collection of cells the luminous depth of life stirs and we see great detail, great adventures.

Nourish each cell as unique, nourish it optimally, says the Wise Woman tradition, and the person will thrive, heal, and become whole as an inherent part of being alive.

With holographic understanding, the Wise Woman way treats each being as a complete and perfect wholeness. With holographic understanding, the Wise Woman way knows that everything we think and do affects the whole: our whole/holy selves, our families, our communities, the earth as a whole, and even the vast universe.

With holographic understanding, the Wise Woman tradition sees each illness as an expression of the ever-changing truth of the full being, and the healing/wholing of the illness to be the wholing of the entire being, family, community, planet, universe.

With holographic understanding, in the Wise Woman way, we nourish and add to each being. Nourishing, we add to wholeness, rather than eliminating "the problem." Adding to, we increase the clarity of the hologram. So each personal problem is seen as an opportunity to strengthen family. Each problem is understood as an opportunity to create community. Each problem is valued as an opportunity to heal the earth. Each problem is respected as an opportunity to nourish the universe.

If we do not nourish the universe and heal the earth and create community and strengthen the family when we cure the pain or the problem, then, to the Wise Woman way of thinking, we have not healed anything at all, even if the patient is well. If we heal the person but disrupt the family, the community, or the earth, then wholeness is not increased, nourishment is not in action, health does not occur, and holiness is forgotten.

In the holographic understanding of the Wise Woman way, you and I are each, no matter how different, a whole picture of the entire universe. Physicists and mystics say this in different ways. We can read the entire universe in each other, though the finer details aren't clear. Our health, our pain mirror and illuminate part of the joy and sadness of the universe. The more of us that think and act in certain ways, the clearer that expression is in the universe.

Each cell is a living entity with feeling and spirit, not just physical substance. Full integration of all parts with all parts is part of the holographic understanding of the Wise Woman tradition.

The Wise Woman tradition knows that individuals aren't just a body, a mind, and a spirit, and even if they were, wouldn't separate the parts.

When we're doing emotional work, we understand that therapy has its emotional, physical, and spiritual aspects. When we are responding to our soul's longings, we are full of feeling, and need to create a physical expression of our heart's desire. When we are engaged in intense physical effort, such as lovemaking, the emotions are more accessible, the spirit closer at hand. All aspects of our being are integrated, inseparable, in the Wise Woman way.

Integration obviates hierarchies. The Wise Woman tradition does not believe that the soul is higher than the body, but that it is in a mutual relationship with the body. All parts of the body (and any part of the body) reflect, holographically, the soul, the spirit.

Optimum nutrition depends on the availability of whole, integrated food and energy sources. Holographically, their wholeness activates the wholeness of each of your cells.

Wild plants are whole, integrated food and energy sources. Wild plants carry spiritual power, emotional power, physical power, and other, invisible, unnameable powers as well. Eat a wild plant, and you're eating wholeness. Wild plants are readily available resonators of health/wholeness/holiness, optimum nourishers to all parts of your being. This is one of the reasons that the Wise Woman tradition herbalist prefers to use wild plants.

In the Wise Woman tradition the body is more than a physical object. Emotional bodies, energetic bodies, dream bodies, soul aspects, and subtle bodies, to name but a few, are just as integral to the hologram as the physical body.

The Wise Woman tradition understands that healing/wholing transformation in the body creates change in the entire being.

With Wise Woman holographic understanding, we learn to see the interconnections and weavings of all ways of being. We learn to perceive and strengthen the weave of ourselves and our lives by walking the way of the flowing spiral and looking for the pattern of the hologram. We begin to see the once-invisible threads of nourishment that weave us in the web of our grandmothers. We begin to notice the story cloak of the ancient ones.

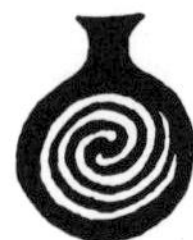

The Wise Woman Tradition Says Health/Wholeness/Holiness is Ever-Changing

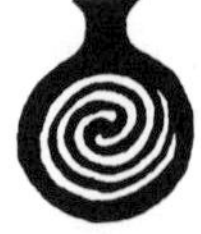

In the Wise Woman tradition, health is flexibility: loose muscles, quick mind, unlimited curiosity. Wholeness is inclusive, pliable, expanding to accommodate. Holiness sees the holiness, wholeness, health, and nourishment in all beings.

So health, from the Wise Woman perspective, includes a lot of people who are considered sick by other traditions. Confinement to a wheelchair, blindness, extreme age, terminal illness, mental retardation, and other disabilities do not disqualify any being from health/wholeness/holiness in the Wise Woman tradition.

Resistance clenches the muscles, causes pain. Resistance prejudices the thought, causes isolation. Resistance says holy must be exactly like this or it doesn't count, and the glory fades from the world.

Flexible, pliable, and ever-changing: that, says the Wise Woman tradition, is health.

Every problem, each pain, disability, disease, is understood, in the Wise Woman way, as a hole for the entry of wholeness, a portal for the arrival of an ally. An ally who opens doorways of transformation. An ally who can protect you. An ally who brings you gifts. An ally who returns your missing pieces. An ally who guides you toward integration, through disintegration. An ally of wholeness, who accepts all of you. An ally who reminds you of your mortality and your immortality.

Healing is not *done* in the Wise Woman tradition. Health is allowed. Wholeness is nourished. Holiness is acknowledged. The wise woman smiles.

The Scientific tradition seeks an objective, impersonal, physiochemical solution to disease. The Heroic tradition seeks to cure by suggesting that you create everything, are responsible for everything, and you can make it all better if you follow the rules from now on. The Wise Woman tradition seeks to understand the personal, social hologram of the disease and to nourish wholeness.

In the Wise Woman tradition, wholeness nourishes wholeness. Fractured or isolated substances, such as drugs or vitamin supplements, create fractured and isolated people, not healthy/whole/holy people. The Wise Woman herbalist pays attention to preserving the integrity, the wholeness, of the plants she uses, rather than to preserving the active constituent or any other single aspect.

Healing/health in the Wise Woman tradition is concerned more with creating meaning than with creating a particular outcome. Healing/health is not dependent on curing, or removing the problem, but on making the problem meaningful, specifically, by finding the gift and the nourishment that the problem brings.

Healing/health, the Wise Woman way, is concerned with the story: the person's story, the family's tale, the community's fable, the planet's myth. When the Wise Woman knows the story (or even a part of the story, in holographic knowing), she can read the story line. She can retell the story, expose deeper roots of the tale, reveal new meanings in the fable, and create anew the myths.

Every personal story has a meaning both special to the one and true for all. By retelling the story, the wise woman weaves wholeness. By exposing the deeper roots of the tale, the wise woman grounds health. By revealing what has been hidden, the wise woman tears holes for holiness. By creating anew the myth, the wise woman offers optimum nourishment.

This is different from finding the lesson or the teaching of a disease or problem. "Learning your lesson" is a thought pattern from the Heroic tradition. Learning the lesson implies that you will never do the same thing again. ("Never doing it again" leads to loss of spontaneity.) Once you learn your lesson, you get well, you are cured. (If you are still sick, you haven't yet learned your lesson.)

The wise woman is impeccably clear of guilt and self-blame (without feeling guilty when she's *not* clear of guilt and blame), while acknowledging herself as creator of her universe.

Receiving the nourishment of the problem, allying yourself with your pain, and loving yourself implies that you are free to continue to have the problem, consensually, as a matter of intent. You can choose to die.

Death is not failure in the Wise Woman tradition. Death may be chosen as a gift of integration and wholeness to self, a gift of optimum nourishment and health to the family and larger community. Disintegration of family and self-respect (and the lost opportunity to strengthen community ties by care-tending the dying at home) is natural when a family member is kept alive in an institution until the family's resources of money, time, and good cheer are exhausted—as is generally the case today in industrialized nations, with Scientific tradition approaches to health.

The Wise Woman tradition can allow death because the Wise Woman tradition is grounded in change. The only thing certain is change. Remember the void? The spiral of life and death is ever-changing and unique, flowing through all possibilities. This is the wisdom of the Wise Woman way.

Do not try to outwit and avoid pain and problems. They can be your means to greater wholeness, to more vital health, to a soaring spirit. They are part of your unique gifts. Fixity is worse than death, counsels the Wise Woman way. Keep on stepping around the spiral. What comes next?

The Wise Woman Tradition is a Both/And Universe

The both/and universe embraces all possibilities. The both/and universe is inclusive. The both/and universe accepts every part of us. There is difference, there is distinction, but not opposition. In the both/and universe, opposites are not compromised and evened out, but united as powerful allies, each with individual uniqueness.

The Wise Woman tradition asks us to nourish all parts of ourselves, and to see our problems as allies, bringing gifts. Sometimes those gifts are the "bad" parts of ourselves. We worry that if we nourish our "bad" parts (bad child, bad parent, bad person, bad lover, bad friend) we'll lose our good parts. We are used to an either/or universe, where one is either bad or good, sick or well, dead or alive.

In the Wise Woman tradition, we are both good and bad simultaneously. We find missing parts of ourselves when we ask to see the gifts, disguised as problems, that our allies bring.

We may discover the bad child, who is an important part of the real child. Following the Wise Woman way, we nourish the bad child. We nourish by listening to this child's needs and answering them. We nourish by allowing, providing, time for communication. And we find ourselves more whole, more holy, more real, more joyous, more alive as a result, not bad (as we feared).

We are both sick and well at the same time, in the Wise Woman tradition. From one viewpoint, we know that different parts of us are healthy and sick. From another viewpoint, we understand that sickness builds health. An immune system unused is an immune system fallen into disuse. People who suddenly die from cancer and heart attacks are often people who were "never sick a day in their lives."

Understanding the gifts of health/wholeness/holiness in every illness, we follow the Wise Woman way and try to nourish ourselves in sickness as in health. How difficult it can be. How little we feel we deserve, how little we love ourselves when we are not well, not able. Even if we are only partially unable, even if we know we will recover shortly, we don't love ourselves as whole, we don't open our hearts to our own holiness.

In the Wise Woman tradition, we are alive and dead at the same time. Each second a million new cells in each of us stir to life. Each second a million more cells expire, die. Breathing in we inspire and live. Breathing out we expire and die. Our death gives life to others. The death of others (plants, animals) gives life to us. Now I eat you. Now you eat me.

Chaos, permeability, and nonsense are honored in the Wise Woman tradition, not instead of, but in addition to honoring order, boundaries, and logic. Life and death co-exist; there is no pitched battle; there are no enemies in the Wise Woman tradition.

The next time you have to make a choice *between,* try this: change the "or" to "and" and look at your decision from a place of inclusion. Let new vistas appear. Let the spiraling path of the Wise Woman tradition become more visible to you.

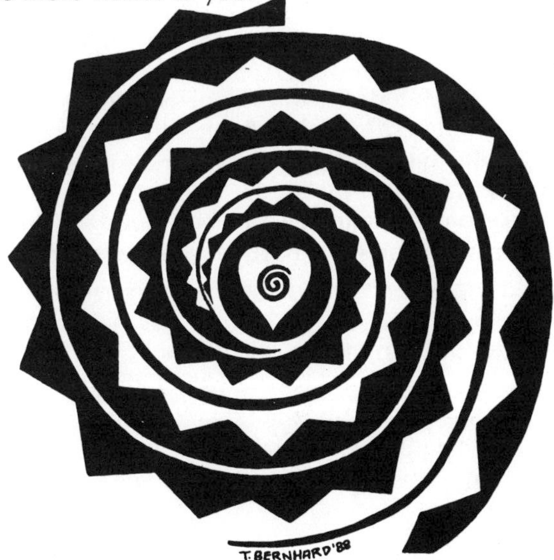

The Wise Woman Tradition is Heart-Centered

In the either/or universe, we know where we stand and how to keep in balance. We strive to keep away badness, sickness, death and we struggle to hold onto goodness, health, life. Holding back the awful things with one hand, we cling to what good we have with the other. It seems such a secure balance. Such a familiar universe.

Where is the balance if we let go of resistance to illness, to death? If we acknowledge our own inability to live up to the standards of thoughts and behavior we set for the perfect person? If life and death co-exist in us, will we choose life? If health and sickness are inevitable turns on the spiral, is exercise and attention to nutrition a waste of time? How is chaos honored without losing all order?

The Wise Woman tradition balances all possibilities in the heart's center, the heart's truth. Balances by simply allowing the heart's truth, the heart's center. There are no right answers in the Wise Woman tradition. The right answer is "I don't know." The right answer is, "I'll have to wait and see." The right answer is silence, wherein the heart's truth rings and health/wholeness/holiness occurs.

The heart's truth is compassion, forgiveness, unconditional self-love. The heart's truth is the both/and universe. In the Wise Woman tradition the focus is on opening the heart, not toward others, but toward self.

Self-love, self-forgiveness, and deep compassion for one's own humanness, nourish the heart and give balance amidst the windings of the Wise Woman spiral. Nourish the individual heart, says the Wise Woman tradition, until the nourishment and love flow out. There is abundant nourishment for every heart when we learn to receive it.

Unconditional love is not for giving, but for taking, claims the Wise Woman tradition. The Wise Woman tradition demands that we learn to receive the abundance of the universe. Learn to receive the blessings of our mother. Learn to receive the ever-changing, ever-different flow of life and death, wellness and sickness, good and bad, with respect and joy.

Learn to accept unconditional love from yourself, says the Wise Woman way. Learn to forgive yourself completely. Even to forgive yourself for causing others to hurt you. Learn to have compassion for your own suffering.

Pain is inevitable. Suffering is optional.

Learn to distinguish, with Wise Woman vision, both/and unconditional love from the sort of unconditional love that's an undercover bargain: *"I'll love you unconditionally: you can do anything and I'll forgive you; I'll always be available to you; and if I fail, you can punish me. In return, you must love me unconditionally: no matter how I behave to you, you must always excuse me, and you must be immediately available to me; if you fail, I can punish you."*

You need love to exist, to survive. In the Wise Woman tradition, love is a crucial aspect of optimum nutrition. Forgive yourself, better yet, enjoy yourself for your attempts to get love. Understand that your fights with your beloveds feel like life-and-death struggles because they are, for certain parts of yourself.

Our attempts to *give* love unconditionally are usually sophisticated strategems for extracting love *from* the universe or another person.

The inner well of need for love and nurturance seems like a bottomless pit when we first gaze down it alone, with no one else to blame for the echoing hollowness. With each act of lovingkindness for ourselves, it fills. Slowly the bottom becomes at least visible. Others don't seem to be sources of pain so often. They, all of them, seem more and more like oneself.

As we love ourselves, and nourish all aspects of ourselves, a rare compassion is nourished, a tender compassion for everyone and everything. We are filled with compassion. We forgive ourselves deeply. And we realize that everyone who ever wronged us was a healer, a teacher, a lover of ours. The heart bursts with compassion. The floodgates of love spill over.

Once we have filled ourselves with unconditional love, once we agree to love and nurture all aspects of ourselves, we emit the energy of unconditional love. We don't do anything particular, yet the beings around us feel this love. Just by being, we resonate love and health/wholeness/holiness.

Some are attracted, some repelled by this vibration of truth, beauty, and love. There is no attachment in us to winning this one or that one, healing this one with love, being adored by that one. No attachment to getting you to accept my love so that I can expect love from you. Right now I love myself, and the universe loves me, and I am in the midst of all this love. If you reject my love, I remember. I remember with compassion the love I rejected before. I remember how vulnerable, how lonely I felt. I love myself as one who has rejected love, and so my love includes you in your rejection of love.

The welling heartsprings themselves are nourished at their sources when we love ourselves unconditionally. This constant inner flow of unconditional love and compassion *for self* creates an axis in the chaos of ongoing life and unwinding death. An axis, a string, a resonant fiber, vibrating wholeness, humming a love song, sounds within you. It flows out from you and touches, sounds in everything.

In the Wise Woman tradition, this strong center of unconditional self-love is a magic carpet, a cosmic surfboard on the turbulent, unpredictable flow of being.

The Wise Woman Tradition Loves Rough

Just as receptive power seems a contradiction in terms to some, so does rough love. Compassion, forgiveness, and unconditional love evoke a sense of squishy soft acceptance to many. In the Wise Woman tradition, love is rough, real, truthful, and unattached to outcome. In the Wise Woman tradition, love says "no" as often as "yes."

The Wise Woman tradition sees compassion as passionate. Passion shared is compassion. Passion is rough; passion is wild. Screams and shouts and tears and touches are part of living with passion, being com/passionate in the Wise Woman way.

Forgiveness is focused on self, in the Wise Woman way, and believe me, that can be rough. Forgive yourself for being hurt, for suffering, and love yourself enough to tell yourself the truth about it. Is it time to say "no"?

In the Wise Woman tradition, forgiving ourselves opens our vision to our limits, to our cramped spaces, to our self-inflicted prisons. Keen-sighted from the truth, we see how to free ourselves by setting boundaries that truly protect our fragile aspects yet are moveable, permeable to nourishment, so we receive the intimacy we desire. Saying "no" leads to unconditional love.

Unconditional love that nourishes the inner being does not tolerate abuse, ugliness, lies. Unconditional self-love brings self-respect and demands it of others. Unconditional self-love knows that it is unloving of anyone, self or other, to allow abuse to continue, no matter their age or circumstances. Loving ourselves unconditionally strengthens our power to say "no" when our heart knows that beauty and truth are not present.

The wise woman understands that, for most of us, saying "no" is hard to do. We're afraid that if we say "no," we won't get enough love. Or worse yet, we won't be allowed to give our love away, and we need to give our love away so we can expect to get love from others. The wise woman understands that we expect love to come from outside, not inside. She knows that this expectation, this assumption, this hope—that love comes from outside—prevents us from speaking our truth when our heart demands that we say "no."

Loving ourselves, generating love from inside, not trying to get it from outside, that is the Wise Woman way, a way that allows "no" to reveal its loving nature.

Become aware of how often you do the expected thing, the good thing, the right thing, says the Wise Woman helper, and acknowledge the part of yourself that is a liar, that is afraid to say "no."

Truth and unconditional love support each other. To love yourself unconditionally, you must tell yourself the truth. You cannot hear your own truth if you are lying to others. Begin to tell the truth in the smallest thing. This brings you wholeness. Tell the truth often and you will be filled with beauty. You will have health. You will walk the beauty way of health/wholeness/holiness. Your truth will bless all you encounter. You will be blessed. Do not be afraid to reveal your own uniqueness, for that is part of your blessing.

The Wise Woman Tradition Insists on Uniqueness

The Scientific tradition defines truth as repeatability. The Wise Woman tradition says nothing is ever the same. Nothing ever really repeats. Everything is unique, is it not? Unique and ever-changing. Uniqueness is the truth of the Wise Woman way.

The Wise Woman tradition does not insist on fixity, does not look for repeatability, and recognizes that there is no such thing as an objective statement or an objective universe. One incidence of something is valid information in the Wise Woman tradition. Uniqueness is recognized and validated in the Wise Woman way. The wise woman knows that change is always moving, fixity is fantasy.

Each person is a unique manifestion of individual and universal consciousness. Each being is unique. Every situation is unique. Every relationship is unique. Each time is unique. Every moment is unique. Each pain, each problem, is completely unique from the view of the Wise Woman tradition. The wise woman looks for the uniqueness, the difference, not the similarity, the sameness. The uniqueness is the hole through which the health/wholeness/holiness is known.

The unique reality of a chickweed flower is far more important in the Wise Woman tradition than a rule for harvesting it, or its chemical composition.

Objectivity is understood as impossible to achieve in the Wise Woman tradition (as well as in quantum physics). Subjective factors are discussed openly and considered in future decisions. When a wise woman measures (length of time before placenta is delivered, normal growth, and so on) she refers these figures to the unique situation, the unique individual, not the norm. Interrelationships are looked for and acknowledged in the Wise Woman way, adding to our appreciation of uniqueness, as we see that everything changes.

The Wise Woman tradition says everything is uniquely connected in an ever-changing spiral web of nourishment and transformation. Uniqueness gives way to more uniqueness. Everything is mysteriously related. The forms keep changing. All things are possible. Trust uniqueness.

The Wise Woman way has no standard other than uniqueness. Uniqueness includes all. All possible treatments, from meditation to surgery, are used in the Wise Woman tradition. For each unique problem has a unique need and a unique gift. Standardized treatments give prompt relief in most cases and are fairly successful in curing or eliminating problems. Unique treatments, such as the Wise Woman tradition uses, nourish the healthy/whole/holy being, the community, and the planet.

The validation of the individual's unique reality is one aspect of optimum nourishment in the Wise Woman tradition. Each being's experience is a unique experience. Support for the individual's unique perspective is a trait of the wise woman. The uniqueness of each being is identified and validated, supported and nourished, in the Wise Woman tradition.

Many unique realities co-exist, each in its truth, in the both/and universe of the wise woman. Your truth does not have to be my truth to be true.

Multiple unique realities exist both within and between beings. An individual being can contain many unique realities, many different ways of experiencing the realms of life and death. Unique and differing realities exist among different kinds of beings as well: rocks, animals, plants, people, devas.

In the moon lodge, in the sweat lodge, realities come and go. Each breath is unique. Each moment is the birth of the universe and myself. Each moment of my existence is a unique experience. In the moon lodge, in the sweat lodge, my reality shimmers and shifts. Each reality has its own unique resonance. Each unique reality offers a special nourishment. Each reality has unique needs. In the moon lodge, in the sweat lodge, uniqueness becomes ordinary. Such is the Wise Woman way.

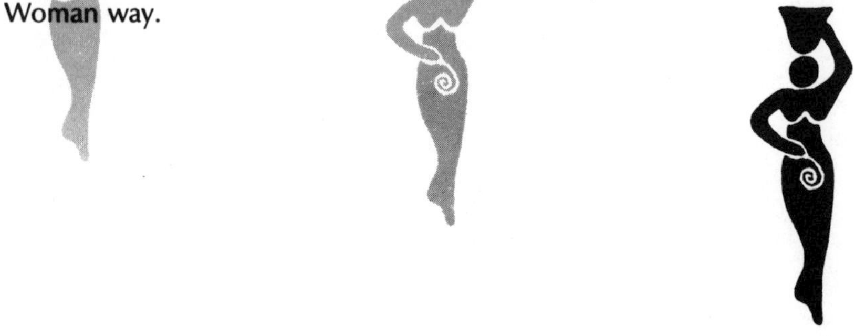

There Are No Diseases in the Wise Woman Tradition

How does someone following the Wise Woman way deal with disease, such as high blood pressure, a fever, cancer? In the Wise Woman way, these words describe things that do not exist. Disease has no existence on its own. Any disease is bound inextricably to the being and setting which expresses and embodies it. In the Wise Woman tradition, disease, pain, and problems exist only within the framework of a particular person and particular society, not independently.

Diseases are certainly recognized, and diagnostic skills are honored within the Wise Woman both/and, holographic, spiraling way. But the focus is on the person as an individual, not on the disease as an entity.

The Wise Woman tradition maintains that the name of the disease is not the disease and that the name of the disease cannot be treated, cannot be healed/wholed. "High blood pressure" is a static, unchanging phrase, and as such can only be eliminated or reduced, not healed. From the Wise Woman perspective, the disease itself is a gift of wholeness to be cherished and nourished, not hastily cured.

Disease does not exist apart from the being manifesting it. Even a typhoid bacterium, a polio virus, is not typhoid or polio without a being to manifest it. And because each being is unique, so each expression of typhoid or polio is unique, and must be treated uniquely in the Wise Woman tradition.

In this way, the being expressing the disease is nourished and becomes healthy/whole/holy in the Wise Woman tradition, whether or not the disease is proclaimed "cured."

The wise woman sees our disease, our problem as an ally of wholeness. Our wholeness comes from disease as well as health in the Wise Woman way.

The Wise Woman Never Asks Why

The Wise Woman tradition accepts chaos. The Wise Woman tradition knows that health/wholeness/holiness is of the void and ever-changing. So the wise woman doesn't ask "why?"

The Wise Woman tradition has no goal but wholeness and inclusion. The Wise Woman tradition accepts uniqueness. The Wise Woman tradition gives up control. So the wise woman doesn't ask "why?"

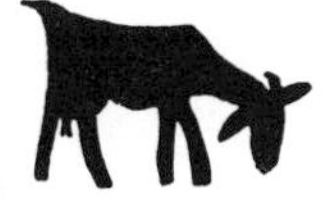

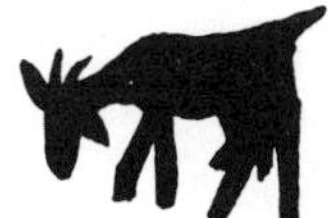

Why am I sick? Why did this happen to me? Why do I feel this way? Why do I have these dreadful menstrual cramps?

The wise woman knows that the answer to "why?" is always "because."

Because I ate the wrong thing. Because the world is a rotten place. Because they were awful to me. Because all the women in my family do.

And that "because" leads to guilt and blame.

And to the setting up of boundaries to maintain control and ensure that the pain/problem never happens again.

So I'll never, ever even think about hot, salty, crisp french fries again. And now I'm on my own and everybody else is out for number one, too, and that's the way it is; don't trust anybody. I'll never feel so much about anyone again. I wish I didn't have a uterus; I wish I weren't a woman.

The Wise Woman way defines health as flexible, encompassing, and vital. How can these attributes be nourished with limits and guilt? How can wholeness be nurtured with blame and boundaries? How can holiness be recognized through fear and separation? They cannot. So the wise woman doesn't ask "why?" The wise woman asks "how?"

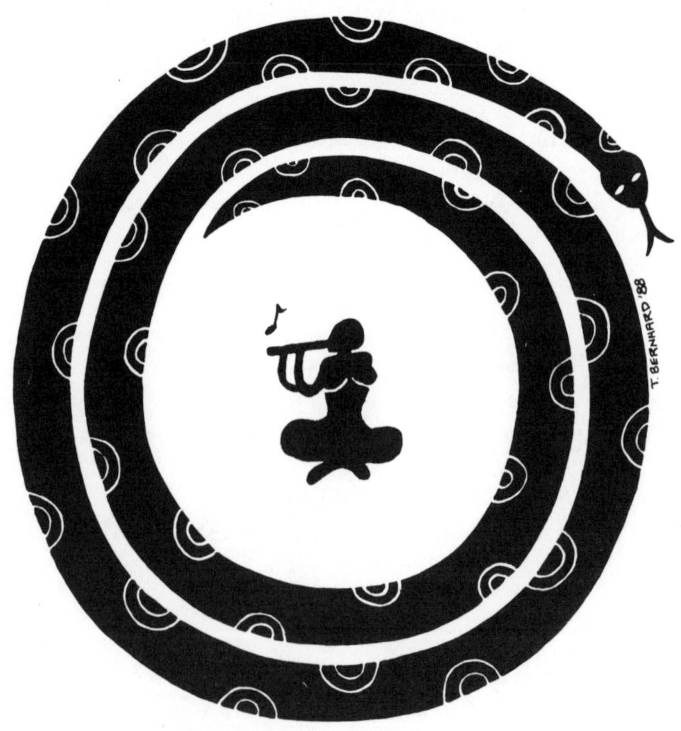

How is this problem my ally?

Menstrual cramps are not an ally.

How does this condition benefit me?

I get no benefit at all from being in pain and sick to my stomach and I resent your implication that I do it to get attention or something.

And the wise woman asks "what?" What does this pain/problem prevent me from doing?

When I'm cramping, I can't cook dinner, I can't drive the kids around, I can't even read.

What nourishment am I given by my pain/problem?

All I can do is curl up in bed or in the bath tub and close my eyes and kinda dream.

What part of myself is revealed there?

I feel like a bad mother and a worthless person if I just lie around and don't do anything.

What nourishment does it need?

I guess I could accept myself. Yeah, maybe it is good to have one day every month for myself. Just for myself. Just for me.

And again the wise woman asks "how?" How can I open to receive the gift of this situation?

You mean, how could I encourage the cramps? No. Oh, how can I have that day to myself, how can I accept a day for myself and not have to be in pain?

How shall I nourish wholeness?

I guess being a bad mother one day a month isn't so terrible. And I found the perfect green ally, Senecio aureus. And I think it will be good for the kids to be more on their own.

What strengthens me, my community, and Mother Earth in this situation?

Women used to believe that their menstrual time was special and holy? I'll have to think that over. Bleeding on the earth nourishes all life? Wow, that's kind of a big responsibility, don't you think. Besides, what if someone saw me? Are you suggesting that my menstrual cramps are the earth's way getting me to love and nourish her? That's weird. Kind of the ultimate recycling. Save a tree and all that, huh? Don't support the multi-billion dollar "feminine hygiene" industry. And it fertilizes plants? No wonder some women have a green thumb. Say, these cramps could be not so bad after all.

There Are No Cures in the Wise Woman Tradition

In the Scientific tradition, curing consists of getting rid of the problem as quickly as possible. In the Heroic tradition, curing consists of allocating guilt, asking for forgiveness, accepting punishment, and learning the rules so it never happens again. In the Wise Woman tradition, there are no cures.

Problems are not cured; they are not enemies to be eliminated.

In the Wise Woman tradition, we do not love our enemies. We make them our allies. In the Wise Woman tradition, we eliminate our enemies. We eliminate them by accepting all their gifts, by feasting on the nourishment they offer. In the Wise Woman tradition, we gain cooperation from our enemies by respecting their unique reality. They become our supporters. In the Wise Woman tradition we honor and cherish our enemies as benefactors of our health/wholeness/holiness; for our enemies force us, as few others will, to be strong and wise.

Problems are not the result of wrongdoing, in the Wise Woman tradition. Problems are allies, powerful presences, who come to help us to wholeness. Sometimes these allies leave when we incorporate them into our compassionate heart. Sometimes, recognizing them as needed helpers, we consent to their continued presence.

Sometimes substances (insulin, antibiotics) or techniques (surgery) strongly associated with the Scientific tradition are used by the wise woman; she understands these substances and techniques as nourishments not cures. It is not the thing done that indicates the tradition, but the thought behind the action.

Getting cured is not the goal in the Wise Woman tradition. Instead, we are healed/wholed/made holy and nourished in our uniqueness.

Outwitting death as long as possible is not the goal in the Wise Woman tradition. Balanced in the heart with the inexhaustible goddess who churns the waters of birthing and dying, we lose our anxiety to be cured or to cure.

Nourishing our wholeness, compassionately embracing our multiple and contradictory self images, unconditionally loving our own neediness, we gradually come to know that the Wise Woman way to health/wholeness/holiness is not by curing our problems, avoiding pain, and living as long as "humanly" possible, but by accepting problems, pains, disease, and death as allies. And by accepting the gifts of our allies.

We mistakenly see our diseases and injuries as other than ourselves. We say our arthritis is bad, not ourselves. My stomach/arm/head hurts, not "me." We fail to see that we have already "embodied" our problems.

Struggling to be rid of the pain and impairment, we paradoxically struggle *against* our own wholeness, our own variety and variability, our own perfection in the moment as a holographic expression of the whole.

Allowing ourselves to find the ally in our problem and accepting the ally's gifts, we validate our own health/wholeness/holiness and nourish ourselves in compassionate transformation. We turn, heart-centered, in the moving spiral of wholeness.

We come to see suffering as resistance and denial, so more and more we open to ourselves, we accept ourselves. And we are filled with joy. What a way to be not cured!

There Are No Rules in the Wise Woman Tradition

The only rule in the Wise Woman tradition is that there are no rules.

Allowing the unjudging flow of compassion, in a Wise Woman way, we are challenged to remember that the perfect wholeness of each moment is ever-changing. There can be no rules. Loving ourselves unconditionally, with Wise Woman roughness and compassion, we are challenged to acknowledge the unique perfection of each pain. There can be no rules. Looking at the both/and hologram with Wise Woman vision, we are challenged to increase the clarity and brilliance of the whole by nourishing—nourishing the web and each of its unique parts. There can be no rules.

In a both/and universe there can be no rules. Any time you think this is exactly the same as before, you're wrong, says the Wise Woman tradition.

Rules make comfortable, secure boxes to hide behind when normalcy stretches its limits and the unexpected occurs. Rules are safe. Rules are not elastic. Rules are visible. Rules are accountable. Rules are regular. Rules are logical.

All rules are made to be broken, says the wise woman.

There Are No Healers in the Wise Woman Tradition

We are all healers in the Wise Woman tradition. Self-healing and self-loving, we co-create healing with our allies. Our allies are our problems; they bring us gifts of wholeness. Our allies are wise women; they support us in our transformation. Our allies are green allies, wild plants: they supply us with optimum nourishment.

The Wise Woman tradition asks us to ally ourselves with our pains and problems, receive their gifts, honor them and listen to them, and to nourish compassionately all aspects of ourselves.

The Wise Woman tradition sees everyone as a potential wise woman, as a wise woman in disguise. Seeking support, we ally ourself with a woman of wisdom. We listen for resonance. We seek ones who can magnify our tone for us, guide us, support us in the vulnerability and chaos of our expansion. We seek the wise woman who encourages, not return to balance or normalcy, but transformation and refinement. We seek the ones who nourish us through the incorporation, not the remission, of the problem.

We go to visit the healer. There is ritual of respect. The healer is welcomed as a visitor to our homeland. We lodge at the healer's home, are treated as honored guest.

Wholeness is accepted, says the Wise Woman tradition, not created. We are precious gifts to each other: for together we are part of the whole universe. Let us love ourselves gloriously and heal each other. Let us see health/wholeness/holiness in ourselves and each other. Let us fall in love again and again. Let our hearts beat and our breath flow at one with the universal pulse: grief/joy, grief/joy, grief/joy.

Having no goals, resonant with truth, beauty, joy, and wholeness, the wise woman does nothing. She is still, sensitive, alert. Like a dolphin she sends out sonar waves to test the frequencies of wholeness. She opens herself to the hologram of this unique being, at this time, in this place.

Having no rules to teach, no morals to preach, the wise woman is silent. She is full in her silence; she is empty in her silence. Her expression is quite clear; she's in love. Her strength is quite visible. She does not reach out. The best helping hand is often the one that touches not.

Energy is visible around the wise woman, sparks and flashes caught in the corner of the eye. Look deeply into her eyes. Feel the energy coil and shift. There is alliance, attunement, acceptance, agreement. Barriers are lifted. Wholeness is revealed.

Blessing the wise woman, blessing ourselves, we part. Savoring the taste of truth-telling, knowing that we empower ourselves, accepting the gifts of the wise woman, we continue our self-healing journey. There are no rules, in the Wise Woman way. There are no cures, in the Wise Woman way. There are no healers, in the Wise Woman way. There are the questions of transformation: "What is the health/wholeness/holiness here? How is it nourished?"

Optimum Nourishment

Nourishment is the keynote of the Wise Woman tradition. Nourishment comes from women. Breast milk is the archetype of nourishment. Now I eat you. Nourishment comes from the earth mother. She gives us abundant nourishment of sweet grains, green allies, and animal give-aways. Now you eat me.

Health/wholeness/holiness is remembered through optimum nourishment in the Wise Woman tradition. Nourishment is a constant need of beingness. Alive or dead, we need nourishment. (Why else are the dead given waybread?)

Optimum nourishment, claims the Wise Woman tradition, is whole, holy, vital, wild, unique, local, common, simple, messy, fresh, abundant, accessible, seasonal, varied, and full of love.

In the Wise Woman tradition, optimum nourishment encourages and supports wholeness, holiness, vitality, flexibility, individuality, intimacy, self-love and self-acceptance, integration, originality, sensitivity, responsibility, creativity, centeredness, and compassion as well as providing physical, emotional, and spiritual sustenance.

Healing and change are best carried out by providing nourishment, counsels the Wise Woman tradition. The wise woman looks at everything from the viewpoint of nourishment. How can optimum nourishment be made accessible, or more desirable, in this unique instance? What nourishment feeds the larger hologram (the family, community, and planet) as well as the individual? Who is starving? How can the one who hungers find nourishment? Who is giving away? "Now you eat me." Who is receiving nourishment? "Now I eat you."

Optimum nourishment, says the Wise Woman tradition, is needed to sustain personal, cultural, and planetary growth. Optimum nourishment, says the Wise Woman tradition, is needed to support the spiraling of transformation, individually and universally. Optimum nourishment is needed, says the Wise Woman tradition, to give the courage and strength to accept our own unique health/wholeness/holiness.

Optimum nourishment? How do we get it?

Appreciate your uniqueness, to begin with, says the Wise Woman tradition. Ally yourself with your problem instead of fighting it. Make yourself available to receive the gifts of your allies: the hidden parts of yourself brought to the surface by your problem allies, the delicious foods prepared from your green allies, the wisdom of your inner and outer Wise Woman allies. Accept these gifts of abundance from your mother. Open yourself to nourishment in the Wise Woman way; open yourself even to nourishment which comes in disorderly, mysterious ways.

Give up blaming yourself for your own problems. Give up blaming yourself for everyone else's problems. Give up punishing yourself. Realize that denying any part of yourself optimum nourishment denies the whole of you, and the whole of the universe as well, from the Wise Woman perspective. Love every part of yourself enough to offer it nourishment. Health/wholeness/holiness are the natural consequences of giving optimum nourishment to every aspect of one's being, according to the Wise Woman tradition.

Remember that the state of your health/wholeness/holiness reflects not only the nourishment available but what you choose to consume, to integrate into yourself. Remember that nourishment, in the Wise Woman tradition, comes in many forms and with many energies. And that health/wholeness/holiness can receive nourishment from every form and every energy. The wise woman knows: the more forms and energies of nourishment you accept, the greater your access to optimum nourishment. There are no food rules in the Wise Woman tradition.

There can be no food rules in the Wise Woman tradition. I am sitting on an airplane, face to the window, crying. I have just had a fight with the stewardess about my carry-on bag, and lost. The older woman sitting next to me reaches into her capacious purse (nearly as big as the bag they wouldn't let me take on!) and finds a wrapped bundle. It is a pastrami sandwich. I am a vegetarian. Smiling tenderly, she catches my eye as I turn to see what she's doing, and offers me half of her sandwich.

With my local vision, I see meat; I ready myself to say "no." Then I look with Wise Woman eyes: She is the goddess, this woman. She is wholeness, holiness, the wise woman. She offers me nourishment, mother love, acceptance in my misery. I feel the openness of my heart.

I offer myself compassion, and smile back at her. I open myself to the sacrament she offers. I accept the nourishment she offers me. I accept the healing gift of pastrami on rye.

Locked into a rule ("I don't eat meat"), how can I be ready to receive the abundance of the universe, the mother's nourishment in its multi-faceted forms? Rules, maintains the Wise Woman tradition, especially about food, generally restrict our access to love and optimum nourishment. Following the Wise Woman way, we find nourishment even in mysterious and absurd places.

Everything offers us both physical and energetic nourishment when we are open to receive it. If we recognize only the form, says the Wise Woman tradition, we open only to nourishment from the form. When we recognize and nourish ourselves with the energy as well, we find health/wholeness/holiness.

There is no pain in the heart but the breaking of barriers to love. As we follow the Wise Woman way, surrender our barriers to self-love and allow ourselves to feed on the mother love of the earth, we notice the various qualities of nourishment available to us. Sitting in a circle is a nourishment. Practiced consistently, this creates a different state of health than always sitting in rows. Daydreaming is a nourishment. And engaged in regularly but not exclusively, this creates a different state of health than chronic logical thought does.

Some forms and energies of nourishment are easy for us to consume; others are difficult. Some warm us, others cool us off when the pressure rises. Some kinds of nourishment allow us to exist in certain environments, other kinds prevent us from experiencing our environment at all. When we give up our rules and recognize our unique place in the hologram of all life with self-love and self-respect, the Wise Woman way, we find it easier and easier to choose the optimum nourishment for ourselves in any situation: shoulders to cry on, chickweed in the pavement cracks, a shooting star that takes away the breath.

Every food offers its special nourishment. Eating wild food is consuming optimum nourishment. Do it frequently, in addition to your regular diet, and your tastes begin to change. The junk foods you couldn't resist before now irritate your tongue, smell offensive, and generally annoy you. The body (as well as the rest of our "selves") prefers the best nourishment it is offered. Hard to believe that most premenstrual women would really rather eat organic kale or cooked nettles than chocolate, but I've seen it many, many times.

Optimum nourishment is craved and sought after. The Wise Woman tradition evokes health/wholeness/holiness by recognizing the opening, the hole, for the desired nourishment to enter. Trauma, grief, pain, disease, and injury create holes. So do safe space, consensual agreement, and respect among beings.

Once there is openness, the wise woman knows that when one being (person, plant, animal, rock) is more compassionate, more self-loving, and more aware of personal and planetary wholeness than another, then fuller integration in the other will be supported and nourished, no matter what the techniques of interaction.

This openness can occur between plants and people (and animals and people, and stones and people, and so on) as well as among people, and is an important key in understanding optimum nourishment. A wild plant nourishes the fullness of your being from the fullness of its being. A cultivated plant nourishes less fully, evokes less integration, wholeness, strength, and energy, according to the conditions of its life.

The Wise Woman tradition *is* nourishment: optimum nourishment from the heart, conscious nourishment of planetary wholeness, in an ever-changing, ever-spinning, mysterious spiral. Optimum nourishment, the Wise Woman way, is simple no matter where on this planet you are.

The Wise Woman Tradition Is a Simple Approach

Simple means easy. Simple means common. Simple means single. The Wise Woman tradition is easy, and singular, and very common; and herbally, the Wise Woman tradition urges simples. In a simple, one herb alone is used.

An infusion of oatstraw, a tincture of dandelion, or a poultice of chickweed is a simple. Simples are usually as effective as compound remedies, far less expensive, and their quality is more easily judged. Using simples has the added advantage of self-teaching the effects of single herbs on your body.

A Wise Woman midwife, for instance, finds birthing tinctures containing many herbs less reliable than a simple tincture of blue cohosh alone, or even blue cohosh, ginger, and black cohosh given simultaneously, but from individual tinctures.

The green gifts of Mother Earth are individual, singular, unique. They each carry a specific wholeness in the form and energy that most suits the particular plant, but they contain, as well, a multitude of lesser abilities. By using simples, we give ourselves a chance to encounter these subtleties in each plant.

Using simples, we experience the uniqueness of each herb. Using simples, we are stretched to become allies, deep friends with each herb. They become our friends in the same ways other beings do: with attention, with love, with care and concern, with time spent together, alone. We come to know, cherish, honor all aspects of each green ally, by being closely and simply together, without distraction.

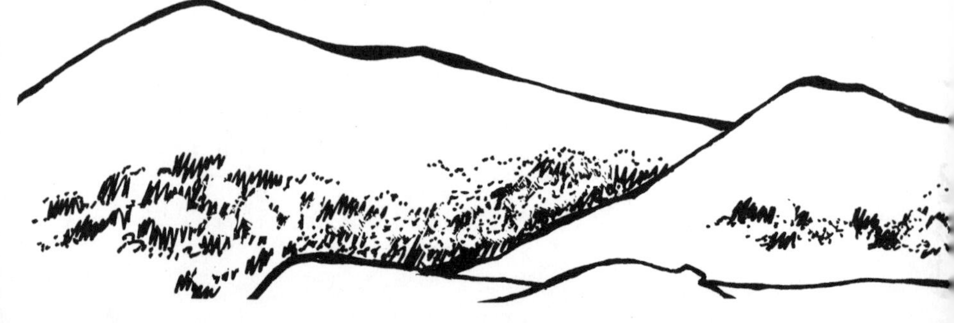

The wise woman may have only a very small group of allies, sometimes only one plant ally. This is part of her invisibility; simple is invisible. She learns, through the use of simples, the ways of her green allies, just as she learns her own ways, her strengths and vulnerabilities, her harshnesses and softnesses, her predictabilities and eccentricities. She becomes so intimate, so allied with those herbs that a handful of them, thirteen or so, suffice for helping her integrate health/wholeness/holiness with the problem at hand, no matter what the problem is, her life long.

How long does it take to make a friend? Start with a year. Choose the herb you want to be friends with. Not an exotic herb, but a local plant, a common plant, a simple weed. Visit . . . sing with . . . draw . . . gather . . . eat . . . experience your herb as often as you can. Every day is not too much.

Not just in the day, at night, too. Not just in the sun, in the rain, too. Not just in spring and summer, in autumn, winter, too.

Keep notes. Write down what you see, smell, feel, hear, experience with this ally-to-be. Invite your herb into your dreams. Introduce your other friends, and your family. Invite your green friend to your parties and celebrations.

Read about your herb. Ask other people about their experiences with this plant as ally. Sleep together. Become available to the emotive force, the physical power, and the holiness of this green ally. Notice what nourishment is available to this plant, and what nourishment it chooses. What are the needs of your ally? Can you hear, sense, feel, know within yourself what is needed? Ah, you are becoming friends.

Ask your new green friend to help you. Rest in her strengths. Make use of her abilities. Call upon your friend. Ask for exactly what you need. Ah, now you are becoming allies.

In the Wise Woman way, we are all herbalists, for we all eat the plants of the earth. The Wise Woman herbalist allies herself with plants that are local and common. Open your door, and there is your ally, waiting to be seen, heard, and cherished, yes, even if you live in the city.

Health/wholeness/holiness, the Wise Woman way, is simple.

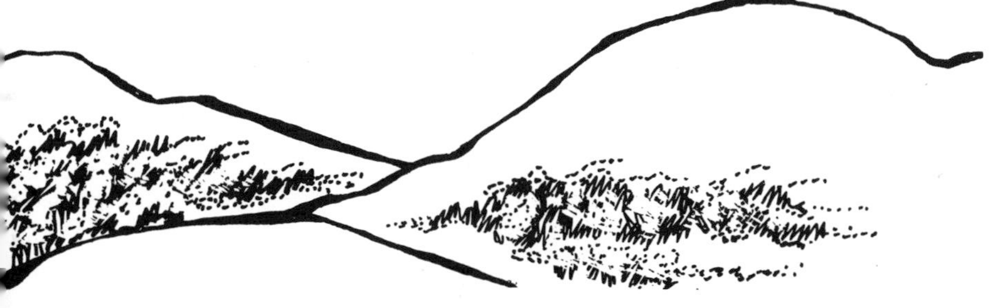

Wise Woman, Witch Doctor, Green Witch

The Wise Woman tradition is natural to women, but not limited to them. Men can be wise women too. Anyone can come to know the wise woman within. Anyone can learn to recognize the wise woman in all other beings. This is the Wise Woman way. A woman whose life is spent in the Wise Woman way may call herself, or be known as, a witch. Witches heal. Those whose special love is the plants, or the green nation, are known as green witches. (Men, of course, may be known as witch doctors when they follow the Wise Woman way.)

Witches heal. Witches are not now, nor were they ever, involved in anything other than the preservation of life and joy. Their blissful delight in life and insistence on honoring the life-giver, life-nourisher, the Mother Earth, earned witches the opprobrium of the Catholic Church, which insisted that life came only from the father and that life and the body were full of suffering.

Witches honor the male principle in the form of a horned animal. How ironic that religions which claim to honor the male cast this image as the very image of the devil, evil incarnate. Pan, horned and hoofed man of the European witches, is full of fun and music, not fire and brimstone, though he does have a reputation for being hot.

A woman learns to be a wise woman by living her life with attention. When she accepts the cloak of her holiness, deeply compassionate for her own wholeness and chaos, and loves herself, she knows herself as wise woman. Each month's stay in the menstrual hut adds to her power and wisdom. At menopause, she becomes the crone, ancient wise one, keeper of the visions. She is wicce, bender and shaper of stories and realities, keeper of wisdom; she is witch. A witch is a woman of power.

A green witch is allied with the green growth of the earth. A green witch is a wise woman whose own heart is as green as the heart of the earth. A green witch is one of the colors of the rainbow of witches, rainbow of wise women, rainbow of women of power.

"Witch doctor" is presently a derogatory term. "Shaman" is used instead. Read "shaman" as "she-man" (though the actual derivation of the word is far from it) and remember that these are men who are connected to their own wise woman within.

Men of all cultures who desire to be powerful train to become wise women. The Wise Woman way is not a natural flow in their lives, so they have learned to copy women's ways, and invent special ones, to find the woman within, who must be present before any man can provide or even support optimum nourishment for health/wholeness/holiness.

Some of the ways a man can find his wise woman within, his womb/man-hood:

- honor and protect all women
- sit alone in a dark place (cave, kiva)
- sit alone on a high point and cry out
- act out pregnancy, birth, and menstruation
- sweat
- fast and pray

Attention to the care of all women brings a man into alignment with his female principle in a natural, invisible way.

Sitting in cave, kiva, sweat lodge, or other small dark place, the man re-enters the mother's womb. The man enters the void. In the dark, no sound but his own breathing, no food, no water, the mother comes to him. She shows him visions of creation, and visions of dissolution. If he is open, she enters and he knows the wise woman within, and becomes capable of giving nourishment and resonating wholeness.

High above even the flight of the hawk, he sits, crying his need with voice or with spirit. How to be whole? How to be nourished? She appears. As her consort, he shares her power, the power to create, the power to include all, the power to weave the strands into a pattern that enriches all.

The sweat lodge follows the way of the moon lodge. In cultures where the Wise Woman tradition persists, the men train to find their wise woman within while the women are in the menstrual lodge. One tale has it that the Native American sweat lodge was given to the men to still their jealousy of the women's moontime rites.

The wise old woman is carved larger than life as the main support of the men's dance hall in Papua, New Guinea. The wise woman smiles from shrines in thousands of cathedrals across Europe and lawns in North America. The wise woman is buried in the ground of every country. The wise woman's robe still flows down your back, centering you in the ever-changing, ever-spiraling mystery.

Everywhere I look, the wise woman looks back.

And she smiles.

References & Resources:

The Wise Woman Tradition

- *Great Cosmic Mother of All*
  Monica Sjöö and Barbara Mor; 1987, Harper & Row
- *Blood Magic*
  Alma Gottlieb & T. Buckley; 1988, U. of California
- *Border Healing Woman*
  Jewel Babb & Pat E. Taylor; 1981, U. of Texas
- Cassandra: Radical Feminist Nurses Network
  PO Box 341 Williamsville, NY 14221
- *A Celebration of Birth*
  Sheila Kitzinger; 1986, Pennypress
- *Crone: Woman of Age, Wisdom, and Power*
  Barbara Walker; 1985, Harper & Row
- *Daughters of the Earth*
  Carolyn Niethammer; 1977, Collier
- *Daughters of Copper Woman*
  Anne Cameron; 1981, Press Gang
- Death, dying, and transitions in the Wise Woman tradition:
  Kubler-Ross Center; South Rt. 616, Head Waters, VA 24442
- *Embodying Experience*
  S. Keleman; 1987, Center
- *For Her Own Good*
  Barbara Ehrenreich & Deirdre English; 1979, Anchor
- "Gray Like Me"
  Pat Moore (with M. Jerome), *New Age Journal,* March 1988
- *Guide Lectures for Self-Transformation*
  Eva Pierrakos; 1984, Center for the Living Force
- "Healing, the Feminine Art"
  Gwynelle Dismukes, *Healer,* Vol II/1 , Feb. 1987
- *In a Different Voice*
  Carol Gilligan; 1982, Harvard University Press

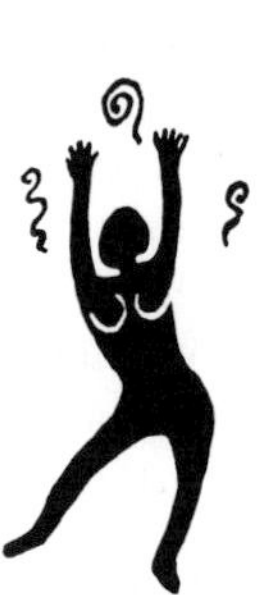

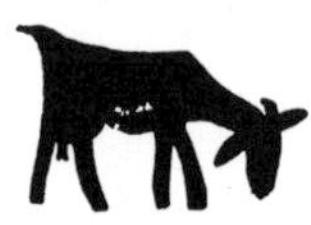

- *Love, Medicine and Miracles*
  B. Siegel, M.D.; 1986, Harper & Row
- *Listening to Our Bodies: the Rebirth of Feminine Wisdom*
  Stephanie Demetrakopoulos; 1983, Beacon
- *Maria Sabina, Her Life and Chants*
  Alvaro Estrada; 1981, Ross-Erickson
- *Matriarchal Mythology in Former Times & Today*
  Heide Göttner-Abendroth; 1987, Crossing
- *Medicine Woman, Flight of the Seventh Moon, Jaguar Woman, Star Woman, Crystal Woman*
  Lynn Andrews; 1981, 1984, 1985, 1986, 1987, Harper and Row
- Native American Wise Woman tradition:
  Yewenode/Twylah Nitsch, 12199 Brant Res. Rd, Irving, NY 14081
- *Not for Innocent Ears*
  Ruby Modesto & G. Mount; 1980, Sweetlight
- *Old Wives' Tales*
  Mary Chamberlain; 1981, Virago
- *Peace Pilgrim*
  Herself; 1982, Ocean Tree
- *Rapture of the Deep: Sacred Land, Sacred Sex*
  Dolores LaChapelle; 1988, Finn Hill, Box 542, Silverton CO 81433
- *Reinventing Eve*
  Kim Chernin; 1987, Random House
- *Shaman & the Medicine Wheel*
  Evelyn Eaton; 1982, Quest
- *Search for the Beloved: Sacred Psychology*
  Jean Houston; 1987, Tarcher
- *Sensitive Chaos*
  T. Schwenk; 1965, Steiner Press
- *Space, Time, and Medicine*
  L. Dossey; 1982, Shambala
- *When Society Becomes an Addict*
  Anne Schaff; 1987, Harper & Row
- *When the Spirits Come Back*
  Janet O. Dallett; 1988, Inner City Books

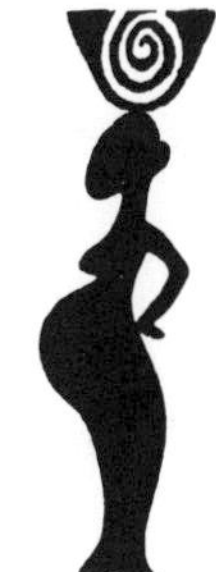

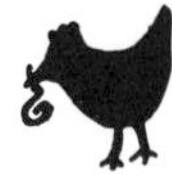

- *Wise Woman Herbal for the Childbearing Year*
  Susun Weed; 1986, Ash Tree
- Wise Woman hospital: Gesundheit Institute
  Patch Adams, MD, 404 N. Nelson St., Alexandria, VA 22203
- Wise Woman tradition midwifery classes:
  Sherry Willis, PO Box 353, Flint Hill, VA 22627
- Wise Woman tradition teaching center:
  Wise Woman Center, PO Box 64, Woodstock, NY 12498

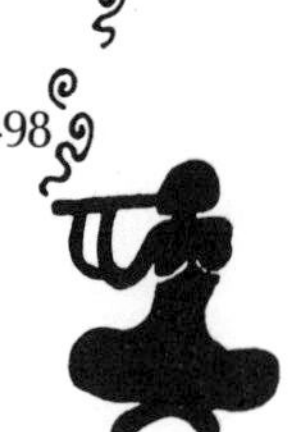

- *Woman: Earth & Spirit*
  Helen Luke; 1984, Crossroad
- *Woman of Power Magazine,*
  PO Box 827 Cambridge, MA 02238

Green Witches and Goddesses

- *Ancient Mirrors of Womanhood*
  Merlin Stone; 1979, Beacon
- *Ariadne*
  June Brindel; 1980, St. Martin's Press
- *The Birth Project*
  Judy Chicago; 1985, Doubleday
- *Book of Goddesses and Heroines*
  Patricia Monaghan; 1981, Dutton
- *Brighde*
  Sinead Sula Grian; 1985, Brighde's Fire
- *Dearest Goddess*
  Eso Benjamins; 1985, Current Nine

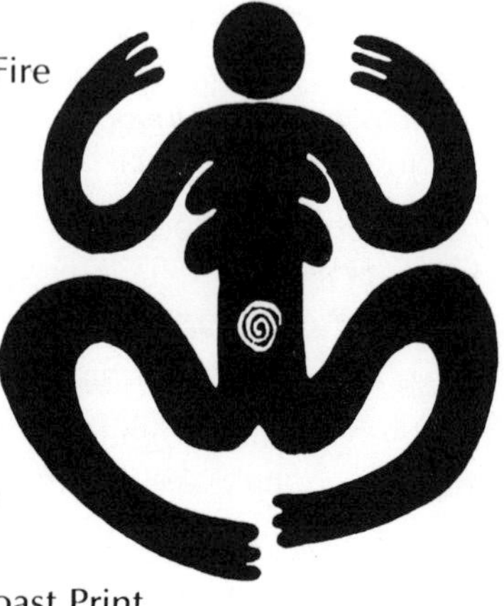

- *Drawing Down the Moon*
  Margot Adler; 1988, Beacon
- *Earth Magic*
  Marion Weinstein; 1980, Phoenix
- *Eight Sabbats for Witches*
  Janet & S. Farrar; 1981, Robert Hale
- *Femaissance*
  Lynne Biggerwomon; 1979, West Coast Print
- *Folk Medicine and Herbal Healing*
  G. Meyer, K. Blum, J. Cull; 1981, Charles Thomas

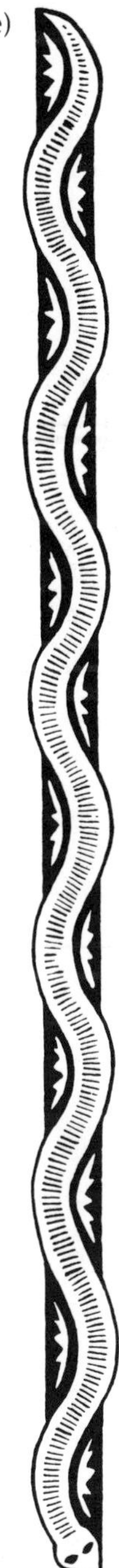

- *The Great Goddess: Heresies Special Issue* (1982 but still available)
  PO Box 766, Canal Street Station, NYC, New York 10013 $8.00
- *Goddesses*
  Mayumi Oda; 1981, Lancaster, Miller
- *Goddesses in Everywoman*
  Jean Shinoda Bolen; 1984, Harper & Row
- *Health Through God's Pharmacy,* pp. 1-51 only
  Maria Treben; 1982, Ennsthaler
- *Her Voice in the Drum*
  Rebecca Beguin; 1980, New Victoria
- *Holy Book of Women's Mysteries,* two volumes
  Z Budapest; 1979
- *Inanna*
  Diane Wolkstein & S. Kramer; 1983, Harper
- *I Send a Voice*
  Evelyn Eaton; 1978, Quest
- *Lost Goddesses of Early Greece*
  Charlene Spretnak; 1978, Beacon
- *Mists of Avalon*
  Marion Zimmer Bradley; 1982, Knopf
- *Plants, Man* [sic] *& Life*
  E. Anderson; 1969, University of California Press
- *Return of the Goddess*
  E. Whitmont; 1982, Crossroad
- *The Sacred Hoop*
  Paula Gunn Allen; 1986, Beacon
- *Secrets of the Tarot*
  Barbara Walker; 1984, Harper & Row
- *Spiral Dance*
  Starhawk; 1979, Harper & Row
- *The Second Ring of Power,* and *The Eagle's Gift*
  C. Castenada; 1977, 1981, Pocket.
- *Way of the Shaman*
  M. Harner; 1980, Bantam.
- *When God Was a Woman*
  Merlin Stone; 1976, HBJ/Harvest.

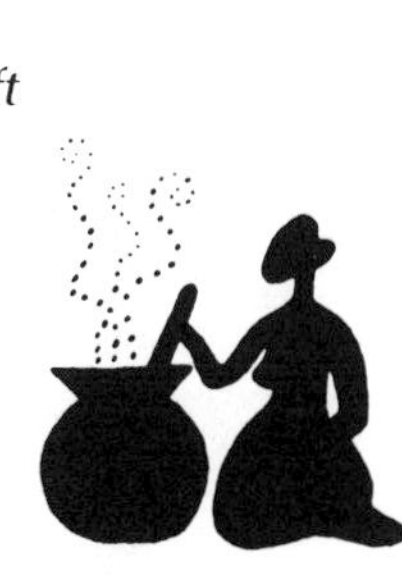

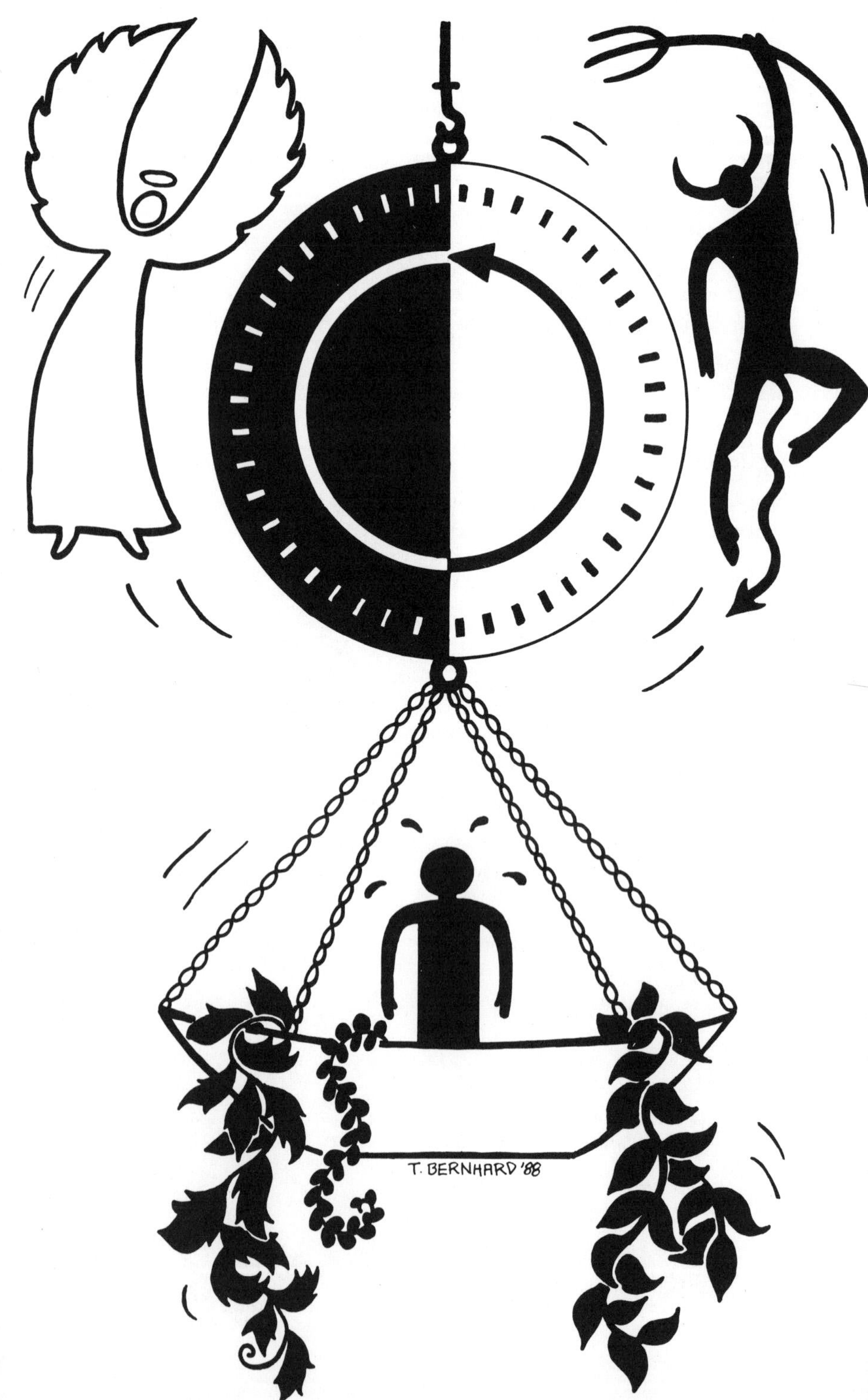
T. BERNHARD '88

Heroic Tradition

There is not one unified Heroic tradition, but many similar traditions known collectively as the Heroic tradition.

In the Heroic tradition, each person has a body, a mind, and a spirit/soul. These three parts make a complete person. Completeness and balance are evoked by the symbol of the Heroic tradition: the circle. The three parts are not equal: the spirit is high and worthy; the body is low and gross; the mind is in between.

Healing in the Heroic tradition attempts to change and clean all three parts of the person. For, according to the Heroic tradition, disease arises when toxins (dirt, filth, anger, negativity, lust) accumulate: the spirit/soul is clouded, the mind is confused, the body is defiled. Healing ourselves in the Heroic tradition often necessitates atoning for our wrongs.

Health itself (typified by a youthful white male) is a delicate balance and a constant struggle: good against bad, light against dark, clean against dirty.

Well-being in the Heroic tradition depends on balance and clarity, which requires disciplining the body and the mind. Guidelines and rules (often strict) for keeping physical and emotional desires in balance are a constant of all Heroic traditions, though the exact rules for correct conduct and correct eating vary from one type of Heroic tradition to another. What all Heroic authors and healers agree on is the absolute need for rules.

"Follow the rules or suffer the consequences." You cause your own consequences in the Heroic tradition. If you have a problem, you caused it. The cure: acknowledge your guilt, ask forgiveness, repent, and accept your deserved punishment.

Today many practitioners of alternative medicine and holistic health think in Heroic ways. Herbal medicine especially is taught and practiced by Heroic tradition guidelines. Most of the world's major religions are strongly Heroic as well.

The Heroic Tradition

Body, Mind, and Spirit

Body, mind, and spirit/soul are present in every being, according to the many Heroic traditions. Healing, full healing in the Heroic traditions, cannot be accomplished unless all three aspects are dealt with: purify the body, control the mind, clear the spirit. Then you will be peaceful, youthful, and healthy.

Body, mind, and spirit are not equal. Your spirit/soul is the highest and purest part of you. Your mind, which includes feelings as well as thoughts, is the intermediary between your pure spirit and your earthy body, which is low, base, material, and dense.

In the Heroic tradition, the spirit/soul is high, white, and free. The spirit is unconcerned with low earthly matters. The spirit is above it all. The spirit comes from heaven and may return there at death. The spirit is clean and white: white light, white skin, good, pure, holy white. The spirit is not bound. It chooses to inhabit a body, but is not the body.

The pure white light of the spirit/soul can be clouded by bad thoughts and wrong actions. The spirit may accumulate bad karma, or be burdened by sin (even ancestral wrongdoing can be inherited). These things are reflected through the soul and manifest as disease in the body.

The spirit/soul, in its innocence and purity, does not create the thoughts and actions which lead to disease. It is the mind that creates them. The mind harbors thoughts and feelings which threaten the health of the entire person. The mind has bad thoughts and bad feelings: greed, anger, jealousy, sloth, lust, vanity, revenge, disrespect, disobedience, violence, and selfishness. Bad thoughts and feelings create disease in the body, says the Heroic tradition, and cloud the soul's purity. The mind cannot be trusted to think clearly or feel freely. When we learn to control our minds we will be healthier and happier.

When we do not keep our negative tendencies in check, they lead us astray, and we inevitably pay the consequences: ill health, bad luck, perhaps an eternity of suffering. Rigorous training, self-control, and discipline enable us to see through the deceptions of mind, ego, emotion, and the body's needs.

The body is the temple, or physical housing, of the soul, in the Heoric tradition. It is, however, an inadequate temple for the soul's purity, whiteness, and highness. It can be made into a proper receptacle by purification and cleansing. The body is filled with primitive emotions, uncivilized urges, and rank needs. The body is full of excrement, frequently dirtied and bloodied, base and low. Because the body naturally tends to act out of its basic filthy instincts, negative consequences can be avoided only by following strict rules and specific guidelines for thought, word, and deed.

The Heroic traditions offer a variety of techniques for freeing ourselves from the everlasting pulls of physical demands and desires. The harsher the rules and the more difficult the techniques, the better. "No pain, no gain."

In the Heroic tradition, we are told that the body will virtually cease to exist when we are in a state of purity. Excretions, such as mucus, urine, feces, sweat, and menstrual blood, will halt completely or decrease noticeably (becoming whiter, lighter, and less odorous), when we are truly clean.

In a state of purity, according to the Heroic tradition, we are undisturbed by sexual desire; we are not subject to the whims of our emotions; we are *in* the world but not *of* it. We will not suffer from sickness when we are truly cleansed. When we are pure, we will have life eternal.

The Circle is the Symbol of the Heroic Tradition

The Heroic tradition sees health as a balance between the pulls of spirit and matter. This balance is a cycle: a cycle of struggle between good and bad, right and wrong, dark and light. The cycle of this struggle endlessly repeats. It is a serpent swallowing its own tail. It is a circle.

The circle is entire unto itself: complete and whole. The circle is predictable, repeatable, reliable. The circle is a closed system. The circle is eternal. The circle is the halo, the pure light of the soul. The circle has no beginning and no end. The circle is not born and the circle never dies. The circle goes around and around, always in balance, always predictable.

The circle is a whole being. And each part of the whole Heroic being is also a circle: three circles interlaced, interlocked in struggle:

the soul circle striving higher, the body circle pulling us down, and the mind circle trying to keep the balance in between.

Punishment as Cure in the Heroic Tradition

When the body wins and drags us down, when the mind fails and gives in to negativity, when the spirit/soul is clouded and our light dims, then we sicken, we suffer, we die. To live, to be happy, to get well, we must clear away the clouds, stay in balance, keep the body disciplined.

Simply put, the Heroic tradition tells us that disease and pain (and even death—death of the soul as well as the body) occur when we do something wrong or bad and do not atone for it. To get well, we must right our wrongs.

How can we right our wrongs and get well? Asking for forgiveness can help right the wrong. And so can punishment. With forgiveness and repentance, we can clear away the wrong we have done. Admitting our guilt in doing the wrong and causing the problem helps prepare us for the punishment. The punishment absolves us and cleanses us and heals us in the Heroic tradition. The punishment balances the wrongdoing and makes way for forgiveness. I have caused suffering; may *my* suffering bring balance.

Punishment is absolution. Knowing that we have caused pain and problems for ourselves and others by our own wrongdoing, by giving in to ever-present temptation, and that we are likely to do it again, we hope to return to (and remain in) a state of grace and health with absolution, with proper punishment. This is the Heroic way.

What is the proper punishment in the Heroic way? Deprivation is a proper punishment, especially deprivation of the flesh. Fasting, strict dietary rules, excessive exercise, and bitter-tasting medicines are proper punishments. Setting strict limits is a proper punishment, especially limits on normal activities. Limited sleep, limited sexual contact, limited stimuli, and limited ease are proper punishments. Withdrawal is a proper punishment: withdrawal of physical contact, of affection, of emotional support, of acknowledgment. Belittlement and negation of individual worth is a proper punishment. With proper punishment, we are ready for forgiveness, ready to regain health and return to the light in the Heroic way.

Forgiveness is dependent on guilt. There must be a guilty party, someone who has done wrong, before we can forgive. We can blame ourselves. We can blame our parents. We can blame the world. But we must have someone to blame, so we can forgive and be well. One of the keys to healing in the Heroic tradition is the establishment of guilt.

"If I hadn't eaten that hot fudge sundae, I wouldn't have this terrible cold." (I am bad and deserve to be punished.) *"At least it's teaching me a lesson."*

"Cancer is repressed emotion, you know, and I bet if you had really told him what you thought you wouldn't be sick now." (You are bad and deserve to be punished.) *"I sure hope you learn your lesson."*

"The universe is a terrible place to be, full of hard lessons. When will I ever learn them all and do everything right so I won't feel so much pain?"

How can we establish guilt? First ask "why?"

"Why did this occur? Why do I feel so bad? Why am I in this trouble? Why does this always happen to me?"

Asking "why?" enables us to establish guilt. Answering "why?" helps us set the rules for future behavior so we won't get hurt and sick again.

Rules and the Heroic Tradition

Rules are vital in the Heroic tradition. Rules help us avoid pain and disease. Rules tell us what is right and wrong, what is good and bad, what is clean and what dirty. Rules establish boundaries. Rules divide the circle of the Heroic way into high and low, white and black, good and bad, pure and unclean, male and female.

Food rules. Feeling rules. Spirituality rules. Hierarchies. Judgments. The Heroic traditions abound in rules, and each individual tradition within the Heroic tradition has its own specific rules. The rules of one Heroic tradition often conflict with the rules of another Heroic tradition. It is not agreement on the rules themselves that constitutes inclusion in the Heroic traditions, but agreement that there must be rules.

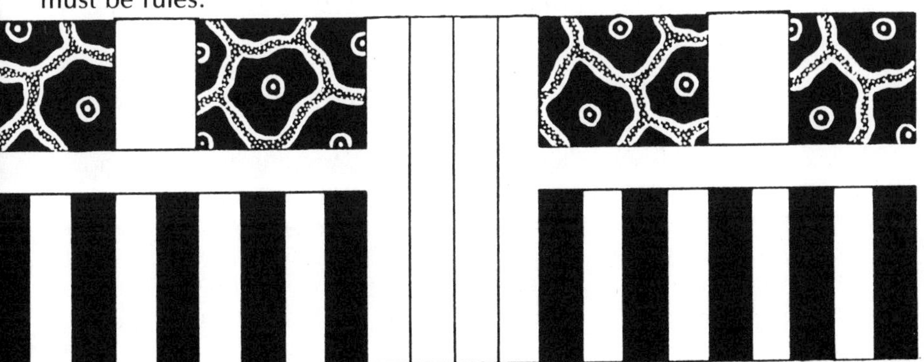

Woman-Hating in the Heroic Tradition

All Heroic traditions have rules about women. Women represent a real and ever-present danger in the Heroic tradition. Women lure us to earthly matters. Women take our minds from the purity of the soul and drag us down into the body, into dirty dishes, dirty diapers, and dirty lust.

We are formed of flesh inside of a woman. We are birthed from between a woman's legs. We are nourished and given life by the love and abundance of women, by women's bodies. But the body is sinful and unclean in the Heroic tradition. So, instead of life-givers, and life-nourishers, women are seen in the Heroic tradition as the source of all problems, all pain, all suffering, all sin.

When women are verbally honored in Heroic traditions, they are then expected to pick up everyone else's shit because they are spiritually higher, or by nature more caring. Putting women on a pedestal is also woman-hating.

The raw-food traditionalists, more obviously than other Heroic traditions, are woman-hating. They are especially adamant: clean women do not menstruate and do not go through menopause. This assertion is not only an indication of woman-hating (since it is usually malnourished women who experience amenorrhea), but promotes woman-hating within the women themselves who then, menstruating normally, view their own unique woman-self cycles as symptomatic of sickness.

Who is This Young, White Male?

This young white male is the embodiment of health in the Heroic tradition. He does not menstruate; his hair is not gray; his face is unwrinkled; his skin is white; his eyes are blue.

The assertion that clean and healthy women do not menstruate implies that a healthy person is someone who does not normally menstruate; that is, a man. Men embody health in the Heroic tradition, as they do in the Scientific tradition. (Traditions based on fixity, repeatability, and rule-following see men as healthier, that is more fixed and predictable, than women.)

Purity and cleanliness imply whiteness. And the Heroic traditions are very clear that white *is* right and good and healthy, while black is wrong and bad and sick. Light skin and light hair and light eyes are seen as more spiritual, more pure, in the Heroic presentation. The Heroic image of health is a white male.

White hair and wrinkles, according to some Heroic tradition writers, are caused by filth in the body. When the blood, liver, and colon are fully cleansed, they claim, the hair will return to its "normal" color and the wrinkles fade away. And the right diet, the right thoughts, the right exercise, and the right prayers (explained however differently through the rules of each Heroic tradition) will keep you young forever.

That Filthy Colon

Youthful long life, promises the Heroic tradition, is given to those who follow the rules, atone for their wrongs, and get clean.

It is especially important in the Heroic tradition to cleanse the body inside and out: to purify the body with austerities and sweats, to clean out toxins with fasts and purges, to clean the blood, clean the liver, and above all, clean the colon.

A widespread belief in the Heroic traditions of health care, especially for the past several hundred years in white-occupied North America, and for several hundred more in Europe, is that diseases arise from filth in the colon.

Many Heroic tradition practitioners recommend enemas and colonics as the first line of defense against every problem from menstrual cramps to cancer. Laxatives and cathartics and all kinds of intestinal cleansings are recommended as daily fare for well-being and optimum health. To some, it seems that the colon can never be too clean. An empty colon is about as close to clean as a colon can be, so frequent or regular periods of fasting are encouraged in most Heroic traditions.

Poke 'Em, Puke 'Em, and Purge 'Em

Cures in the Heroic traditions are usually through dramatic and heroic means. Purity is to be achieved at any cost. If the treatment is part of the punishment, so much the better. Poking, puking, and purging (or bloodletting, emesis, and catharsis) satisfy all the requirements, and thus many Heroic healers offer some form or combination of this trinity. Stimulants and sedatives also cause dramatic physical changes, and so are greatly favored by many Heroic tradition healers.

While visiting a Heroic tradition school, I heard a lecture given to a graduating class of healers. The speaker, an experienced practitioner, said: "Eighty percent of all your patients will get better by themselves. It is up to you to give them something powerful or do something dramatic (and the faster-acting the better) so they will believe you have been the agent of their return to health."

Poking techniques involve dramatic manipulations of the patient, as seen in some Heroic tradition psychic surgeons, sucking doctors, bone-crackers, and others. This type of dramatic technique ensures that attention is focused on the healer and that the patient will correctly identify the healer as the one who caused the return to health. (And if there is no return to health, in most Heroic traditions it's the patient's fault.)

Puking techniques usually involve the use of harsh substances or physical manipulations resulting in the expulsion of the contents of the stomach and upper portion of the small intestine. Reflexive action in the lungs, liver, and adrenals can prompt dramatic cures from this type of treatment, though the stress to these organs is often severe and can result in death as well as cure.

Some bulimics I've met tell me they were encouraged initially by Heroic tradition literature to vomit and use laxatives, and that they continued (to excess) in the hope that once all the toxins and waste were removed from their bodies, they would be perfect; that is, thin, disembodied.

Purging involves the emptying of the colon and is accomplished with cathartic substances and manipulations such as colonics. Again, reflexive action, especially in the liver, can cure or cause dramatic and rapid improvement, or can end in liver failure and death.

Purging still maintains currency as a much-recommended Heroic tradition health practice. Since constipation is defined by some Heroic tradition authors as fewer than three bowel movements a day, laxatives (actually cathartics, in many cases) and enemas are clearly needed by the vast majority of the public.

While bloodletting, catharsis, and emesis are dramatic techniques long associated with the Heroic tradition, it is important to remember that no particular technique or remedy belongs to any one tradition. The use of a specific health care technique does not predicate the thought patterns (Scientific, Heroic, or Wise Woman) of the person using it.

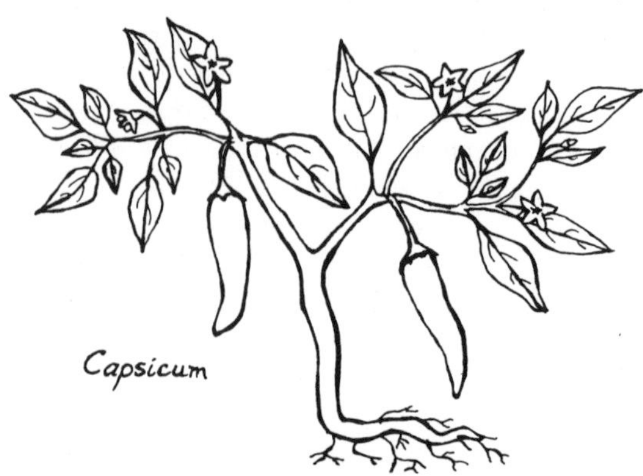

The Heroic Tradition Heals The Masses

With knowledge of the rules, of the means to eternal life and perpetual health, the Heroic traditions are concerned with helping the masses, with saving the people. Remedies and techniques which affect a broad range of people are preferred over individualized treatments in the Heroic tradition.

Combinations of substances (such as different herbs, herbs and flower essences, or herbs and vitamins) and combinations of techniques (the business cards of many Heroic healers list six or more techniques they "specialize" in), are believed to expand the scope of the remedy, and enable it to affect the largest number of people. These combinations become closely-guarded secrets: "patent medicines."

The result of such combinations, however, is often confusion in the patient as to what was effective, thus keeping her/him hooked on the "patent remedy."

The Heroic Tradition: From the Far Corners of the Earth

Ad copy: *"We travel to the far corners of the world gathering herbs to cleanse your system."* Picture: In the foreground, a youthful, though gray-haired, white male; and in the background, a kindly herb gatherer, also male, but older, smaller, and with darker skin.

Rare substances and occult techniques are favored in the Heroic tradition. Anything hard to get, foreign, rare, or out of the ordinary is prized in the Heroic tradition. Secrets abound among Heroic healers. The cost of these things is, of course, commensurate with their availability. But, then, in the Heroic tradition, we do not expect to achieve good health cheaply.

Health and happiness are rare, claim the Heroic tradition. We must search ceaselessly for them, we must endure hardships to find them, we must earn them. They are costly prizes.

Health and happiness are not given freely, as a grace, in the Heroic tradition. They are precious treasures, closely guarded treasures which must be wrested from the universe with struggle. We must fight for them; and we can only win them by resisting and countering all our natural tendencies. Health and happiness must be taken by force from a universe which offers mostly pain and sickness, negativity and dirt, chaos and imbalance.

The Heroic Healer Knows Best

In the Heroic tradition, disease begins in the spiritual realm, moves through the emotional realm, and finally manifests in the physical realm.

The enlightened and aware Heroic being never gets sick, never experiences pain, for sickness and pain imply that s/he is not only physically impure, but unmindful, and possibly in spiritual trouble as well. In the Heroic tradition, someone who is sick is no longer valid; they need help, the help of someone who knows how to remove (and avoid) pain and sickness. They need someone to lay down the law and shape them up.

Health and happiness are not easily available to the individual in the Heroic traditions; healers, helpers, and intermediaries who are wiser and higher are needed.

When we are thinking in Heroic tradition ways, we see the healer or helper as big daddy.

Daddy makes the rules for us. Daddy decides on the punishment. Daddy tells us how to be in balance.

Most of the time this works just fine, but we don't always want to follow daddy's rules. We haven't yet decided where we stand with daddy, either. We know he is mortal, though he claims not to be, and he is ever so much wiser than we are. Better play it safe and follow the rules.

Heroic Herbalism

The Heroic traditions of herbal medicine are the most common forms of herbalism in the western world. Most of the easily available and widely distributed herbals are written from the viewpoint of the Heroic tradition. Jethro Kloss, Arnold Ehret, and Dr. Christopher are well-known American writers and herbalists in the Heroic tradition. Because herbal medicine in the Heroic traditions is so widespread, I think it important to take a look at its practices and characteristics.

Heroic tradition herbalism is characterized by reliance on some of the vilest-tasting, strongest-acting stimulant and sedative plants in the herbal nation (that is, herbs that are as druglike as possible), a penchant for exotic herbs, and an emphasis on herbal combinations.

Foul-tasting brews are the hallmark of Heroic herbalism. Bitter as the taste of poison, we could rightly say, for Heroic herbalists often use plants that heal by poisoning slightly. *"The worse it tastes, the better it is for you."*

Since the herbs most favored in Heroic herbalism are the most dramatic ones, and therefore have the highest potential for severe side effects, combinations of herbs are always used, and single-herb remedies (the Wise Woman way) are generally considered inferior.

Carefully chosen modifying herbs must be included to buffer the effects of such herbs as the Heroic herbalist's big three: cayenne *(Capsicum frutescens)*, goldenseal *(Hydrastis canadensis)*, and lobelia, also known as puke weed *(Lobelia inflata)*.

Cayenne is a circulatory stimulant, or stimulating tonic; that is, one that tonifies by cracking the whip. Like any stimulant, such as coffee, it must first be used in small doses until the body learns to accommodate the stimulus. Excessive amounts, which for some individuals may be less than a gram, can cause severe irritation of mucus membranes, bleeding, and serious gastrointestinal damage.

Goldenseal, usually classified as a digestive tonic, is also a stimulating tonic. Goldenseal pushes liver functioning; it pushes kidney functioning; and it alarms the immune system. That's a *normal* dose. A large dose can cause vomiting, diarrhea, or death from respiratory failure. (Goldenseal actually kills by depressing the nerves; this dual, contradictory character is not uncommon in stimulant and sedative herbs.)

Lobelia is also both a stimulant and a sedative, depending on the dose. A dose of fifty milligrams of dried lobelia herb, or one milliliter of the tincture can provoke stupor, convulsions, and death. A normal dose may cause vomiting.

And then there are the exotic herbs from far-away lands or inaccessible peaks: *pau d'arco. . . dong quai. . . osha. . . false unicorn. . .* The list is long and constantly growing in the herbal pharmacies of westernized nations where the wealth of the planet is ours (so we assume) for the taking. But it is often only the wealthy heroes who can afford the exotic prices these herbs and their staggeringly complex combinations fetch. In addition, the use of rare or foreign herbs in formulae and patent medicines makes it exceedingly difficult for the remedy to be duplicated. The patient helped by a Heroic combination herbal remedy is not encouraged to go out and make it personally, but to return to the healer for more of that special, hard-to-get brew.

Combination remedies, especially many plants ground together and put in gelatin capsules, obscure the actual plant nature of the healing substances, lending a druglike credibility to Heroic herbalism, and offering the patient the opportunity to believe that health comes from a pill or a bottle or the doctor, not the earth. Thus Heroic herbalism is familiar and reassuring to us, especially if we have been brought up (and most of us have) in the Scientific tradition of health care.

Voices of the Heroic Tradition

- *"Food is the earliest addiction, starting with the newborn's first mouthful."*
- *"The fall from God consciousness came from eating forbidden food."*
- *"Overeating poisons; undereating is the most important factor for health."*
- *"You must select and prepare foods properly, and eat them properly as well."*
- *"Periodic fasting keeps the body (the temple of the spirit) clean."*
- *"Teach correct ways of eating and living so they can avoid ever being sick."*
- *"In most humans, the digestive tract is filthy."*
- *"The purpose of a cleanse is to eliminate mucus and toxins from the body."*
- *"The mind must be controlled, trained, and directed."*
- *"Real things are of the spirit . . . daily life is impermanent and continually changing, and so unworthy of much thought or excitement."*
- *"When the stomach works, vital force is centered in digestion, not spirit."*
- *"If human beings consumed only radiation, if radiation were never polluted, if the procreative function remained dormant, sickness would be unknown."*
- *". . . enables one to get away from the gross and intoxicating nature of food."*
- *". . . menstruation has its origin in the inflammatory condition of the uterine mucus membrane due to the toxic condition of the intestines."*
- *"The toxicity of menstrual blood has been well substantiated . . . the blood plasma, milk, sweat, and saliva of menstruating women contain a substance that is highly toxic to the protoplasm of living plants."*
- *". . . menstruation is unnatural and pathological."*
- *"If the female body is made perfectly clean, menstruation ceases."*
- *"If a woman stops her monthly loss at an early enough age, her reproductive capacity will persist into centuries."*
- *"In the healthy woman, menopause occurs, if at all, late in life."*
- *"Unless you change your lifestyle, you may anticipate the gods' vengeance."*
- *"The most aggressive health care available today: fasting, frequent enemas, the combining of herbs to make effective remedies, and controlled diet."*

References & Resources:
The Heroic Tradition

- *Back to Eden*
  J. Kloss; 1939, J. Kloss. Also 1983, Woodbridge
- *Green Pharmacy*
  Barbara Griggs; 1981, Viking
- *Guidebook for Living*
  G. Oshawa; 1968, Macrobiotic Foundation
- *Herb Lady's Notebook*
  Venus Andrecht; 1984, Ransom Hill
- *Herbally Yours*
  Penny C. Royal; 1976, BiWorld
- *The Herbalist*
  J.F. Meyer; 1960, Rand McNally

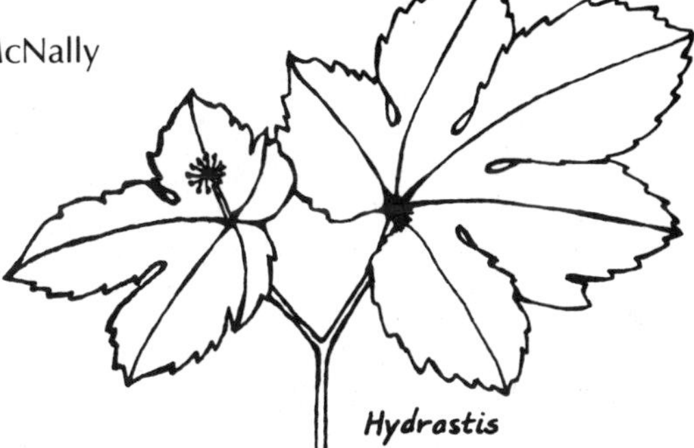

- *Mucusless Diet Healing System*
  A. Ehret; 1920, Ehret Lit. Pub.; 1976, Lust Pub.
- *Nature's Healing Agents*
  R.S. Clymer, MD; 1963, Dorrance
- *School of Natural Healing*
  J. Christopher; 1975, Provo
- *Seven Herbs, Plants as Teachers*
  M. Wood; 1986, North Atlantic
- *Survival into the 21st Century*
  V. Kulvinskas; 1975, Omangod

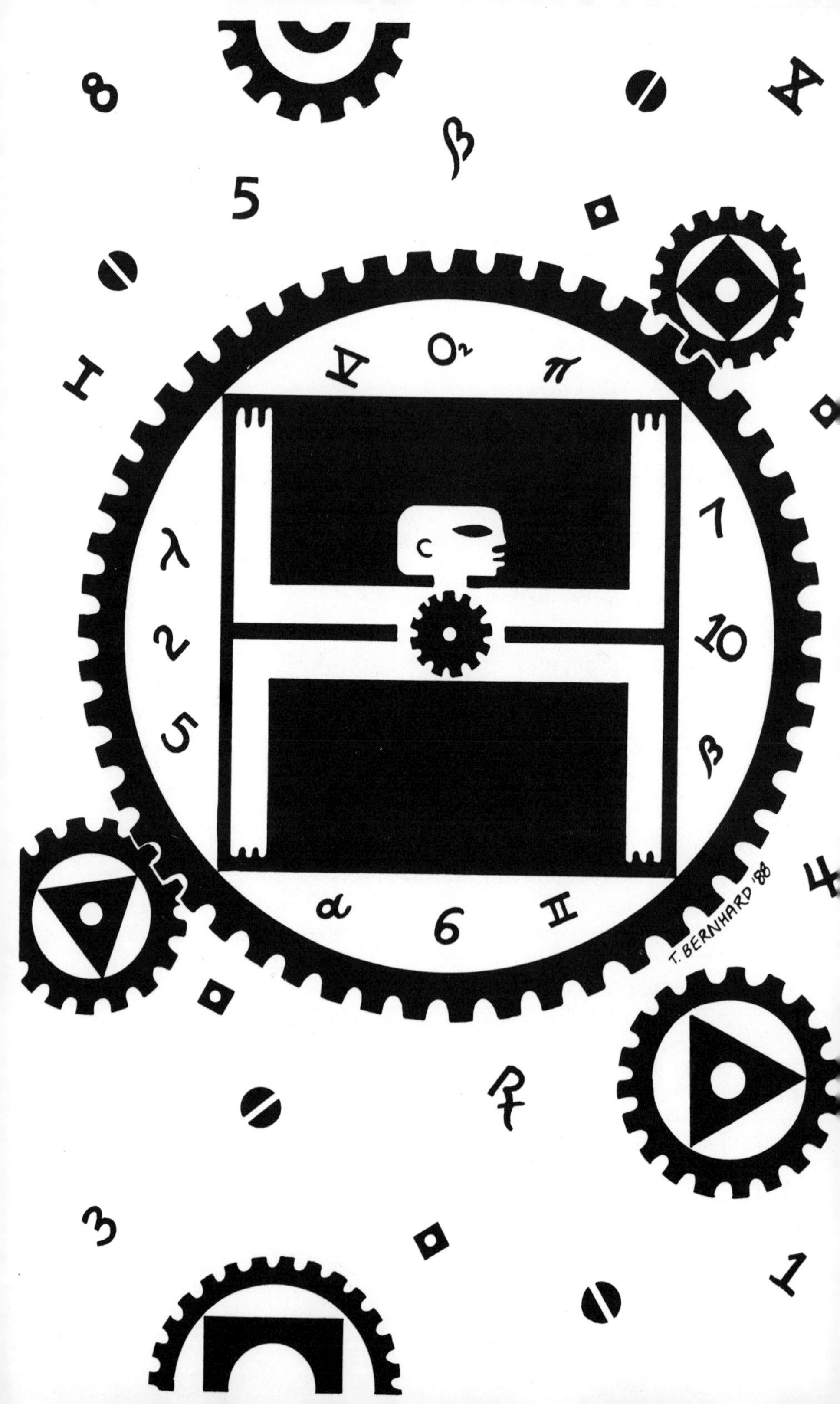
T. BERNHARD '88

Scientific Tradition

The Scientific tradition sees healing as fixing. The line is its symbol: linear thought, linear time. Truth is fixed and measurable. Truth is that which repeats.

Newton's universal laws and the mechanization of nature are the foundation of the Scientific tradition. Bodies are understood to be like machines. When machines run well (stay healthy) they don't deviate. Anything that deviates from normal needs to be fixed or repaired. We must take measurements to determine deviation and assure ourselves that everything is normal. Regular diagnostic tests are critical to maintaining proper functioning and ensuring utmost longevity in the Scientific tradition.

The Scientific tradition healer finds and fixes deviation. Fixity is health.

Health is the absence of disease in the Scientific tradition. Health—exemplified by a fully-functioning, white-skinned male—must be maintained, with a proper diet (by the numbers), the proper exercise (at the target heart rate), and regular check-ups by professionals.

The Scientific tradition health care professional must be highly trained since his preferred healing techniques (drugs, surgery, and machine-enhanced diagnosis) are extremely dangerous. You don't know enough to treat yourself safely, so it is best to leave the technical stuff to the body mechanics whose high-tech eyes and magic bullets can kill disease and conquer death.

All plants are potential drugs: they can kill you in their unpredictable crude states; they are potent helpers when refined into synthesized drugs. Herbs and herbal medicine are ineffective as well as dangerous. It's best to leave such things to the experts.

The Scientific Tradition

The Straight Line of the Scientific Tradition

The straight line measures.
The straight line is static.
The straight line separates.
The straight line is stable.
The straight line defines.
The straight line is phallic.
The straight line makes a mark.
The straight line is a boundary.
The straight line slashes and cuts.
The straight line is the sword of the warrior.
The straight line has two opposite and opposing ends.
The straight line is the sign of the Scientific tradition.

The straight line: linear thought, linear time. Linear thought, inherently static, remains energized by opposition and conflict. Life against death. Good against bad. White against black. Light against darkness. In the Scientific tradition we fight to stay alive. Death tries to extinguish life at every opportunity. Death is the enemy, the enemy we must fight.

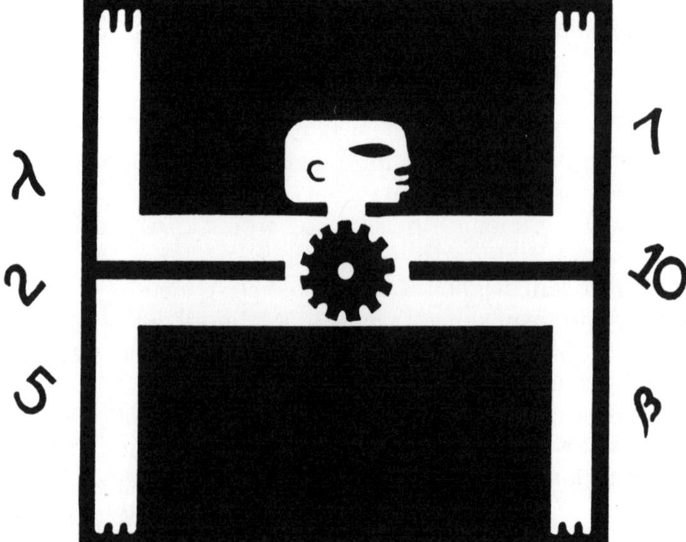

The Struggle to Survive in the Scientific Tradition

In the Scientific tradition, life is a struggle to outwit death. Life is a struggle to maintain fixity in the face of endless assaults. Life is a struggle to stay warm and fed and win the battle. And there is never enough warmth and food to go around.

There are laws in the struggle. There are laws that must be learned and remembered, that are vital in battle.

Hold tightly to what you have.
Put up your best defenses.
Stay on top.
Keep an eye out for the bad guy, the enemy, the other.
Don't expose yourself.
Change is the vanguard of disaster.

Death sends against us teeming, deadly bacteria, greedy and opportunistic invaders always ready to sicken us and kill us. Death sends viruses to gain entry slyly and attack from within the cell, weakening us, destroying our defenses. Death sends temptations of all sorts to destroy us.

Our defense against death is the immune system, helped by modern scientific medicine. The immune system wages war on the enemy's troops. The Scientific tradition offers new killer drugs, new micro-spies, and continually newer, better, stronger protection on every battlefront. Is it any coincidence that General Electric and Hewlett-Packard, among others, produce both medical and military products?

In the Scientific tradition, life fights against death, health fights against sickness, good fights against bad; there *must* be a fight. If there is no fight, the enemy wins. The enemy doesn't believe in co-existence. Keep away death and disease with all your power, says the Scientific tradition. Hang on to life and health with all your strength. And stay just like that: half of you holding off the enemy and the other half hanging on to what you've got.

The Scientific Tradition: Fixity

Truth is that which remains constant and repeats, says the Scientific tradition. Constancy, fixity, that is truth. The universe runs according to laws forever set and never changing. Fixity is health: steady, reliable, dependable, accountable, knowable.

In the Scientific tradition, we want to keep things ordered, arranged, and set—ever so exactly—to assure repeatability. Without fixity, repeatability is difficult. How can we know if this works if we can't repeat what you did? How can you guarantee the safety of this plant when you know its constituents are variable? How can you give the right answer if you don't memorize it? How can you know what you're doing if you can't measure it?

In order to eliminate the variables inherent in crude plants that thwart repeatability and confound measurability, the Scientific tradition researcher identifies the active ingredient (usually an alkaloid) in the plant, maps its molecular structure, and then synthesizes it. In this way, the variable plant medicine is fixed. This fixed substance is called a drug. The standard dosage can then be established. Repeatability is assured. Measurement is possible.

The Scientific Tradition Measures

According to the Scientific tradition, measurement leads to truth. By measuring (repeatedly) we can determine what is real, what is fixed, what repeats, and therefore, what is true in the Scientific tradition.

The universe and the body, as machines, can be discovered and known by measurement, says the Scientific way. Since they cannot be measured in their entirety, they must be measured part by part.

Although living organisms consist of interrelated and interdependent parts, the Scientific tradition measures and treats each part as independent. Each independent part is measured separately and treated separately.

Once the individual parts are measured, the particular part responsible for the problem can be determined. The part which deviates from the "norm" (by the standards of the Scientific tradition) is considered broken and when it is fixed, health is restored.

Interrelationships are difficult to measure and quantify, so they are routinely ignored in the Scientific tradition. For example, experts from the Scientific tradition assure farmers and consumers alike that the safeguards for individual pesticides are unchanged when several pesticides are used concurrently on a crop, though no studies confirm this.

In the Scientific tradition the whole is understood to be comprised of its many parts. But some parts are more important than others. The more active a part is, the more important it is. The most active part of a whole is understood to be identical to the whole in the Scientific tradition.

The vitamin C complex, for example, is composed of many interrelated factors, ascorbic acid being only one of them. However, those in the Scientific tradition treat ascorbic acid as though it were the complete vitamin C complex; no distinction is made between the whole and the part. When the amount of vitamin C in a food is measured, only the ascorbic acid is measured, not the entire vitamin complex.

Measuring the part leads to an emphasis on the part. The Scientific tradition, in its molecular theory of disease, looks to the smallest measurable part and tries to fix the problem from there. Since some part must be responsible for the breakdown of the whole, much of Scientific tradition medicine consists of looking for the responsible part and measuring it to determine how best to fix it.

Numbers don't lie, claims the Scientific tradition. The implication is that everything else does, including feelings, intuitions, hunches, and memories. Numbers are true because they are constant, they quantify, and they repeat. Feelings and such must lie because they are changeable.

In the Scientific tradition, we even eat by the numbers. So many grams of protein, so many units of vitamin A, so many calories, so many milligrams of sodium and calcium, and so on. It doesn't matter whether these numbers come from a plate of fresh vegetables or a bowl of fortified Jello. The important thing is to get what science has determined to be the right amount of amino acids, carbohydrates, minerals, and all other necessary nutrients into your body every day.

The ascorbic acid molecules in this tablet are exactly the same as the ones in that fresh, wild salad, except that the tablet is clean, white, pure, reliable, and repeatable, while the plant, you must admit, is dirty (do wash it!), multicolored, crude, and variable.

Body as Machine in the Scientific Tradition

Machines eat by the numbers too. It is vital that the can of oil you put in your engine has the right number on it. The wrong measure in a machine is a problem. Repeatable, reliable results, numerical results, scientific truths, are most easily obtained when the object under consideration is a machine. So the universe is a machine. The body is a machine.

The Scientific tradition healer physically and chemically manipulates the patient's body (or surroundings) with the aim of mechanically changing behavior and eliminating the problem.

"I've had a lot of bladder infections, a chronic cystitis. And the drugs always stopped the worst of it. But now, after 25 years of recurrent infections and drug treatments, my kidneys are failing. Dialysis is just

ahead. Dialysis! I don't believe I can bear to be on a machine. I treated myself like a machine and now I feel like I'm becoming one."

Machines are too complicated for the ordinary person to fix, and dangerous besides. What if something should short-circuit? You could get hurt. Fixing (that is healing) of delicate machines (bodies) is best left to the experts, the Scientific tradition experts, who are highly trained to measure, find, and fix the dysfunctional part with equally delicate (and expensive) machines.

Scientific Tradition Healers: Mechanics and Gods

The expert, the healer, following the Scientific way, is a godlike mechanic of the human body, at least in part by virtue of lengthy and rigorous training and access to costly and restricted substances and machines.

Mechanical diagnostic and health-care procedures are required by the Scientific tradition, so the healer must be a skilled mechanic. Drugs, surgery, machine-enhanced tests, and imaging techniques such as x-rays, sonograms, and CAT scans (favored means of finding and fixing problems in the Scientific tradition) require mechanical skill.

In the Scientific tradition of healing, remedies are chosen based on their repeatability and their ability to restore normalcy, not because they are life-enhancing. Most people feel awe, a mysterious fear, in the presence of these godlike machines and the master mechanics who run them and understand how to decipher their messages.

The training of the Scientific tradition healer/mechanic includes a sizeable amount of time on mechanics of people, especially sick and injured people, yet gives little time to the study of healthy/whole/holy people. Cases, diseases, the minutiae of the physical body are memorized and treated, but the healer, godlike, no longer notices the populace. One doctor trained in the Scientific tradition commented: "How am I supposed to create, or even recognize, health? I didn't see it once in the six years I was in medical school."

The healer/mechanic is as dependent on the accuracy of the machines as the patient/machine. They both put their trust in the new gods, machines. But the patient identifies the healer with the machines and comes to see him as a god, as well. The Scientific tradition healer understands that all this is confusing; he's sometimes confused, too. Thank goodness for the machines: they're never confused.

As a patient in the Scientific tradition, I put off going to the doctor/god because I'm afraid of what will be discovered. I ignore my little aches and pains. I put off going to the healer/mechanic because I don't have the money. I put off going to the healer/doctor because I don't want to take drugs, and I'm afraid of surgery.

As a patient in the Scientific tradition, I desensitize myself, becoming a foreigner in my own body, becoming more like a machine. I don't notice the signals that indicate something is wrong with me until it is *very* wrong. I know I'm most likely to be abused by modern medicine when I wait until the situation is critical, yet I resist going to see the mechanic/god. I've been told that the healer/mechanic/god can fix anything. But what if they can't fix me?

When my car breaks down, I take it to a Scientific tradition mechanic. I describe the problem and leave it there. He doesn't want me hanging around while he fixes it, so I leave. When he's done, he calls me and I go pick up my car. The bill is always more than I think it will be. If it's fixed and not a problem to me anymore, fine. If it isn't fixed, I sue. It's the mechanic's responsibility to see to it that there aren't any problems. I just drive the machine.

Both These Machines Need To Be Overhauled

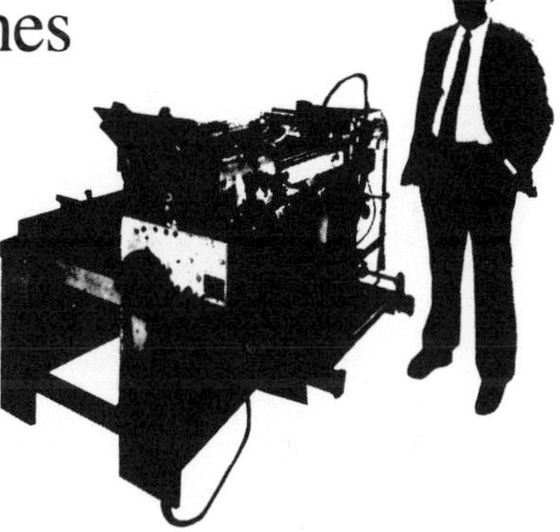

I'm not in charge of myself, in the Scientific tradition of health. I run the body/machine. I feed it the right numbers. If it breaks, I want it to be fixed as fast as possible. I want to be normal again.

Normal Health in the Scientific Tradition

Normal health in the Scientific tradition is found in a computer print-out of statistics on a normal, fully-functioning, young white male.

Normal health in the Scientific tradition is defined by numbers and verified by tests. Machines monitor the invisible physical processes for regularity and repeatability, measuring and testing the components of the blood, the resistance of the blood pressure, the electrical activity of the heart, the folds of the digestive system, the thickness of the bone, and much more, allowing the Scientific tradition healer/god to look deep inside.

The Scientific tradition healer looks with precision at the smallest molecule of your being. The Scientific tradition can take it to pieces, measure it, and judge it for deviation or normalcy.

Normal health, in the Scientific tradition, wears white skin. Most scientific tests are calibrated to reflect the normal ranges of white males. Racism is rampant in Scientific tradition health care in the United States. In 1986, for instance, three times as many black women (16.3%) as white women (5.9%) died during pregnancy and childbirth. Potential benefits of sickle cells (they help prevent malaria) are rarely mentioned. One friend tells me she's sick of explaining to (white) healers that her build is typically black and she does not intend to try to change it to conform to their (white) standards.

Normal health in the Scientific tradition means youth. Problems of the old are often disregarded, dismissed as senility, or regarded as typical of old age and therefore not worth dealing with. Machines don't get old, they just get out of date, and old-fashioned. Best to retire them before they break, or overtreat them with polypharmacy. Estrogen replacement therapy speaks to women's fear of growing older and offers them Scientific tradition health: eternal youth.

Normal health, in the Scientific tradition, means full functioning, with or without assistance. If you can't see normally, you wear glasses. If you can't hear normally, you wear a hearing aid. If you can't walk normally, you get an artificial hip, or foot, or whatever you need. There is no excuse not to be normal. The benefits, and gifts of blindness (such as acute sensitivity to non-visual stimulae) or other disabilities are not considered healthy or normal by the Scientific tradition.

Normal health in the Scientific tradition is "male": strong, powerful, rugged, predictable, fixed. Sickness in the Scientific tradition is "female": weak, vulnerable, delicate, erratic, unpredictable, and constantly changing.

Normal female physical functions such as pregnancy and lactation, menopause and menstruation are regarded by the Scientific tradition as dangerous, painful, frightening, weakening, and unsustainable without help. The male standard of Scientific tradition medicine in the United States is especially visible in the hundreds of thousands of unnecessary hysterectomies, episiotomies, caesarean sections, and radical mastectomies. Conservative sources estimate half of these operations are unnecessary; radical sources claim ninety percent are unneeded (closer to the fact, I believe).

Unhealthy, not normal, out of whack, abnormal, out of kilter, beyond reasonable limits, irregular, illogical, dark, old, broken? Time to be fixed.

Get Fixed Fast with Active Ingredients

The best way to get fixed is to get fixed fast. The active ingredient is the one with the power to fix, fast. The active ingredient is the one that does the real work. The active principle is the one that matters. Doing is more important than being in the Scientific tradition.

Active ingredients in plants make plants dangerous from the perspective of the Scientific tradition. Any plant may have active ingredients. Active constituents of plants are potential drugs. Drugs can kill.

Herbalists in the Scientific tradition (sometimes known as experts in pharmacognosy) concern themselves primarily with identifying and measuring plants' active constituents: tannins, terpenoids, steroids, saponins, essential oils, and alkaloids. Any of these constituents, used in a large enough single dose or accumulated in body tissues over a period of time, can cause acute and long-term trauma and dysfunction. Large enough doses of most of them can kill.

"Any plant strong enough to heal is strong enough to kill," says the Scientific tradition. And if we agree that the active part, looked at in isolation, *is* the equivalent of the whole, then that's a true statement.

Plants are valued for their active constituents in the Scientific tradition; plants are equated with their alkaloids or essential oils, their active ingredients.

Inert materials and passive constituents (which the wise woman regards as carriers of subtle and specific nourishments) are largely ignored and regarded as unworthy of scientific scrutiny. (And, in fact, the energies available from these passive parts is not measurable, especially by machines, as research on psychic states at Duke University revealed many decades ago.) Mechanically-assisted studies of plant energies, or plant intelligence, are generally regarded as unscientific or pseudo-scientific.

Current Scientific tradition research with plants focuses on extracting, duplicating, and testing (on laboratory animals) the amazing array of alkaloids and active ingredients found in plants. While this has yielded some remarkable drugs, and interesting insight into the active energies of plants, such research has cast what I consider unwarranted suspicion on the crude plants themselves, imputing ability to inflict severe damage.

Comfrey is now suspected of causing precancerous liver changes in humans (some articles have even claimed "liver cancer") since research done with pyrrolizidine, an alkaloid present in comfrey but not extracted from it for this particular study, showed hepatic (liver) cell changes in laboratory animals fed pyrrolizidine by itself and in massive doses.

Similiarly, sassafras root cannot be sold legally for human consumption on the suspicion that internal use will cause precancerous changes. Scientific tradition researchers did not use sassafras root in their study, nor did they test it internally. They used extracted (and thus highly concentrated) sasfrol, the essential oil found in sassafras root, and injected it under the skin of laboratory animals. This caused carcinogenic changes.

There is no question that pure alkaloids and essential oils, sometimes in one small dose, sometimes in cumulative doses, can cause cancers and precancerous changes, severely injure, and even kill. However, the Scientific tradition claim that the crude plant itself is harmful, not just the oil or alkaloid, is questionable.

In fact, folklore and much rich personal anecdotal material have convinced me that both sassafras and comfrey are especially helpful nourishers of health/wholeness/holiness when cellular changes/cancers/tumors are present in a person.

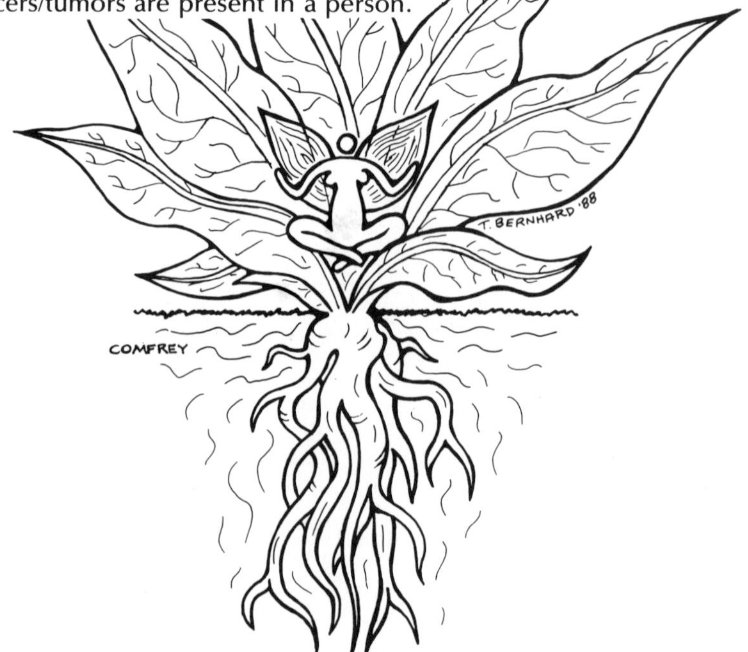

Doctors and Scientists and the Scientific Tradition

The Scientific tradition includes scientists and follows scientific ways, but it is neither restricted to, nor fully representative of, all scientists and all of science.

The Scientific tradition in general agrees with Isaac Newton (1642–1727) that the universe is a machine, operating according to identifiable rules or laws, even if we don't know them yet. There is little evidence that Newton's ideas were specifically applied to health until the beginning of the twentieth century.

The Scientific tradition of healing was not in existence in North America until 1910, according to biologist Joshua Lederberg. Lewis Thomas, MD, says it wasn't until 1937 that the "profoundly ignorant" practice of medicine began to change into a technology based on rigorous science. Other writers argue that medicine is still not fully scientific, though bedside manner has become but a memory as the twentieth century closes.

Scientific tradition thought patterns and reliance on machines for diagnosis and treatment is not limited to MDs and the established medical profession. Alternative health care practitioners can heal and fix in the Scientific tradition, too.

Scientific tradition chiropractors tend toward X-rays, hair analysis, and concentrated, drug-like supplements. Scientific tradition midwives insist on the value of synthetic vitamin and mineral supplements, sonograms, and blood work in pregnancy. Scientific tradition acupuncturists use an electrical machine to stimulate points rather than the usual hair-fine needle inserted into the point (tsubo).

Even psychic skills can be learned and practiced in the Scientific tradition: laboratory dream studies, biofeedback, and psychoactive drugs given by psychiatrists are examples.

Nor does use of machines, or drugs, or surgery necessarily imply the Scientific tradition. Chemotherapy and radiation are the allies of Bernie Siegal, MD, who uses them in conjunction with non-scientific (Wise Woman) ways to help individuals with cancer to health/wholeness/holiness. His written and recorded statements clearly indicate his understanding and use of Wise Woman tradition healing, and this in no way conflicts with his choice of healing techniques and substances.

New science and quantum physics, as explained by Einstein, Bohme, Prigogene, and others, is a science that speaks to us of Wise Woman ways: immeasurable time and immeasurable space in constant change; the energy of chaos; the inability to separate observer from observed; the futility of trying to find fixity and predictability; and the great joy and freedom that arise from these recognitions.

Voices of the Scientific Tradition

- *Not "herbal medicine" but "botanical therapeutics."*
- *"Herbal teas are dilute sources of drugs."*
- *"Herbs are crude drugs of vegetable origin selected and utilized by laypersons for treatment of disease or to maintain health."*
- *"The only way to gain a real understanding of herbs or their uses is through the scientific method. All other methods lead to delusion."*
- *"The hazards associated with herbal medications are quite numerous."*
- *"Lack of definite knowledge regarding the constituents and pharmacology of herbs renders their use imprecise at best, and dangerous at worst."*
- *"Prominent experts will speak on biochemical pharmacology of alkaloids and the production and ecology of secondary plant products."*
- *"When I saw her vomit violently, I realized the plant had great potential as a medicinal drug."*
- *"The herbs of which you speak belong in a lab with qualified professionals, not in a teapot in someone's home."*
- *"The risks of injury from herbal medications is much too great to warrant experimentation in this relatively unexplored field."*
- *"A scientific body of experimentally-based and rationally-arranged knowledge has nothing in common with traditional lore based on symbolic connections."*
- *"Herbal teas have no therapeutic value that cannot be more safely and effectively obtained from a specifically targeted modern drug."*
- *"It is impossible to distinguish between drugs and poisons; drugs given in excess will cause death; poisons are valuable remedies in small doses."*
- *"It is essential that the amount of the active principle given in any dose be uniform and of known potency."*
- New England Journal of Medicine *reports:*
(1981) 36% of hospital admissions caused by previous medical treatments.
(1983) rate of correct diagnosis dropped 20% from 1960 to 1980.

References & Resources:
The Scientific Tradition

- *Green Medicine: The Search for Plants that Heal*
  Margaret Kreig; 1964, Rand McNally
- *Guide to Medicinal Plants*
  P. Schauenberg & F. Paris; 1977, Keats
- *Herbal Medications*
  D. Spoerke, Jr.; 1980, Woodbridge
- *The Honest Herbal*
  V. Tyler; 1982, Stickley Co.
- *Magic & Medicine of Plants*
  1986, Reader's Digest
- *Major Medicinal Plants*
  Julia Morton; 1977, C. Thomas
- *Medical Botany*
  Memory Elvin-Lewis & W. Lewis; 1977, Wiley
- *Science of Herbal Medicine*
  J. Heinerman; 1980, Biworld
- *The Youngest Science*
  L. Thomas; 1983, Bantam

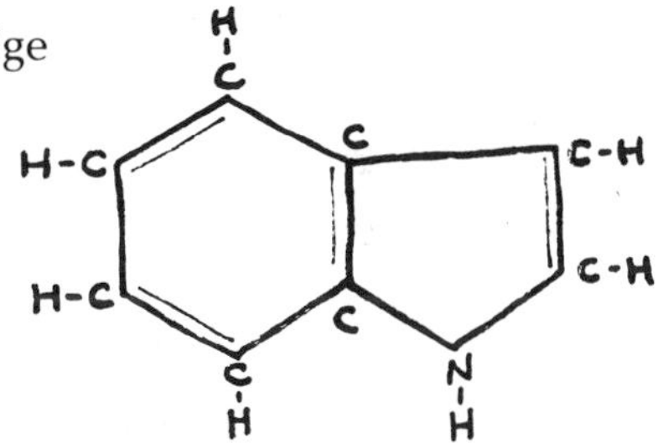

Journals

- Harvard Medical School Health Letter, PO Box 10944, Des Moines, IA 50340
- Herb Research Foundation, PO Box 2602, Longmont, CO 80501
- Journal of Natural Products, Lloyd Library, 917 Plum St, Cincinnati, OH 45202
- Journal of Ethnopharmacology, Elsevier Pubs., 52 Vanderbilt Ave., NY, NY 10017
- Medical/Aromatic Plant Abstracts, CSIR, Hillside Rd, New Delhi, 110012, India
- Planta Medica, Thieme Medical Publishers, 381 Park Ave. South, NY, NY 10016
- Phytotherapy Research, Heyden & Son Ltd, Spectrum House, Hillview Gardens, London NW42JQ, UK
- Quarterly Journal of Crude Drug Research, Swets & Zeitlinger, BV, PO Box 825, 2160 SZ Lisse, The Netherlands

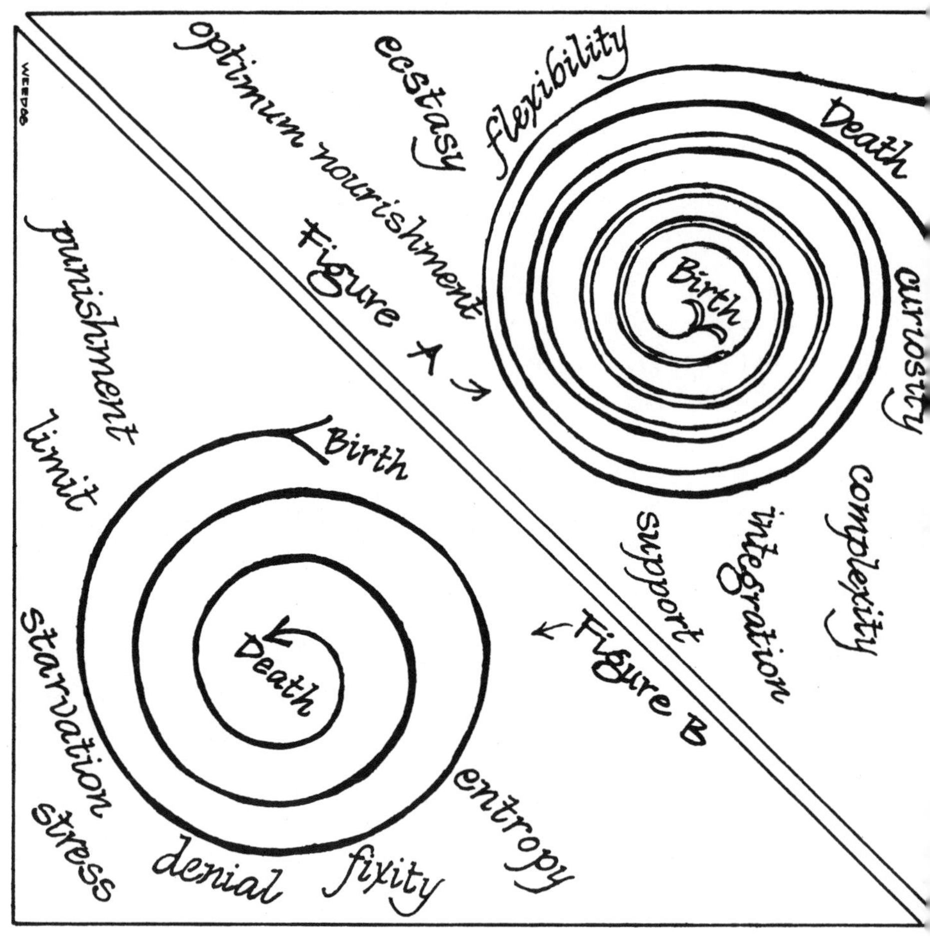

Spirals of Transformation

How does my life look if I see myself from the viewpoint of each health care tradition? Where do I come from? Where do I go? And what of the accidents and ill fortune I encounter on my way?

I will symbolize my life as a spiral—a moving line of vital vibration—and follow my way from birth to death through well (joy, ease, health) and hurt (pain, injury, disease) as seen by each tradition.

Two motions of the life spiral are shown. Figure A: Increasing the vitality of the individual increases the vibration and thus the spiral

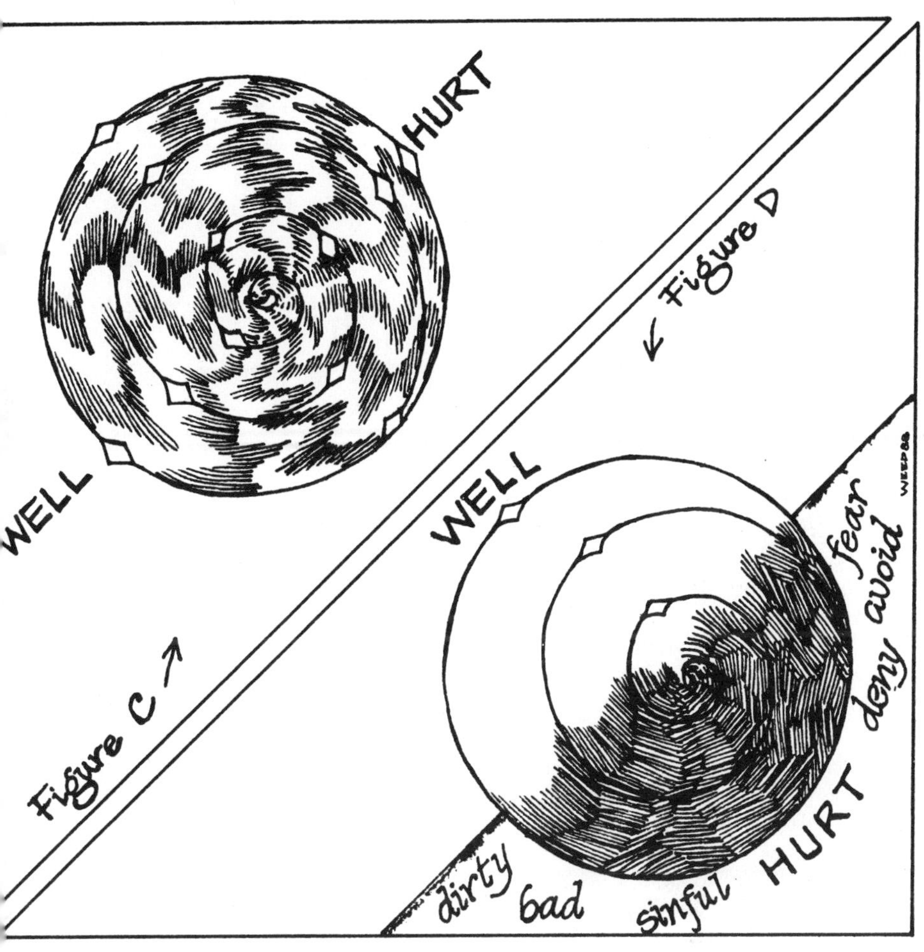

expands. This is typical of Wise Woman tradition nourishing/healing. Figure B: Damping down the vitality of the individual slows down the vibration and contracts the spiral. This is typical of Scientific tradition fixing and Heroic tradition cleansing/balancing.

Two ways of viewing the relationships between well and hurt are also shown. Figure C: Well and hurt are equal. Both are visible, speakable, and knowable. One is not avoided in preference to the other. This is typical of Wise Woman tradition thinking. Figure D: Well is superior to hurt. Well is visible and speakable. Hurt is hidden and quiet. Hurt is to be avoided as much as possible. This is typical of Scientific and Heroic tradition thinking.

Scientific Spiral

The pointing finger of God comes to spark the conception of my life spiral in the Scientific tradition: from the heavens into form (Figure 1).

I am born to be a precise and perfect replica of divine form in the Scientific tradition. Yet I slide down the curve of the spiral and come to the low point: disease, injury, pain. I am broken. I must be fixed. I need to be repaired. I want to be up on top where I belong (Figure 2). Quickly!

The fastest way up is to make a smaller curve—takes less time to get back to the top that way. And fixing makes it easier. When I get fixed, my vibration is more fixed, more limited, so I have less energy, less range of resonance available. Good thing it's faster to make my curve smaller, moving back to health. I'm not so sure I could find the vitality to make it all the way back to the very top again (Figure 3). Now that I've been repaired, I'm not quite as good as new, you know. But at least I can still do my work.

And so it goes, sliding down into despair and disease, being fixed with drugs and surgery, feeling my vitality shrink and become denser, less flexible. Needing the fast fix now more than ever. Fighting off the enemy, spying on the enemy (preventive medicine),

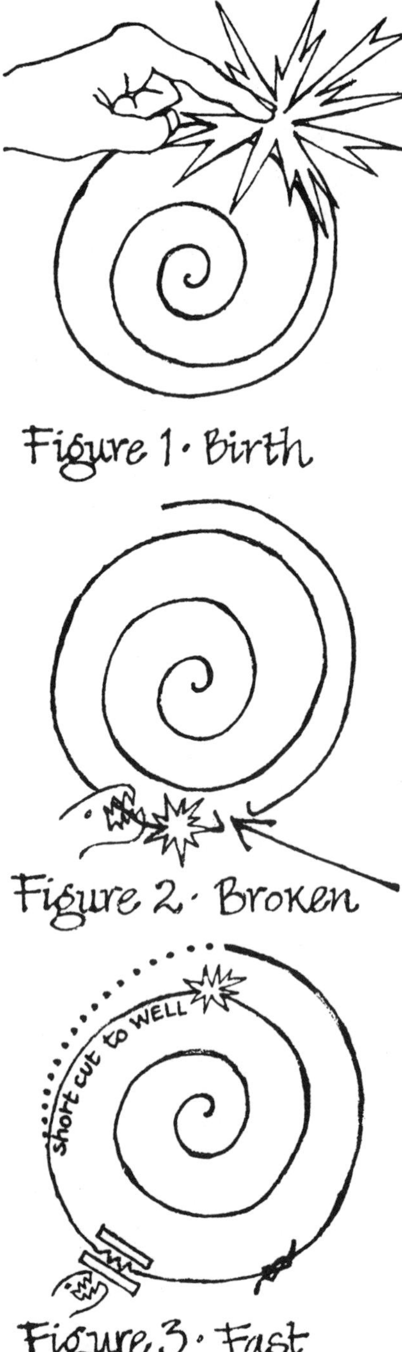

Figure 1 · Birth

Figure 2 · Broken

Figure 3 · Fast

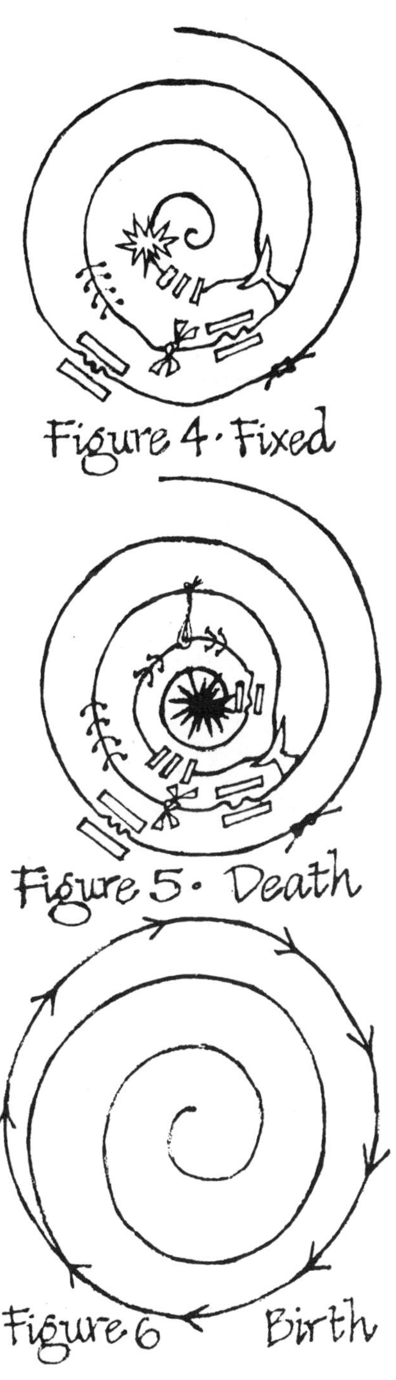

keeping death at bay, going in for regular checkups, waiting for the test results, being a patient, submitting—and with each submission, a diminution of self-worth and vital force, a loss of flexibility. I sense myself continually needing props: glasses, vitamin pills, and x-rays to begin, then to strong drugs and innumerable corsets of mind, heart, spirit, and body—all designed to fix me up. Fast. So fast that I never even know I'm sick or sad or confused. I can't complain (Figure 4).

Faster and faster around the spiral I go, but I've convinced myself I'm static, unmoving, unchanging. I stay the same, always well, always content, always on top. I don't notice the toll of vitality and joy taken by each fierce battle to stay on top. I stay in control takes until death slips in, until the day when there's no difference between top and bottom, up and down; nowhere to go. That's it—I lose: lose out to death. Fall down the dark hole void in the center of the spiral (Figure 5). Lost. Dead. The end?

Paint my cheeks and lips red, like life. Fix me up once more so I can be seen in death, well dressed, serene. Enclose me now in steel or concrete to keep away the earth changes that would mold me (spare parts in good working order have been salvaged). The end. Better to have it end than change.

Heroic Spiral

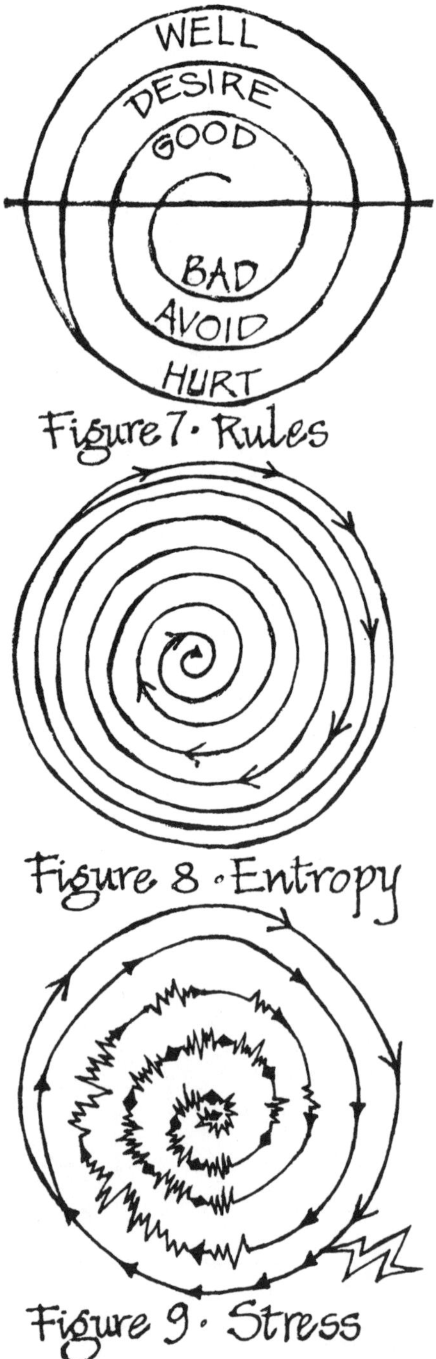

Figure 7 · Rules

Figure 8 · Entropy

Figure 9 · Stress

My life from the view of the Heroic tradition begins when my soul slips from perfection and falls into form. Immaculately conceived as a cosmic circle/egg of completeness, I should be able to continue on endlessly in perfect balance (Figure 6).

But I am born in sin. My body and mind are not to be trusted. So when I follow the Heroic tradition, I put my hope in following the rules (Figure 7).

The rules help me keep clean and clear. When I break the rules I get punished: get sick, break a leg, lose my sweetheart, get a traffic ticket. I try to learn my lessons, the teachings of my pain, so I'll never have to experience bad things again.

Even in perfect balance, doing only the right things, I cannot repeat my circling cycles into immortality; entropy quietly takes a bit of my vitality as I go round the spiral and this alone slowly unwinds me into death, unclean death (Figure 8). Trying to outwit death with rigorous cleansing measures, I move my spiral more rapidly inward. As I constrict the space of my self-love, I stress kidneys, liver, and colon, thus decreasing reserve energy (Figure 9). The more rigidly I adhere to the rules, the less flexibility I have and the less vitality flows through me. Thus, the spiral turns in, quickly in to unruly death's realm—failure. The horrible grief of failure. Dirty death—winner at last of the balancing game, the be-good game—the way of all flesh, dust to dust.

I atoned for all my sins, Father. May I live forever as pure and good and white? Clay to clay, but my spirit never dies. Pray for me.

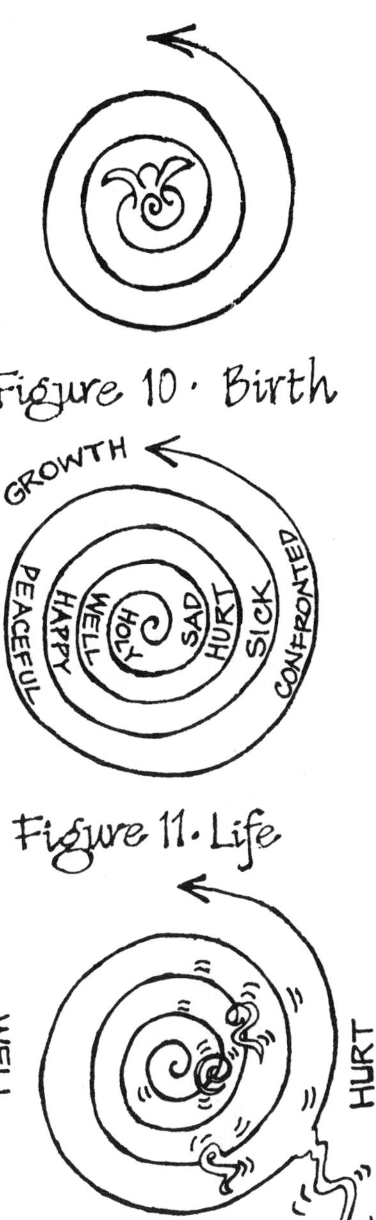

Figure 10 · Birth

Figure 11 · Life

Figure 12 · Nourish

Wise Woman Spiral

I begin at the center, says the wise woman seer. I come from the chaos and the completeness at the center of the spiral (Figure 10).

I am vital, moving, growing, unrestricted in resources, as I am born in the Wise Woman tradition. In the natural flow of my expansion and enrichment, I encounter pain; I lose control; I die. In the natural flow of my curiosity and play, I discover joy and wisdom. I am born. Pain is inevitable, suffering optional in the Wise Woman tradition (Figure 11).

When I hurt (when my heart hurts, when my head hurts, when my shoulders hurt) I nourish myself: I nourish my heart, my head, and my shoulders (Figure 12). I nourish myself and am strengthened, transformed and deepened; my vibrational rate increases.

I expand. I open my spiral. I ask myself, "How can I make this problem my ally? What is the gift of health / wholeness / holiness here?" I gain energy with each sickness or problem. My range of resonance and my capacity to receive and to share increases every time I encounter pain and loss and make it my ally. I ally myself with all that I resist and thus become whole. I regain my holiness. Every time I nourish myself in pain, honor my distress, and love my uniqueness, my vibration is vitalized and the spiral gets bigger and more open, more forceful (Figure 13).

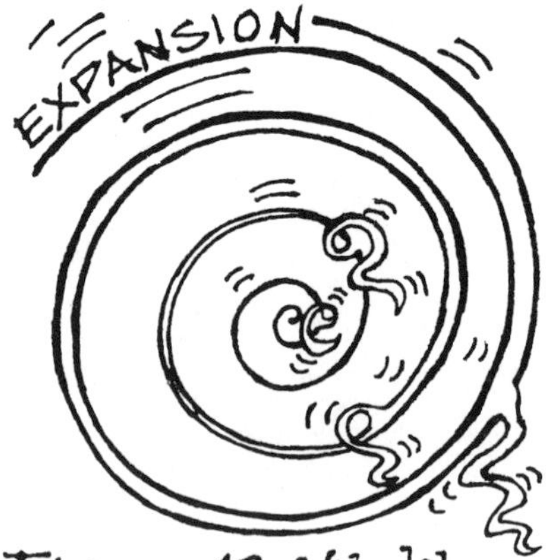

I may walk the widening arcs of the spirals slowly, chewing well all the nourishing bits, or I may slip round spinningly fast, like a stone twirled round and round in a sling. Eventually I become so big and so vital that I can no longer contain myself. Too rich to be bound in matter. My every disease a transformation, death now another (how extraordinary) transformation (Figure 14).

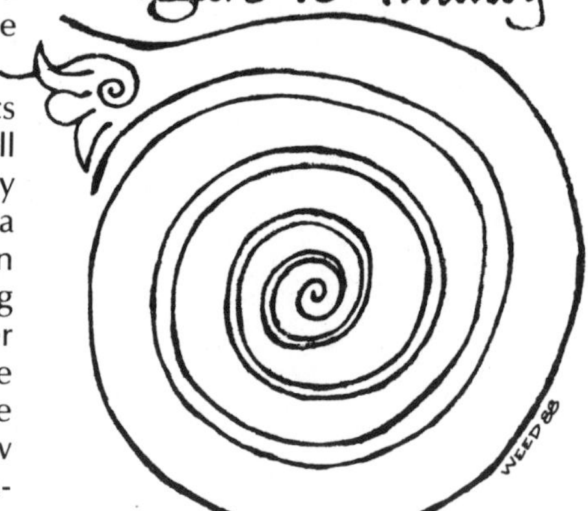

Yes, this death is part of my whole self. I expand, compassionate, confident, successful. I let loose, flying off into death, birth, void, full. I let go to transformation. I become completion. I am one with the beloved again! She died laughing. She died in ecstasy. She died with her eyes wide open.

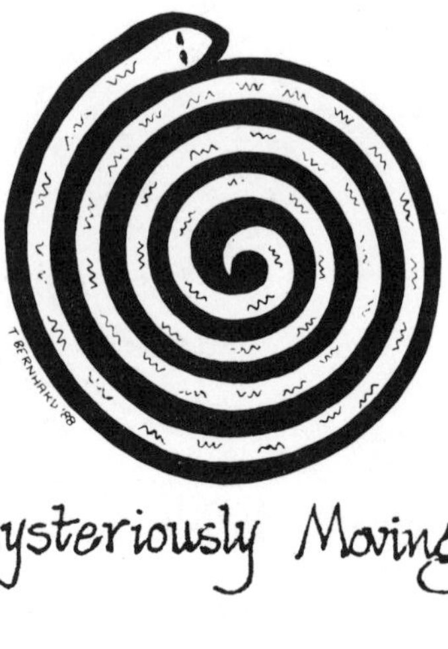

EXPANSION

Figure 13 · Vitality

Figure 14 · Death

Mysteriously Moving

MEDICINE WHEEL of the WISE WOMAN TRADITION

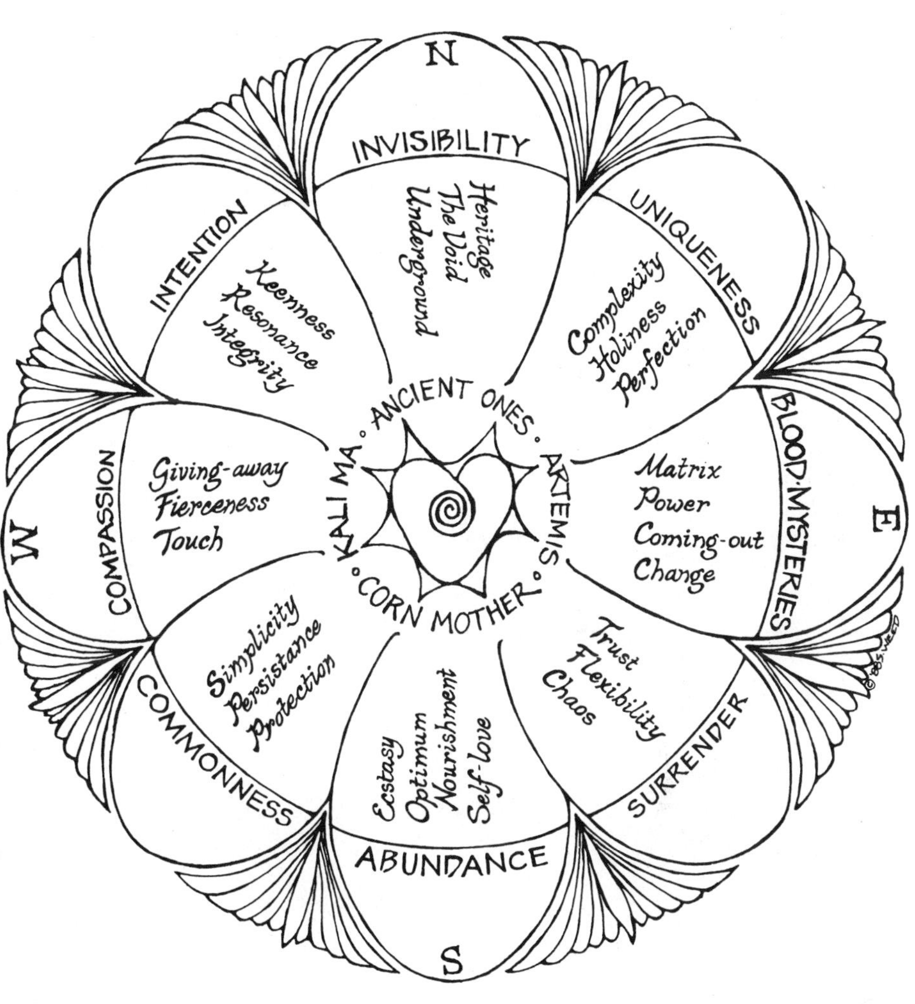

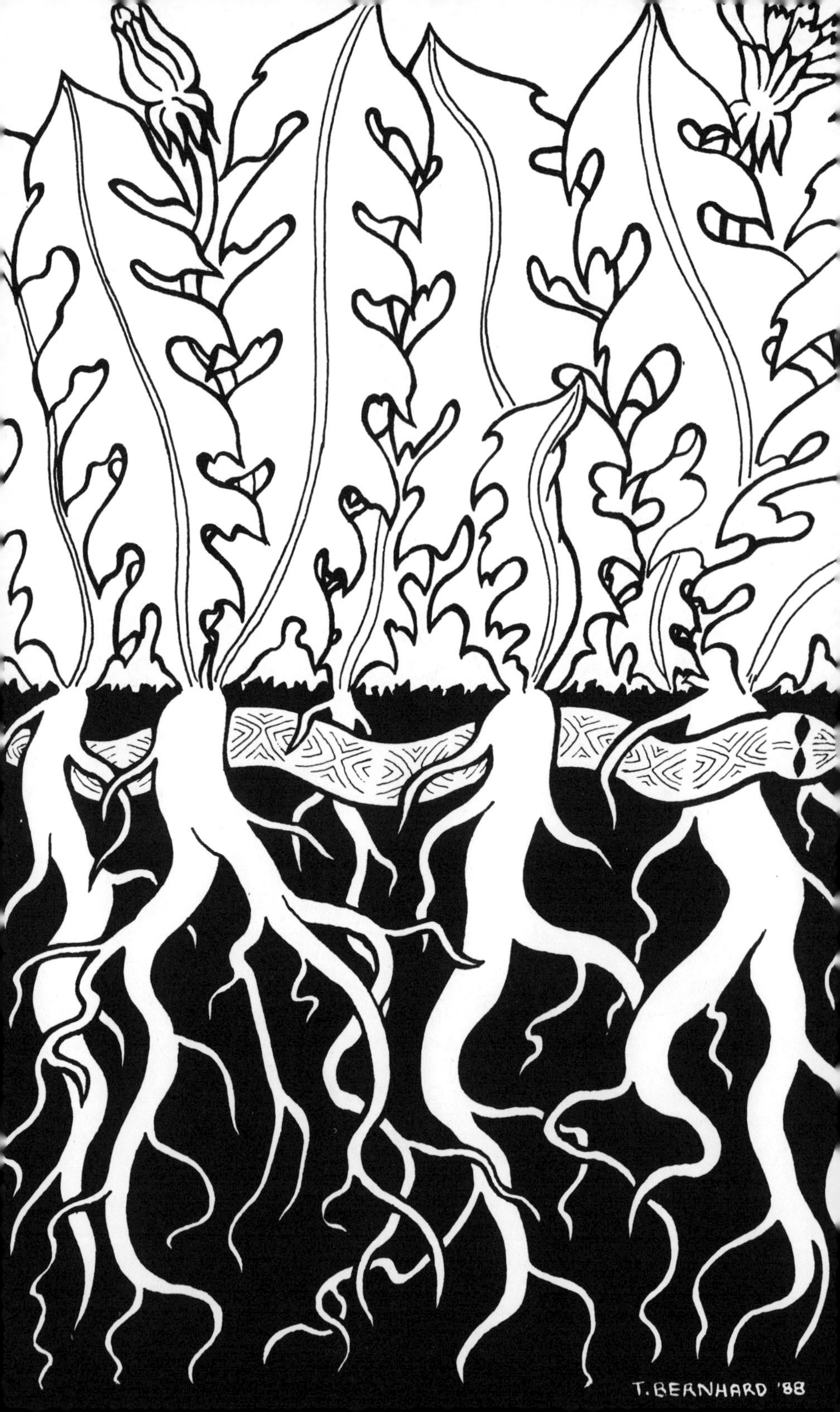
T. BERNHARD '88

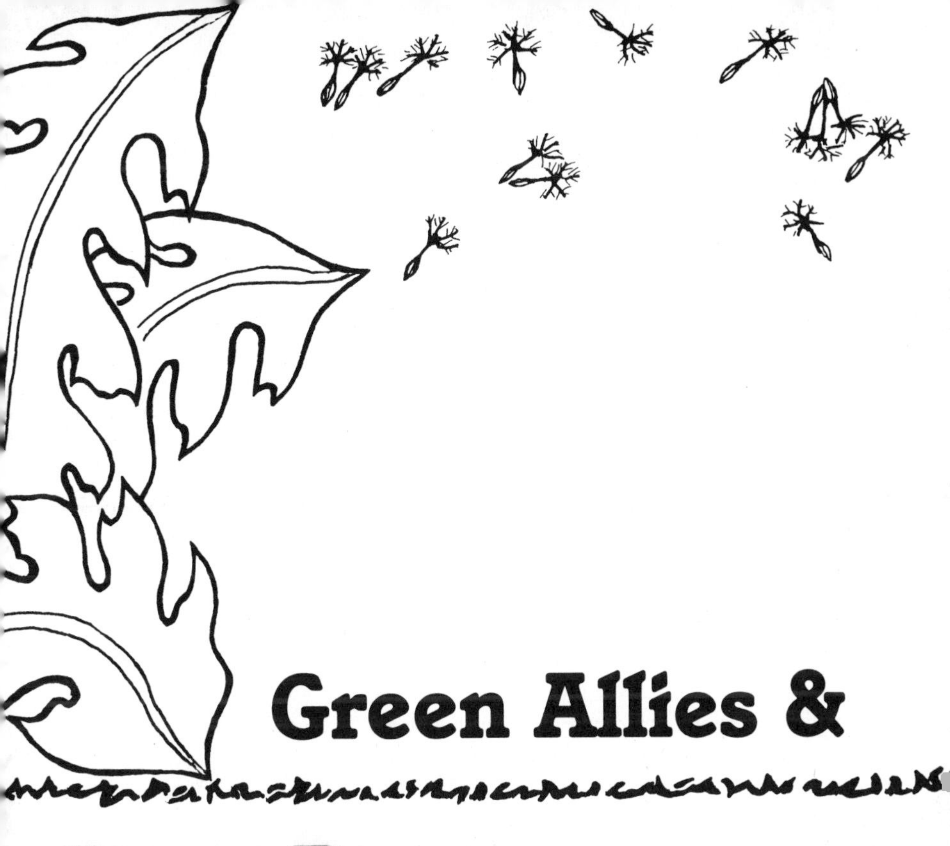

Green Allies & Deep Roots

Those who heal and teach in the Wise Woman tradition claim that we can improve our health/wholeness/holiness by allying ourselves with common, abundant, wild plants, that is, weeds.

But how can we do this? Where does one begin? Who will introduce us to these weeds, these green allies?

Begin right here. Let me introduce you to some of my favorite green allies.

The seven green allies presented here are common, abundant weeds found virtually everywhere on our planet (though not in tropical or desert areas). These weeds are some of my closest friends: ones I know I can count on when I feel terrible, and ones who share the daily joys of life with me.

I introduce them to you in a special way, to activate all of your brain/mind and allow you to learn at an accelerated pace.

Your intuitive aspect (said to be focused in the right brain) is engaged immediately by the illustration of each herb with its deva or fairies, then nourished as you read **The Green Ally Speaks.**

Your analytical aspect (said to be focused in the left brain) is engaged by **Green Ally Facts,** a one-page summary of the names and uses, the habitat, range, and characteristics, and possible toxic effects of each weed.

Now both hemispheres of your brain/mind are ready to work together. Come on a **Weed Walk** with me, where we will encounter our green ally at home. You will sense her in your imagination as I speak of her particular powers.

Then the left brain is strongly activated with **Green Ally Properties and Uses**. This section begins with a list of the properties of the plant (there's a glossary in the back of the book to help you decode the unfamiliar words), a brief summary of the green ally's uses, and dosage recommendations. Because the wise woman can use any *single* plant for *all* her needs, if need be, I present you with many properties and uses of each plant, not just the major ones. This section is dense, replete with the myriad ways I and others have allied ourselves with this plant to nourish health/wholeness/holinesss. There is vast potential available in even the most ordinary weed. You'll discover new uses every time you open this book.

To keep the left brain from becoming too dominant while you study **Green Ally Properties and Uses**, I've provided nourishment for the imaginative right brain by inserting quotes along the bottom margins of the pages. These quotes bring you the thoughts and impressions of others (from many times and places) who know this green ally well. Look out for fairies flitting among the pages.

Then we take the left brain to the kitchen for the **Green Ally Pharmacy** where special preparations are explained. For most preparations mentioned in the text, such as infusions, tinctures, oils, and poultices, consult the last chapter, **The Herbal Pharmacy**, where you'll find complete directions for making your own simple, effective herbal remedies with green allies.

In the kitchen, the right brain is thinking food and your mouth is watering. Go straight to the recipes. Yes, recipes. **Green Ally Kitchen** shows you how to invite a green ally in for breakfast, lunch, or dinner. Wouldn't you do that for any new friend you want to get to know better?

The last part of each chapter, **Green Ally Fun and Facts,** engages the whole brain/mind, and the humor ganglia, too. Here you'll find funny facts about the green ally, literary mentions (Shakespeare often calls upon green allies), and references and resources unique to the plant.

For complete bibliographical information and access to herbal preparations by mail, consult the appended lists of **Resources** and **My Favorite Mail Order Sources for Herbs**. For further information on **Nutritional Values**, consult that appendix.

Green Blessings!

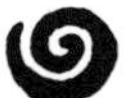

Special information for those wishing to be green witches:

To deepen your alliance with these green allies, try this.

Read aloud, or have someone read to you, the **Green Ally Speaks.** Go no further than this at first. Read this section several times, both silently and aloud, over several days, especially just before going to sleep. Tell the plant you want to know her, want to honor her, want to become her friend. Sleep deeply.

Special dreams may come or not. Pay attention if they do; fret not if they don't.

When you feel ready, read over the **Green Ally Facts**, then go on to the **Weed Walk.** Get a field guide (check **Resources**) or a knowledgeable friend, and go out on your own weed walk. In all likelihood you'll find the green ally growing close to you (yes, even if you live in the city).

Time to get some hands-on experience. Harvest some of the plant you've found and make a meal or a medicine out of it.

Check your intentions before you begin to use your green ally for healing. Are you using this hoping to fix what ails you? (Scientific tradition intentions.) Are you hoping to clean up your diet and become more spiritual? (Heroic tradition intentions.) Are you hoping to nourish and love your health/wholeness/holiness? (Wise Woman tradition intentions.)

Experiment with your green ally on yourself, your beloveds, your friends, and your pets. For greatest effect, keep notes on your successes and failures. When approached from the Wise Woman perspective, healing with green allies will provide you with amazing results and profound insights into the interconnections of self with self, family, community, and world.

Keep notes too on your frequent visits to your green ally. Weekly visits for at least a year will expose you to the full solar cycle of each weed. Put up your medicines and cook meals with your green ally in every season. Before long you'll find your alliance is strong, available to you without particular thought, a part of your own being. Ahhh.

Green Blessings indeed!

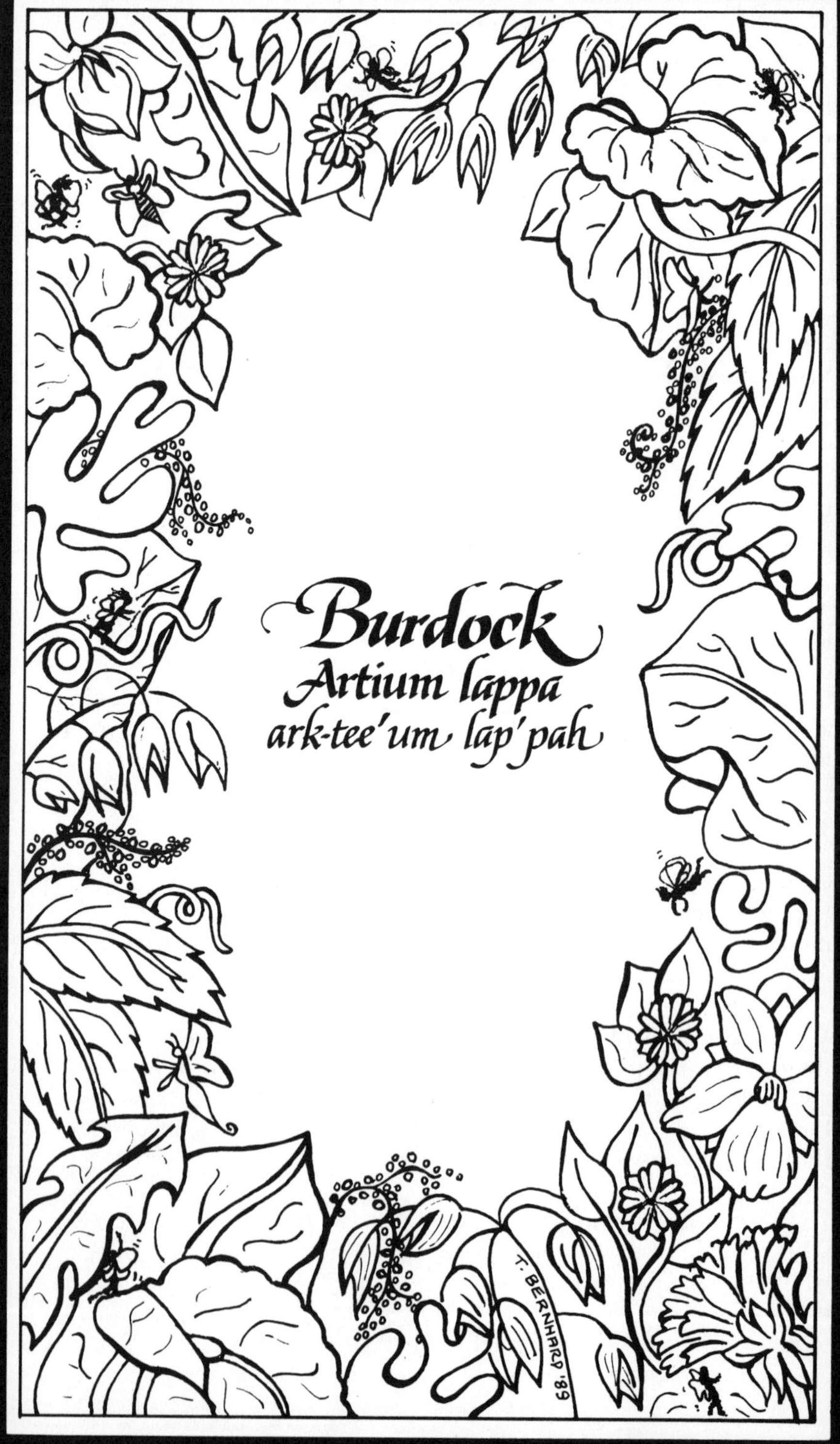
Burdock
Artium lappa
ark-tee'um lap'pah
T. BERNHARD '89

Burdock Speaks

Hey, you. C'mere. Yeah, YOU! Hey! I'm talkin' ta you. C'mere so's I don't hafta shout . . . not that I mind shoutin'. Just get yourself over here closer a bit. OK? OK!

Say, are ya comfortable? You can use one of my tremendously large leaves as a cushion if ya wanna sit. Huh? A sunhat? Sure thing. You're not too hot now, are ya? Me, I like it here . . . plenty of sun, plenty of rich soil, and a nice big rock or two to get a good grip on. Yeah, yeah, you're right; the neighborhood is kinda run-down. But still it's a fine place by me; beauty's more than skin deep, ya know. Wadda ya think, huh?

Hey! Now don't go away. Hey! OK. OK. I know ya think I'm a good for nothin'. A hassle, a pain, a problem. Ya no doubt heard I'm a shiftless stranger, coarse and crude. A worthless pest, a ne'er-do-well. I know, I know. Ya think I'm a torment to little girls. And a tangler of dogs' tails. And a menace to fine wool. In short, a rank and obnoxious weed. I know. I heard it all before. But ya don' know the half of it, the other half of it. Ya ain't heard my side. Ya ain't heard from me.

What? Ya say I'm difficult to hear from? Get down. Just get down, now, cuz I work deep down. If you wanna hear from me you're gonna hafta get down, go slow, and chill out. I'm not just a surface phenomenon, ya know; I'm deep. Ya hear me? Deep. I work behind the scenes, in the depths. Kinda like a housekeeper, or a janitor, or a plumber. I work under the skin, from the inside out, ya know.

I take on the unsavory stuff: the rough work nobody else wants to touch. Call me names; curse me like the others do; look down on me and deny my goodness. But still I am the mighty burdock, and I stand in my truth. My truth is my heavy-duty nourishment and my penetrating power. My nourishment dat hits on your depths just like my root plunges down into the earth. And my power, like a sword of health/wholeness/holiness. I cut the shit, if you get what I mean. Toxic waste . . . negativity . . . useless junk . . . garbage . . . I cut it out. And I nourish my helpers: your liver, your kidneys, and your lymphatic system.

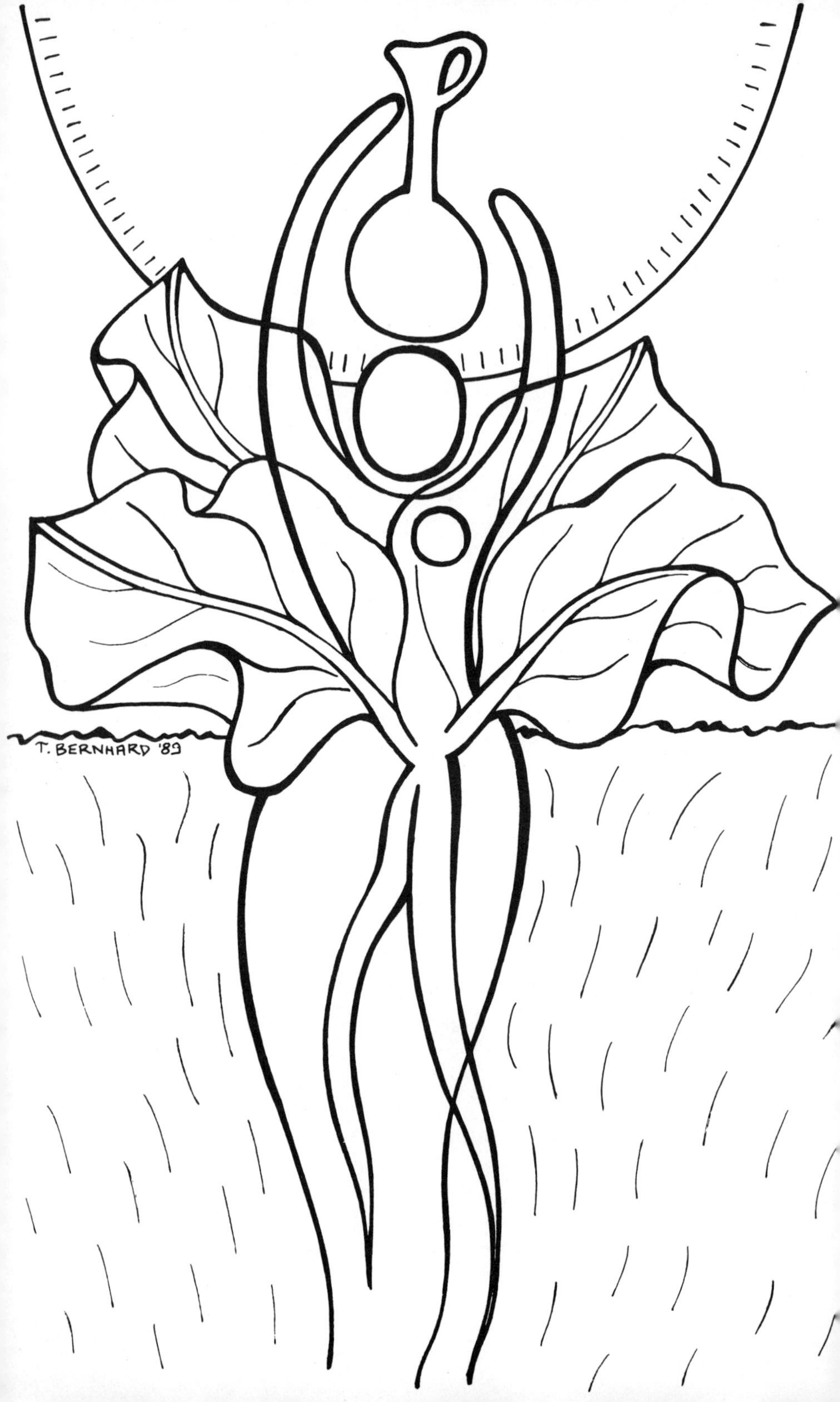
T. BERNHARD '89

Now, does that make me a hero or an outlaw? I ask ya. M'self, I think my work is grand. I'm proud of my ability to clean up your messes and strengthen your innards. But you, you people make laws against me. Revile me. Abuse me. Say that I am a pesky cousin of thistle. Call me a rank immigrant. Claim that I'm degenerated from a good herb! Degenerated? Look who's talking! It's a wonder I even consent to talk to ya dumb primates.

Hey, hey, I'm sorry. Listen, I'm sorry. C'mon. Sit down again. I may be bitter on the outside, but inside I'm a real sweetie, believe me. Hey, si'down!

I can tell you're different, right? Maybe you's one a those mackeys. Yeah, that must be it. Mackeys love me awright. Or maybe you's oriental? Maybe chinee? Orientals love me, too, ya know. Here in America they call me gobo. Great name, huh? Gobo, da root of energy. Strongest of da strong. Whooee! Wadda ya think? Ain't I tuff? Ain't I yang? Get down.

I'll get ya going; just let me at 'em. I'll get ya movin' and groovin' and sweatin'and stokin'. I'll get ya moanin' and pissin' and groanin' and grindin'. I am burdock, a cool head in a pinch and a boogie baby in da easy times.

Why don' you get to know me better? Ya know I'm a favorite of Venus, and she's full of love medicine. I'm known for my staying power, baby. I say, get down. Ain't I robust looking? You can tell I'm full of get-up and ready to go. If you dares ta try me, know that you's in for an extended play. I ain't no one-night stand, oh no. I'm in for the long haul and I got endurance, too. Some swear I can make your womb do somersaults. I ain't jivin'.

'Course, that don't mean I'll be around forever, ya know. I'm fulla seeds and I scatter 'em where I can, it's true. And I never stick around long enough to see their second birthdays.

The only long-term relationship I got goin' is wit' Doctor Dandelion, my chéri. But she gets around too, dig me? We got this open thing, ya know, but we're real sweet on each other. We each got our own lives, and our own work ta do. But we get together on the harder jobs, ya follow?

So dat's my story. Now ya heard the other side, my side. Now ya heard from me, burdock.

Burdock Facts

Botanical name: *Arctium lappa*; Arctos (Greek) means bear; lappa (Celtic) means hand or to seize. ***Other useful species:*** *Arctium minus, A. tomentosum*. ***Natural order:*** Compositae/Daisy family, Dandelion tribe. ***English names:*** Love leaves, beggar's buttons, cockle buttons, thorny burr, stickers, stick tight, burs, burrseed, harebur, cuckoo button, cloth burr, clotbur, fox's clote, personata, hare-lock, turkey burr, bat weed, hardock, woolly dock, happy major, prosopium, philanthropium, bardona, gobo, lappa. ***Chinese names:*** Wu shih, niu bang, niu-tzu, ta-li-tzu, sheng-ma, niu-ting pao, niu-bang-tzu. ***French names:*** Bardane, grande bardane, glouteron. ***German names:*** Klette, Grosse Klette. ***Italian names:*** Bardana. ***Russian names:*** Repeinik, lopuh. ***Old English names:*** Herrif, aireve, airup. ***Fiber uses:*** Velcro fasteners are actually based on burdock burrs. ***Food uses:*** Root sold in specialty markets and stores, especially Chinese, as "gobo"; leaves and stalks pickled; cultivated in Japan, Hawaii, and occasionally in the New England states. ***Medicinal uses:*** Root sold dry and tinctured; burr seed oil occasionally sold. ***Soil uses:*** Restores minerals to topsoil: burn or add to compost. ***Animal uses:*** My mother taught not to say anything if I couldn't say anything nice. What shepherds and dog owners have to say about burdock's clinging burrs is rarely nice. ***Habitat:*** Moist, fertile soils in the temperate zones, especially abandoned sites, roadsides. ***Natural range:*** *(A. lappa)* throughout Europe and Asia; *(A. minus)* most of North America. ***Current range:*** Throughout the temperate zones of Asia, China, Europe, North America, Australia, Tasmania, Japan, and Hawaii. ***Toxicity:*** *Externally,* one case of contact dermatitis from leaves has been reported. *Internally,* burdock is quite non-toxic; there are no known alkaloids or saponins in the root; occasional reports of double vision have resulted from contamination of dried root with poisonous plants; extended or sudden extensive use may initiate loose stools. ***Best identified by:*** Very large (up to three feet/one meter long and nearly as wide) leaves with reddish stalks and woolly undersides; bitter taste left on fingers after rubbing leaves; *!#!@*!! burrs.

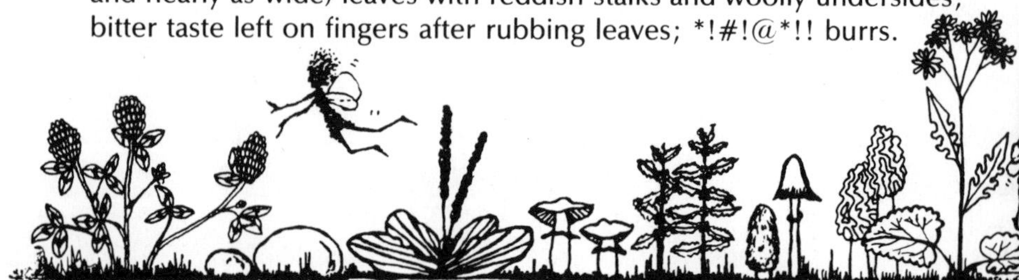

Burdock Weed Walk

Look at the glorious fall colors! Let's go for a walk. We'll go down to the abandoned farm and harvest some burdock roots and seeds. Grab a sweater; it'll be chilly by the time we start back. Let's take the spading fork, and these bags. And the hand trowel. And gloves. We're likely to need them all. Burdock roots are hard to dig out.

There's lots of burdock here along the way. But we'd never stand a chance of loosening it from this roadside. No more chance than I'd have had if I'd tried to harvest the biggest burdock plant I ever saw. It was in Toronto, on a street corner. Out of a crack between the cement sidewalk and a brick building grew a flowering burdock higher than my head and wider than my arms could stretch!

Burdock is a plant that takes two full years to complete its life cycle. See here: these are the first-year plants. We'll dig their roots. They have leaves only, no flower stalk. They'll flower next year and then they'll look like these, filled with the burrs that follow the flowers. The burr-y second year plants are nearly dead now. All the life has gone from them into the seeds, so we'll gather some seeds as well.

The first-year plant develops such enormous leaves that it is easily mistaken for some kind of rhubarb. The reddish, purplish leaf stalks and veins add to the mistaken identity. But the dense white undersurface of the leaf is quite distinct, as is the exceedingly bitter taste left on your fingers after rubbing the leaf briskly between thumb and forefinger. Here, try it.

Turn down this dirt road. See how much bigger even the roadside burdock gets as we get down toward the river, where the soil is richer and wetter? Let's start digging here.

The burdock root develops by growing straight down, sending out lateral holding roots wherever it finds a sufficient anchor, such as a rock. These lateral anchors and the propensity of the burdock leaves to break off when you pull on them, make it impossible just to pull up the burdock root. We're going to have to dig, a lot, to harvest these roots.

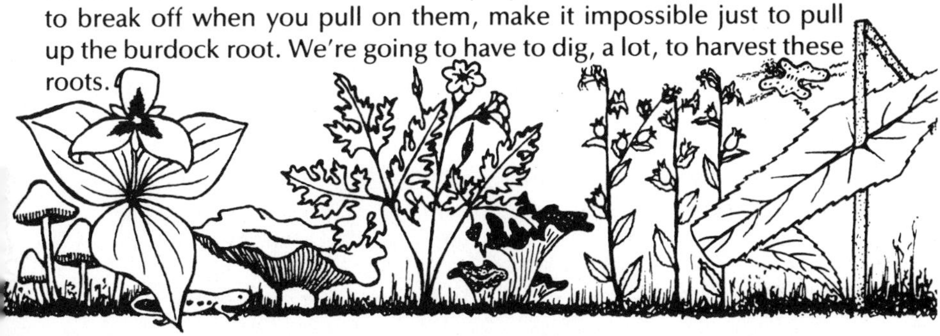

We've been broadcasting our intentions to these burdocks as we walked here, so let's begin without further ado. Today is excellent for digging medicinal roots. The frost last night signaled the plants to put energy down into their roots, and the new moon strengthens that flow down and in. I've been harvesting roots to eat since the middle of July, but waited until now to harvest roots for medicine. The tincture we make from this will be good for drawing out fluids: urine, sweat, menstrual flow, inflammation, infection.

I'll come back next spring, no doubt, to get more of these same roots for soups and, if needed, for more tincture, though their energy and medicinal value won't be nearly as strong then as they are now.

This plant looks healthy: the leaves are as long as my arm and nearly as wide, a greyed green, and broadly wavy at the edge, undulating softly. The size of the leaves doesn't always tell the size of the root, but I suspect this one will be worth our efforts.

Notice the rough texture of the older leaves, and the velvety smooth fuzzy surface of the young leaves. And how the fuzz extends down the leaf stalk, or petiole. Once we dig up the root, we'll take off the leaves. We'll cut off their stalks/petioles, and take those home for dinner, leaving the leaves here to decompose, which they do remarkably fast.

Start in the east and made a plunge straight down with the spading fork right next to the root. Here, I'll hold the leaves away.

This is called great burdock: *Arctium lappa*. See how the petioles are grooved with a u-shaped gouge on top? And solid? Here, break this one off.

Arctium minus, the slightly smaller sister plant, has hollow leaf stalks, as though the groove had grown together. Her flowers are stalkless, while the great burdock has stalked flowers. Essentially, though, they are the same plant and used in exactly the same ways. And you'll find interbreeds, too: at least eight distinct ones are already recognized. Don't worry; they're all burdock, stubborn root.

How's this stubborn root coming along? Great. Good work with the fork. A shovel will cut through the root, that's why we don't use one. Now take the fork and go straight down again, only this time in the south. And now in the west. Rock the spading fork from side to side before you take it out of the earth. And here in the north. Good. Now go around again, and again. As you loosen the soil, I'll get it out of the way with the hand trowel so you can go deeper with the fork on your next round.

Whew. Well, we're down past the leaf base. It's quite the trick that burdock has, keeping so well buried that the first several inches of digging only brings us to the top of the root. Go around some more with that spading fork.

Aha. There's the first lateral root. That one going off to the side and under a rock, no doubt. Let's see if we can pull it loose. Oops, broke it. Smell it. Earthy . . . open . . . cool . . . faintly aromatic . . . deep, deep, slow. Yes. Yes. Have a taste. Like it? It's such a surprise to find the root so sweet after tasting the bitterness of the leaves, isn't it? That piece that stays in the ground will grow a new plant next year, so I'm glad it broke off.

The young root is entirely white when it sprouts, but as it grows, the outer layer attains a dark-brown-to-black coloration which, in the second year, becomes a thick, distinct layer. Under that, the burdock root is a beautifully striated white, with a dense inner core.

OK! We're down nearly as far as I can reach and we still haven't come to the end of this burdock root. Put your feet in the hole here with me and hold on to the root. Now envision it loosening from the earth and giving away its firmness, its wholeness, its abundance, to us.

And gently, slowly pull . . . pull . . . yes, that's it! We got it. Let's do another one.

Next year flower stalks will grow from the roots we leave undisturbed. Besides being certain to leave enough roots here to ensure an ongoing supply of burdock, we want to leave enough so I can harvest flower stalks next summer. It is the choicest edible of the whole plant, both because the flavor is so good and because the effort involved in harvesting it is so minimal.

I have a funny memory about burdock stalk. The first time I harvested it I was on my own. I remembered it was edible, but nothing more. Not wanting to carry the whole stalk home with me, I decided to take only the choicest bits. I knew that most wild plants were tastiest and tenderest in the new growth, so I carefully cut off and saved all the little branches and threw the big stalk away. Was I ever chagrined when I got home and checked in my books to discover I'd discarded the best part!

It was really too late for gathering stalk, anyhow. The flowers were already opening, and burdock stalk is at its best before the flower buds even form. Seems like it takes only a few days for that stalk to grow from nothing to shoulder high. And the bigger it gets, the bigger a knife you need to cut it. In places where people war against burdock and cut it off repeatedly, the stalk still persists, branching furiously and even flowering at ground level if need be.

What are the flowers like? Imagine little purple thistle flowers on top of these prickly round seed capsules and imagine that the capsules are green: like a fuzzy purple ball on a denser fuzzy green ball. And all these little hooks you see here on the mature seed capsule are there on the young green ball, but flexible, not ready to hook you yet.

The green burdock burrs don't disintegrate when you handle them, the way the ripe brown ones do, so they're fun to play with. I've made all sorts of pretend characters from green burrs, and even put on shows with them, much to the delight of my young friends (and the fairies).

The leaves on the flower stalk are different from the leaves you see here now. These basal leaves have wavy borders, are huge, roughly heart-shaped, and are on long leaf stalks (called petioles, you recall). The leaves on the flower stalk next year will be more oval, much, much smaller (some no longer than your little finger), without petioles, and not wavy at the edges. You can see some of them here still on this dying second-year burdock.

It's late autumn of the second year of its life, and the great burdock is nearly dead: the seed-filled burrs are brown and ready to break away from the stalk when barely touched; the leaves are withered; and even the sturdy root can now be wrested from its earth socket, for it has shrunken and is ready to let go of its grasp.

Here, try it, carefully. Tug on it. Envision it coming loose. There it is! I wish the first year roots could be removed with so little exertion. But look how withered and rotten this root is. All the good stuff is in the seeds now.

Oh, I see you've already started to gather burrs. You'll really find it much more convenient to put them in the bag than sticking them to your arms and legs and back and hair like that.

Ready to go? We still have a lot of work ahead of us at home, but I want to take the long way back through the woods. None of this burdock harvest is perishable, so we can afford to dawdle and enjoy the autumn show.

Once home, we'll jump up and down on our bags of burdock burrs, or roll them with a rolling pin to loosen the seeds. Then we'll sieve out the little fiberglass-like white hairs intermingled with the seeds. We could let a pan of water be our sieve too: the hairs float and the seeds sink. We'll put some seeds up in oil (wet ones won't work for that) and the rest in vodka. I've kept the seeds dried once or twice, but they always seem to hatch out crawling, wiggling things if kept until spring.

And we'll clean and tincture the roots, too. But that's later. *Now* is this exquisite autumn afternoon. What a beautiful sunset. What brilliant colors. How abundantly we are cared for by the earth. Doesn't it make you happy to be alive?

Burdock Root Properties and Uses

- ***nutritive tonic,*** antiscorbutic, hypoglycemic
- ***alterative,*** exthanematous, depurative, anti-onchotic, anti-tumor
- ***anti-pyretic,*** anti-rheumatic, antibiotic, anodyne
- ***rejuvenative,*** aphrodisiac, estrogenic cholagogue, pulmonary
- ***stomachic,*** carminative, aperient (varies, may bind), astringent
- ***urinary tonic,*** diuretic, demulcent

Fresh burdock root is also

- ***bacteriostatic,*** fungistatic
- ***diaphoretic,*** febrifuge
- ***strongly diuretic,*** tonic

With so many abilities to offer, it is no wonder that burdock is a beloved ally of wise women and herbalists everywhere. Burdock's action is most profound on the **lymph, sweat,** and **oil glands**, though its influence is felt in the **liver, lungs, kidneys, stomach, uterus,** and **joints.** Medicines made from the fresh burdock root are always preferable and superior to dried root preparations. Burdock is not for people in a hurry, or most acute problems; burdock works thoroughly and **slowly**.

Use burdock root as a nourishing tonic, a skin clearer, a super cooler, a slick trick in the guts, and a guardian of your inner flows.

- Dose of *fresh burdock root tincture* is 30-240 drops a day, in water.
- Dose of *dried burdock root infusion* is ½-2 cups/125-500ml a day.
- Dose of *burdock root decoction* is 1-9 teaspoonsful/5-45ml a day.

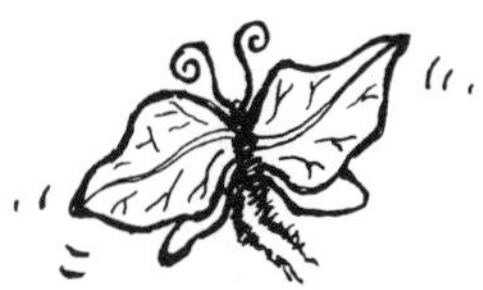

"Burdock is a widely used blood purifier and alterative, stronger than sarsaparilla but less energetic than echinacea and with little of the intestinal effects of yellow dock." M. Moore (1979)

Burdock Root is a Nourishing Tonic

(Numbers indicate milligrams per hundred grams burdock root)

Even occasional use of burdock root, or any part of the plant, will help provide optimum nutrition to the glandular and immune systems, liver, kidneys, blood, lungs, and nerves, as well as providing overall power and emotional stability to the whole being. Burdock nourishes the most extreme, buried, and far-reaching aspects of ourselves. Burdock breaks the ground for deep transformation.

Longevity, steady energy, sexual vitality, and freedom from chronic disease and cancer are a few of the reported effects of long-term, frequent use of burdock. Given the ways and talents of burdock, I would say these are modest claims.

Burdock root is very high in chromium (2), iron (5.1-147), magnesium (537), silicon (22.5), thiamine (1.1), and inulin (27-45%).

Burdock root is also high in cobalt (12), phosphorus (247-437), potassium (766-1680), sodium (127-152), tin (2.1), zinc (2.2), carotenes expressed as vitamin A (7500 IU), protein (10.6-12%), fiber (70%), and mucilage (5-12%).

Burdock root also supplies aluminum (23), calcium (212-733), manganese (6), selenium (1.4), and lappin, a glucoside.

Burdock root is low in calories (205-379) and fat (.4-.7). Fresh root contains enough vitamin C to be an oft-reported cure for the deficiency, though analysis of the dried root detects only traces of ascorbic acid.

Burdock Root is a Skin Clearer

Burdock root preparations are highly regarded by wise women of all centuries, and verified by recent tests, as an ally for healing those with skin diseases (blemishes to tumors).

Poultices or frequent applications of burdock root oil or freshly grated burdock roots are a wise woman's ally for healing and easing the pain of those with inflamed, reddened, heated skin conditions: boils, abscesses, pimples, acne, chronic rashes, eczema, cysts, infected wounds, burns, itchy skin, leg ulcers, frequent fever blisters and cold sores, herpes outbreaks, tumors, breast cancers, rheumatic joints, swollen legs, and back pain. The effectiveness is increased if burdock root tincture or infusion is taken concurrently and for several months after the noticeable problem has cleared.

Try frequent light applications of burdock root oil as part of your Wise Woman ways when helping anyone with cold sores, hemorrhoids, acute rashes, fungus infections, psoriasis, impetigo, and menstrual pimples.

Burdock root tincture and infusion are effective allies for the wise woman healing herself or those with acne, psoriasis, dermatitis, erysipelas, chronic allergic hives, and nervous rashes.

Try baths and soaks of burdock root infusion to ease those with swelling from sprains, broken bones, bursitis, arthritis, rheumatism, sciatica, varicose veins.

The dried, powdered root is sufficiently astringent to close open wounds and ulcers when applied directly.

Even the scalp benefits from burdock's skin-clearing ability. Try the infusion as a hair rinse to check dandruff and ease itchy scalp.

Burdock Root is a Super Cooler

Hot conditions calm down when burdock root is added to the diet as a cooked vegetable or taken as infusion or decoction. If you are laid back, lethargic, frequently feel chilled, and crave warm or hot foods, burdock is *not* the ally for you.

If you are ambitious, fiery, full of energy (sometimes to excess), occasionally aggressive, struggling with jealousy or rage, and known as "hot stuff," burdock can show you a thing or two about how to use all that energy to good advantage.

Cool off those with infections, excess nervous energy, rheumatic joints, gout, pulmonary catarrh, feverish colds, herpes pain, scalding urination, rage, and resentment, from the inside out, with Wise Woman ways and burdock root.

Soothing and cooling to all mucus surfaces, burdock root is a respiratory system ally frequently chosen by wise women around the world when healing themselves and others with chronic colds, smoker's cough, dry sore throat, emphysema, wheezing lung problems, deep, dry pulmonary congestion, pleurisy, and swollen respiratory membranes. Try frequent teaspoonfuls/15ml of burdock root syrup, or frequent sips of the infusion.

"Herbalists all over the world use Burdock. Such an effective and ultimate blood purifying plant has well earned its unpretending authentic value. . . . It [works] slowly but steadily." Alma Hutchens (1973)

Burdock Root is a Slick Trick in the Guts

The sticky fiber in burdock root energizes the peristaltic muscles as it soothes and nourishes the mucus surfaces of the intestines. This mucilaginous fiber also absorbs chemical residues, metabolic breakdown by-products, and metal contaminants, then binds them and escorts them rapidly through the large intestine. Burdock root can neutralize and elimininate poisins and toxins in the digestive tract.

Try the fresh infusion or tincture of burdock when fasting to help maintain intestinal peristalsis, and prevent ketosis and acidic overload in the blood.

Try fresh burdock root as a cooked vegetable once a week or more; or the fresh root tincture, 20-30 drops, in water up to four times daily. Least effective for those with intestinal problems, but still helpful, is the infusion of dried burdock root.

Intestinal flora respond to fresh burdock root preparations quite favorably; try burdock, along with your other Wise Woman ways, for helping those with candida/yeast overgrowth, chronic stomach aches, colitis, and colon cancer.

"Burdock is like a cleaning woman or a garbage collector: essential to modern life, but underpaid and undervalued. She's the old black rag-a-muffin of herbs." Ellen Greenlaw (1988)

Burdock Root is a Guardian of Inner Flows

Burdock energizes and organizes the lymphatic and immune systems, encourages the kidneys, sweet-talks the liver, turns on the flood gates of sweat when fever rises, and helps the uterus and the wise woman to move with truth and strength in the flow of birthing.

Burdock's old reputation for being "blood cleansing" is more accurately described as "immune strengthening." I used to envision little street-sweeping machines moving through my blood vessels gobbling up debris. But blood cleansing is actually done by the kidneys and the liver and the immune system. By nourishing and strengthening these systems, burdock does seem to clean the blood. Note that other blood-cleansing herbs stimulate these systems. While stimulation shows fast results, it does not promote health/wholeness/holiness in the Wise Woman way.

Burdock is slow, and steady, and ready to nourish you deeply as you transform and heal.

Try infusion or fresh root tincture when healing yourself or helping others with slow-growing cancers, herpes infections, chronic venereal infections, diabetes, and rheumatism.

Burdock seed is known as "the unfailing kidney ally," but the fresh root, infused, tinctured, or steeped overnight in wine, also soothes, nourishes, and prompts the kidneys. Try it, with other Wise Woman ways, when helping those with gravel, dropsy, bladder irritation, back pain from kidney distress, nephritis, edema, and hypertension from water retention.

In the liver, burdock root promotes secretions, nourishes and tonifies, moderates sugar swings, and tickles gall stones loose. Long-term use of burdock root, a dropperful of tincture three times a day, or a cup of infusion daily, used with Wise Woman wisdom, stabilizes blood sugar levels in hypoglycemics and helps moderate them in diabetics.

Try burdock root also when helping those with headaches centered in the forehead and top of the head (this area corresponds to the liver), and frightening premenstrual rages (also associated with the liver). And don't forget how much burdock and dandelion like to work together on these tough cases.

To use burdock as your ally when helping those with fevers, including childhood fevers, nervous fevers, jealous fevers, vengeful fevers, fevered imaginings, and fevers of eruptive diseases, pertussis (whooping cough), tonsillitis, and the flu, brew up several fresh roots in a quart/liter of boiling water. Add ten dropperfuls of echinacea tincture. Store in a tightly-lidded jar and sip every ten minutes or so, reheating as needed, until an easy sweat is achieved. Keep well wrapped up while sweating; sleep afterwards.

Native women in the Cherokee and Meskwaki nations, and probably many others who did not reveal their knowledge to white writers, used burdock root to strengthen their wombs before and after birth, to give themselves, as well as their wombs, stamina in birth, and to nourish (even during the birth) their ability to be stable, yet still flexible and available to the enormous flow of birthing energy.

In England, midwives help women heal acute uterine prolapse with frequent small sips of a brew made by soaking fresh burdock roots overnight in wine or hot water.

". . . without irritating or nauseating properties. It [burdock] will slowly influence the skin, soothe the kidneys, and relieve the lymphatics."

Henrietta Rau (1968)

Burdock Seed Properties and Uses

- ***diuretic,*** alterative, tonic
- ***vulnerary,*** demulcent, relaxant

Powerful **kidney** action is initiated by burdock seed remedies; take care not to overdo it. All parts of burdock have a beneficial influence on the **skin** and **hair**, and burdock seed is no exception. Easier to collect than the roots, burdock seeds often provide the novice wise woman with her first means of meeting the great green ally burdock.

Use burdock seeds as a loving friend to your urinary system and as a smooth touch.

- Dose of *burdock seed tincture* is 20-160 drops a day, in water.
- Dose of *burdock seed infusion* is ½-3 cups/125-750ml a day.

Burdock Seeds are a Loving Friend to Your Urinary System

Burdock seeds are cherished the world 'round for their unfailing ability to strengthen and encourage kidney action. The diuretic action of one cup of the cold infusion is prompt and remarkable.

Use burdock seeds as part of your Wise Woman nourishment when helping yourself or others heal chronic urinary and kidney problems, including dropsy, cystitis, and an irritated or weak bladder. Try sipping a cup of cold infusion throughout the day or take it all at once. Or drink a cup of any liquid with a dropperful (25-30 drops) of burdock seed tincture.

Burdock seeds not only increase urine flow, but also reduce urinary tract inflammation, soothe bladder, kidney, and urethral irritation, relieve scalding and burning urination, and help remove mucus and infection from the entire urinary system.

Those troubled with water retention during the latter part of pregnancy, whether simple or associated with kidney stress or pre-eclampsia, can be helped with Wise Woman ways and burdock seed infusion or tincture.

Take care: the "get 'em going" approach of burdock is not helpful in the early stages of pregnancy. Though by no means an abortifacient, fresh burdock used in sufficiently large amounts will initiate menstruation; therefore any burdock usage in the first trimester of pregnancy is contraindicated for women with a herstory of miscarriage.

Burdock Seeds Are a Smooth Touch

Burdock loves impeccably smooth skin and lustrous, thick hair. What a powerful ally to have when you want to create them, or prevent them from fading with advancing age.

The hot infusion, made by grinding 35-40 seeds and steeping in a cup of boiling water until cool enough to drink, is taken by the half cupful/125ml, up to six times a day. In addition to using this for everyday beauty, try it to break a fever, cool off a steaming system, and help prevent skin damage in those with extensive burns, acne, eczema, and eruptive diseases such as chicken pox, measles, scarletina, and typhoid.

Burdock seed tincture (20-40 drops, taken up to four times a day) is more convenient than infusion, and just as effective, when helping yourself or others heal chronic skin and joint problems. Burdock seed tincture, often in conjunction with burdock leaf poultices, is a Wise Woman favorite in many parts of the world for helping those with inflamed joints and extremities (gout). By increasing the urinary output of uric acid, burdock seed also helps prevent bouts of gout.

Those with chronic lung problems, especially due to smoking or chemical exposure, or with a nervous cough, also report benefit from daily alliance with burdock seeds.

Burdock seed oil (*Repeinoe Maslo* in Russian) is used daily as a strengthening, nourishing tonic to the hair follicles. If your hair is thinning from stress, try this: rub a cupped palmful of oil into your scalp (not hair), cover with a hot, wet towel for at least an hour, then shampoo. Repeat once a week as needed. Those with hair loss and thinning due to lack of optimum nourishment are well advised to include internal use of burdock, any part, in addition to rubbing their heads.

A facial steam from burdock seed infusion helps clear blackheads and whiteheads from the face and back.

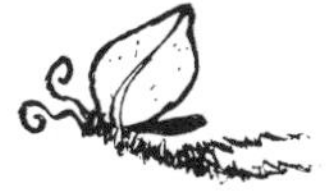

"Burdock leaves are so rank that man, the jackass, and caterpillars are the only animals that will eat of them." C. Millspaugh (1892)

Fresh Burdock Leaf Properties and Uses

- ***vulnerary,*** discutient, keratolytic
- ***tonic,*** cholagogue, diuretic, depurative

Use burdock leaf as a knuckle-buster fixer, and a cooler, you bet.

- Dose of *fresh burdock leaf tincture* is 10-100 drops a day, in water.
- Dose of *fresh burdock leaf tea* is ½-4 cups/125-1000ml a day.

Burdock Leaves Are a Knuckle-Buster Fixer

Fresh burdock leaves fix busted knuckles and virtually every other knock, abrasion, eruption, or mishap your exterior covering will encounter. This tough fighter is knowledgeable in the ways of healing wounds, not making them.

Try a hot, fresh burdock leaf poultice to relieve, repair, and resolve your inflamed wounds, sprains, swelling from broken bones, bruises, leg ulcers, bed sores, joint aches, boils, cysts, mastitis, eye irritations, conjunctivitis, and sties.

Fresh bruised burdock leaves, applied frequently, help soothe and heal your hot and irritated skin when troubled by poison ivy, poison oak, heat rash, prickly heat, scalds, burns, and ulcers. An old wives' cure for those with extensive burns includes dressing the burn with fresh raw milk and covering it with burdock leaves, in addition to other Wise Woman ways of encouraging health/wholeness/holiness.

Try a burdock vinegar poultice (see **Burdock Pharmacy**) when helping yourself or others with scabies, ringworm, painful joints, backaches, varicose veins, and swollen legs.

"Prosopium *in Greek means masked, and in Latin* personata *means one who is masked. . . . Further research disclosed the fascinating information that the large heart-shaped leaves of the humble, now ignored burdock were once used as masks in ancient Greek drama to cover the faces of actors when they performed!"* Maida Silverman (1977)

Burdock Leaves Are a Cooler, You Bet

Internally, burdock leaf tea, made by steeping fresh leaves for several hours, cools the inner works and increases your ability to deal with elevated temperatures, burning issues, hot situations, and all manner of irritations.

The intensely bitter leaf tea, taken hot and seasoned with tamari, strongly affects the sebaceous (oil) glands and sudoriferous (sweat) glands of the skin and scalp, encourages perspiration, relieves irritated liver disorders, brings on the menstrual flow, eases pounding headaches, and soothes burning stomach pain.

The same brew is used with Wise Woman wiles to help those clearing the lingering cough of pertussis, any dry hard cough, and coughs associated with smoking.

When you're hot under the collar and pissed off, try a dropperful of fresh burdock leaf tincture. And chill out.

Burdock Pharmacy

Burdock Vinegar Poultice

Roll up some big green burdock leaves. Soak them overnight or longer in apple cider vinegar. Use them as poultices to ease pain anywhere, but especially in the joints. Heat the vinegar-soaked leaves, as warm as can be tolerated, before applying them to sore areas. Try heating them in the oven, out in the sun, by steam, or in boiling water. The vinegared leaves may be returned to the vinegar and reused if no infection is present.

Parsnips Love Burdock

a bio-dynamic fertilizer

3 pounds/1.5 kilo manure*
3 gallons/12 liters water
½ pound/240g fresh nettle
1 lb/475g burdock leaves
2 ounces/60g dry kelp

*goat, rabbit, or horse

Combine all ingredients in a tightly covered container (a tofu bucket or compound container is ideal). Let sit six weeks. Sprinkle wood ashes around your parsnips and then water with this brew, diluted at least by half. This bio-dynamic combination grows fat, sweet parsnips.

Burdock Kitchen

Collect burdock **seeds** in the fall. Soak them overnight, drain, and sprout like radish or alfalfa seeds for a fresh bitter bite in winter salads.

Collect burdock **leaves** that are as small as your hand, preferably from first-year plants. Parboil as below; no need to soak. Serve with vinegar to cut the bitterness, or try in place of dandelion in any of the dandelion greens recipes. Italians, Scandinavians, and French enjoy the bitter taste so much they put young leaves in salads and soups. Larger leaves take the place of aluminum foil when cooking fish, game, potatoes, and so on in campfire coals.

The long **leaf stalks/petioles,** best picked when a handspan or less in length, are good in "Chicken Fried Burdock." Rub "wool" off and cut into small pieces before parboiling as below. Add cooked petiole pieces to omelets, quiches, and casseroles.

Use first-year burdock **roots** only, or roots collected very early in spring of the second year. If peel is tough, remove it, though it is not bitter and can be eaten. The taste of fresh burdock root is sweet, the texture, a little sticky. Soak and parboil as below. If very young, burdock roots can be grated into salad or cooked in "The Fast Root" without parboiling. Dried burdock root can be added to beans, rice, soups or stews. Burdock root mixed in equal amounts with dandelion root and sprouted grain, all dark-roasted and ground, makes a popular coffee substitute.

Collect burdock **flower stalks** as they emerge, while leaves are still unfolding and well before the green burrs are visible. Take care to peel all the bitter skin off. Basically, just the pith is sweet enough to eat. Eat raw, with salt, or soak and parboil, as follows. Taste/texture resembles broccoli.

To Soak and Parboil Burdock

a preliminary step in many of the following recipes

After harvesting and cleaning, cut roots or stalks into pieces and soak in water with a splash of vinegar added. A fifteen minute bath prevents discoloration, speeds cooking, and helps the burdock retain a crisp succulence even after cooking.

Meanwhile, boil a quantity of water. Put soaked burdock roots or stalks, or fresh, very young leaves, into half the boiling water and cook for 10-20 minutes. Drain. Then cook in the other half of the boiling water until tender (10-30 minutes). Drain. Serve as is, or try the following recipes. Extras store at cool temperatures for up to a week.

As your taste for wild foods grows, you'll find yourself dispensing with the water change, which does leach out minerals and vitamins as well as bitterness. When you need extra optimum nourishment for extensive transformation, you'll even find yourself drinking the cooking water.

Burdock 'n' Brown Rice

serves 4-6

1 burdock root 4 cups/1 liter water 2 cups/500ml brown rice pinch salt	Clean burdock root; cut into 6-8 pieces and soak. Bring water to a boil in tightly covered pan. Add rice, salt, and burdock. Return to boil with lid on, reduce heat; cook without peeking (!) for 40-45 minutes.

Preparation time: One hour. A traditional macrobiotic food/medicine to increase yang and metal energies, this dish is exceptionally strengthening to the intestines, prostate, ovaries, and uterus.

"Chicken Fried" Burdock Stalks

serves 4

2 cups/250ml burdock stalk 2 tablespoons/30ml tamari 1 egg 4 oz/125ml nutritional yeast 4 tablespoons/60ml olive oil	Soak cooked burdock stalk (or root) in tamari while you beat egg, put nutritional yeast in a plate, and begin to heat the oil. Put large spoonfuls of tamaried burdock into egg, then into yeast, then into hot oil. Turn once. Cook until brown. Serve with vinegar and salt as table seasonings.

Preparation time: 90 minutes: an hour to harvest, peel, and cook burdock stalk; 30 minutes to coat and fry it. Youngsters love to help harvest burdock petioles to prepare this way. Tofu can be "chicken fried," too. Serve with a huge wild green salad.

Japanese Sweet & Sour Gobo

serves 4

4-5 burdock roots
2 tablespoons/30ml tamari
2 tablespoons/30ml honey
2 tablespoons/30ml vinegar
4 oz/125ml water
2 Tbs/30ml sesame seeds

Cut burdock roots into very thin diagonal slices. Soak and parboil. Add tamari, honey, vinegar, and warm water to burdock root. Simmer 5-10 more minutes. Add more water if needed. Put in serving dish with liquid; garnish with sesame.

Preparation time: Only 15 minutes once you've dug and cooked the roots, which can take the better part of a day. Those who live near oriental markets can buy gobo (burdock root). In that case, soaking, parboiling, and cooking take only an hour.

The Fast Root

serves 4

1 tablespoon/15ml olive oil
1 burdock root*, grated
2 carrots, grated
1 parsnip, grated
1 Tbs/15ml dark sesame oil
1 teaspoon/5ml tamari
handful water

*or salsify, sunchoke, wild carrot root, turnip, or cattail roots.

Heat oil. Add shredded or grated roots. (Soak burdock in vinegar water before grating; do not parboil.) Sauté while stirring for five minutes or so. Then toss in water, tamari, and sesame oil. Cover well and cook until tender, roughly ten minutes more.

Preparation time: 30 minutes. Grating or shredding fresh roots before cooking increases their already abundant energy. This food/medicine gives optimum nutrition for great strength, staying power, rooted energy, and creativity.

". . . and the governor told me that its tender shoots are eaten in spring as radishes, after the exterior part is taken off." Peter Kalm, Swedish naturalist, recalling a visit to Ticonderoga, NY (1772)

Herbed Burdock

serves 6-8

4 cups/1 liter burdock root
3 tablespoons/45ml olive oil
3 tablespoons/45ml butter
4 oz/125ml fresh herbs
2 cloves garlic
2 Tbs/30ml lemon juice
2 tablespoons/30ml tamari

Soak and parboil burdock root or stalk. If you use chilled, already cooked burdock, warm it. Heat oil and butter. Add burdock, then minced garlic and herbs. Stir and heat together for a minute, then add tamari and lemon juice. Serve hot.

Preparation time: With precooked burdock, 15 minutes at the most. Add another 45 minutes to soak and cook burdock.

Burdock Stalk Marinade

serves 15-20

4 cups/1 liter burdock stalk
2 cups/500ml green beans
1 c/250ml mushroom slices
1 tsp/5ml dried thyme
1 tsp/5ml dried marjoram
1 tsp/5ml dried mint
1 cup/250ml olive oil
3 Tbs/45ml herb vinegar
6 Tbs/90ml tamari
½ tsp/3ml garlic powder
2 c/500ml cherry tomatoes
1 cup/250ml black olives
8 Tbs/125ml fresh chives
8 Tbs/125ml fresh parsley

Soak and parboil burdock stalk pieces. Cut beans in half and cook until tender. Mix mushroom slices and dried herbs in a large bowl or jar with warm beans and burdock. Combine oil, vinegar, tamari, and garlic powder. Mix well and pour on. Let marinate in a cool place all day or all night. Add cherry tomatoes, olives, and fresh herbs just before serving.

Preparation time: An hour to set it up to marinate, plus 10 minutes just before serving. Try this at your next lawn party or cook out!

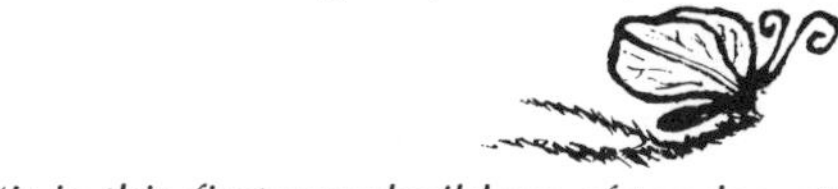

"It is this first year build up of tender, stored energy that we gustatory botanists want to cash in on. The first year plants are fine anytime after they obtain a good size in early summer, but I have had my best tasting burdock roots in the autumn and early winter." D. Eliot (1976)

Spring Tonic Soup

serves 13-15

2 c/500ml onion, chopped
4 tablespoons/60ml olive oil
2 c/500ml fresh burdock root
1 c/250ml fresh dandelion
1 c/250ml fresh yellow dock
4 ounces/125ml seaweed
2 c/500ml carrot, sliced
6 c/1500ml potatoes, cubed
4 quarts/4 liters water
salt

Cook onion in oil in soup pot until golden. Add soaked, but not parboiled burdock root slices. Chop fresh dandelion leaves and roots; add. Chop fresh leaves and roots of yellow dock (Rumex crispus) and add. Add all remaining ingredients. Bring to a boil; reduce heat and cook covered at least an hour.

Preparation time: Collect the necessary weeds while preparing garden soil. After that, it will take roughly 45 minutes to get everything into the pot, and an hour to cook.

Summer Flush Supper

serves 2

1 onion, chopped
2 cloves garlic, minced
2 tablespoons/30ml olive oil
1 c/250ml cooked grain
1 c/250ml burdock stalk
2 c/500ml diced tomato
4 oz/110g grated cheese

Sauté onion and garlic in oil in heavy skillet or casserole. Add cooked grain and heat through. Layer parboiled burdock stalk pieces, diced tomato, and lastly cheese on top of grain. Cover and cook on stove top, or cook in oven uncovered at 350 F/80 C, until cheese is melted.

Preparation time: 25-30 minutes. As the days get longer, supper comes later and later and I look for fast dishes to get us fed before we realize how late we've been out playing.

"This herb [burdock] is burnt between the time it flowers and seeds, in a hole in the ground and not allowing the flame to escape; three pounds of ashes produce about one pound of a fine white alkaline salt as good as the best potash."

T. Green (1850)

Burdock Fun and Facts

• Is it beurre-dock, a leaf used to wrap beurre/butter? It is.
Is it bourre-dock, a big woolly leaf? It is.

• *Cyclopedia of Horticulture,* a well-respected reference, actually recommends burdock as a fast-growing foliage mass to provide a visual barrier.

• By the time European settlers had the time to write down native uses of herbs, burdock was well established as an excellent herbal medicine among the Cherokee, Chippewa, Menominee, Meskwaki, Otos, Abenaki, Omaha, Ojibway, Iroquois, Nanticoot, Penobscot, Potawatomi, Mohican, and Delaware.

• A single burdock plant can bear 400,000 seeds, and of these, as many as 30,000 harbor and nourish insect larvae.

• Burdock was well known to Shakespeare and is mentioned in *Troilus and Cressida, King Lear,* and *As You Like It.*

• Thanks to Deborah Hoog, in *Nature's Uncultivated Garden,* for inspiring "The Fast Root" and "Burdock 'n' Brown Rice" recipes.

• Burdock root was official in the US Pharmacopia from 1831 to 1916 and in the National Formulary from 1916 to 1947.

• *The Herbalist*, one of the first herbal magazines I ever read, featured burdock in June 1978 in an article by U. Bentlov: "The Great Burdock."

• "Tumor growth inhibiting substances of plant origin," by S. Foldeak and G. Dombradi, in *Acta Physiology & Chemistry,* 10, 91-93, 1964, mentions burdock.

• *The Chemical Constituents of Oriental Herbs,* published by Oriental Healing Arts Institute in Los Angeles, California, has an extensive section on burdock.

• "The Biology of Canadian Weeds 38; Arctium minus & A. lappa," by R. Gross, et al., in the *Canadian Journal of Plant Science,* 60: 621-634, has good drawings and interesting information.

• Japanese research into burdock properties is frequently reported in various professional journals. For example, see "Two Polyacetylenic Phytoalexins from Arctium Lappa," in *Phytochemistry,* volume 26, number 11, pages 2957-8.

• According to *Medical Chemistry,* by C. M. Suter, 1951; John Wiley Pub., Arctium minus inhibits the growth of gram positive bacteria (such as staph and strep).

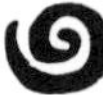

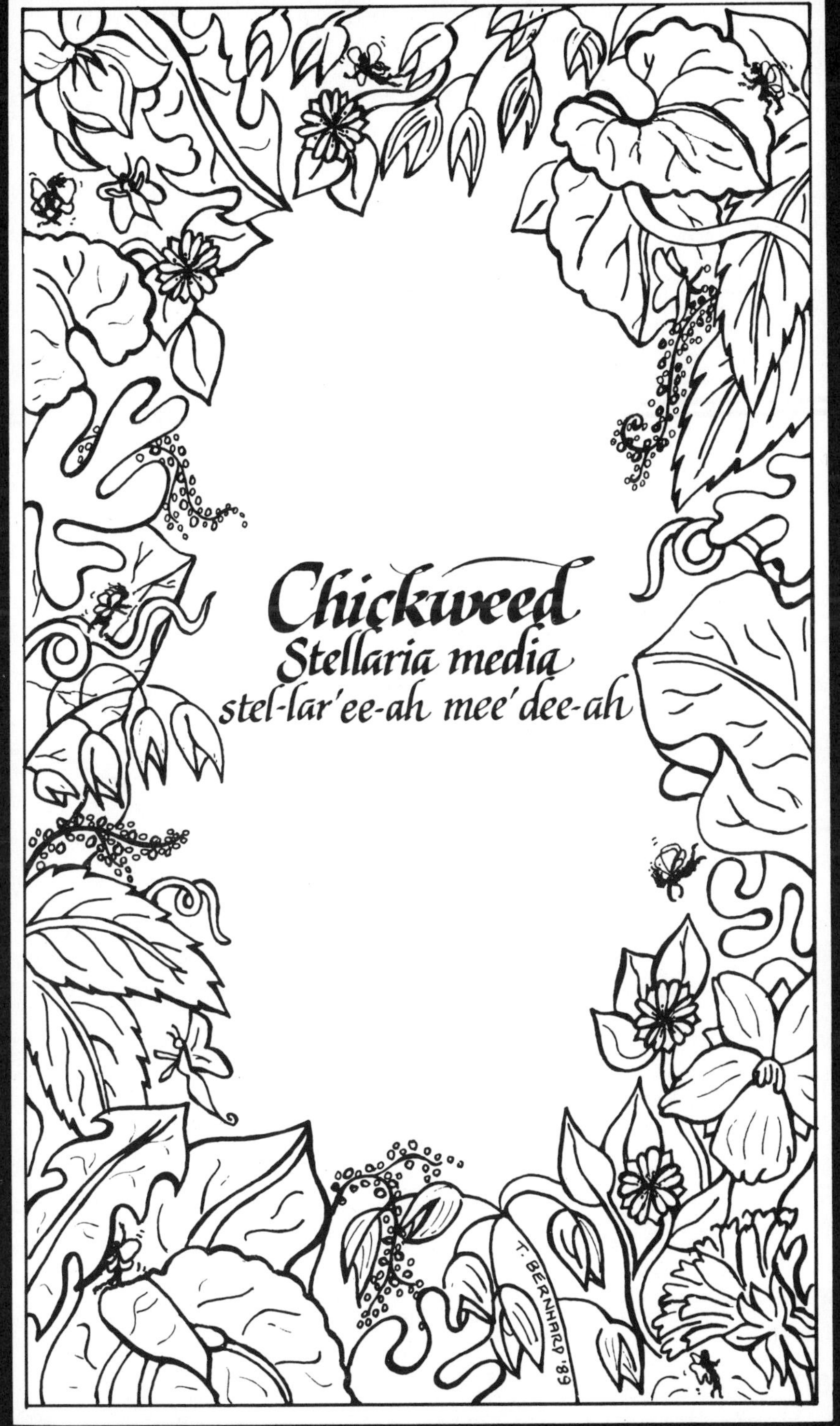
Chickweed
Stellaria media
stel-lar'ee-ah mee'dee-ah
T. BERNHARD '89

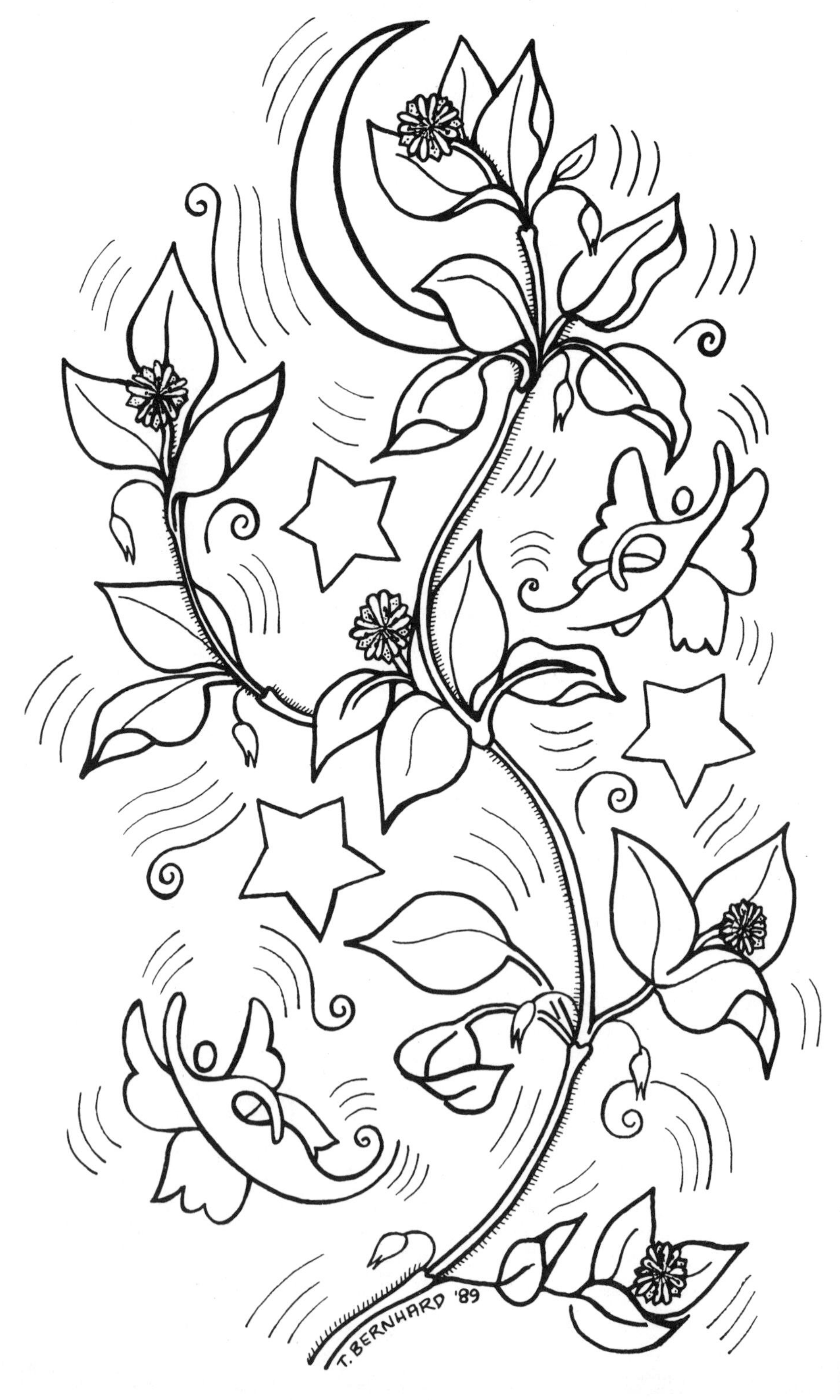
T. BERNHARD '89

Chickweed Speaks

Hi. Hi! Come play for a while. Come play with the fairies and me. Come play with the fireflies and me. Come play in the star fields with me.

I'm a cool chick, chickweed, indeed. No, no, not chicory. Call me stellaria, the little star lady, if you like, then you won't confuse me with that bold thing, chicory, so unladylike.

What do you want to play? Do you want to play moon and stars? Why so puzzled? Oh! You can hear me but you don't see me. *There's a laugh like the twinkling of the heavens.* Of course. You're used to looking in the sky for stars, aren't you? But I'm the little star lady of the fields. I spread my little stars at your feet.

Sit down here now, for a minute. We'll play moon and stars later, if you like. Can you see me now? Reach out and put your hand among the mosaics of my flowers, my mandala stars. Feel the energy of the stars in you. Let yourself become available to the energy of my stars, and through them, to all the stars in the cosmos.

Yes, become available to the energy of the cosmos. That's how we begin another game I love to play: leaky margins. *There's a chuckle like moon-struck icicles vibrating.* It's a game of becoming more than you know you are. It's a game of removing boundaries. When I play it with your cells, the cell membranes thin, your lungs release fluid, intestinal absorption increases, bacteria become highly vulnerable to white blood cells, and instant optimum nourishment is available to every cell that I contact, especially injured ones.

Leaky margins is a game I play a lot. Do you want to play? Do you want to experience for yourself the joy and perfection, the grief and chaos that stream through the universe? Any time you want to, I'll play with you. Just let me know.

How do I play leaky margins in your cells? Oh. I am a *lady*, you know. *There's a sigh like the sound of snowflakes sliding on pine needles.* The little star lady. And ladies do not tell certain things. The slippery, soaplike way I have of sliding into everything and sponging up the spills is really very private. The way I replace fat with protein and mineral salts is not for public discussion. Please!

Have you noticed how smooth I am? Smooth and cool? Smooth and cool and sleepy, some say. *There's a laugh like a ripple of ice sounding in the frozen lake.* Do notice my points. I am not altogether without an edge. I do have some sharp abilities.

I do not sleep in, as some suppose from seeing my flowers opening so late in the day. I stay in meditation, that's all, and so don't open my flowers 'til mid-morning. What of it? I'm not lazy. My inspiration is not the sun, if you want the truth. I am the little *star* lady, remember. Though the sun is a star, I admit, I find it a star too near, too fierce, too hot, too drying.

How I love the rainy days when I lie close to the earth and bend my flowers' ears to her song. I love the short days of winter. I love long twilights. I love the relieving shade. I love cool corners. *There's a murmur of shade settling softly into place.*

Yet one must pollinate. That's another thing we ladies don't speak about, so don't ask. If I didn't desire pollination, I wouldn't show my delicacy to the sun at all. But my life is short and I want to leave children, so I must set seeds, and pollination is needed for that. At least no sticky footed insects lap at me. And I do it wearing white lace. A lady can remain pure even in such circumstances, I believe.

Let us talk more of my sharpness. Look closely now at my tiny white petals and see how very like sharp knives they are. Each petal is slit almost in half, leaving a thin, sharp blade of white. And each parted petal is backed up by a green lance. My stars are points upon points of sharp light. *There's a whistle like the keen edge of a wing slicing the air.*

I am sharp like a needle, to repair your rips. I am sharp like a knife, to cut through your problems. See how skillfully I can sew together the traumatized flesh, the broken self, the torn weave of your being. See how I can cut away obstacles: infection, limitation, resistance, rigidity.

Do not fear to bring me into frightful and messy situations. There is this about ladies: though we don't like to admit our own juiciness (and I am *very* juicy), we don't mind mucking about in anybody else's fluids. I am quite inured to the horrors of war, accident, and disease.

I can be tender as well, it's true. See what tender care I take of my new leaves and flower buds? See how securely I protect them in the embrace of my leaves? I am so tender and careful with myself.

I may look weak and pale to some, inconspicuous and insignificant to others, but I assure you, I am worth the effort to get to know. For I grow everywhere and offer you abundant nourishment and prompt healing. And I do mean everywhere. We little star ladies get around. City or country, north or south, the little star lady is on the scene, ready to play.

Now, about our game of moon and stars . . .

Chickweed Facts

Botanical name: *Stellaria media*; stellaria (Latin) means little star; media (Latin) means "in the midst of." ***Other useful species:*** *S. pubera*; the unrelated look-alike, carpetweed/*Mollugo verticillata* is used similarly. ***Natural order:*** Caryophyllaceae/Carnation family. ***English names:*** Starweed, tongue grass, winterweed, satinflower, white bird's eye, adder's mouth, starwort, stitchwort, clucken wort, skirt buttons, chick wittles, chickenyweed. ***German names:*** Vogelmiere, Hühnerdarm, Augentrosgräs. ***French names:*** Stellaire, mouron des oiseaux. ***Maori names:*** Kohukohu. ***Food uses:*** Once hawked on the streets of London, chickweed is now only occasionally sold at all, and then, only dried. ***Medicinal uses:*** Most powerful fresh, chickweed does not lend herself to commerce and is rarely seen for sale as a medicine. ***Soil uses:*** Helps soils retain nitrogen; indicates fertile, mineral-rich soil. ***Animal uses:*** Esteemed food for caged songbirds, as well as barnyard fowl, homestead rabbits, and the kids' guinea pig; most ruminants eschew it, although lambs may overeat of it. ***Habitat:*** Cultivated land, rich, moist soil, open but cool environs. ***Natural range:*** The world. ***Current range:*** Wherever people disturb the soil: throughout temperate North America, Europe, Australia, Tasmania, New Zealand, southern and central Asia, even within the Artic Circle. ***Toxicity:*** *Externally,* chickweed has never been reported to cause reaction; her wind-blown pollen may contribute to hay fever. *Internally,* "Human cases of temporary paralysis have been reported from large amounts of the infusion, although there is no recent evidence to indicate that chickweed presents a toxic hazard." (D.G. Spoerke, 1980) ***Best identified by:*** Many very small starry white flowers, with five petals so deeply divided they appear to be ten petals; growing in low, dense, vibrant-green mats; single line of hairs on smooth stalk.

> *"This small herb, often classed as a troublesome weed, is one of the supreme healers of the herbal kingdom and has given me wonderful results."*
>
> Juliette Levy (1966)

Chickweed Weed Walk

Put on your warm coat, and boots, and your hat, and come out with me to pick some chickweed. Yes, it is the middle of January! No, I'm not crazy. The sky has cleared and we'll have some good foraging down where the river widens and seeps toward the sea.

I have the basket and some scissors. There's no dirt to wash off if we carefully cut an inch away from the ground, like giving the plants a haircut. Come on, already; you won't need gloves. It's warm out today.

I love chickweed. It's my favorite salad green. And not just because I can harvest it fresh all winter long. The taste is exceptional: clean, bright green without a trace of bitterness, but just a little salty. Umm!

Umm . . . smell the fresh sea air. There's our supper. Ready to be cut. Snip, snip. We'll be like the hairdresser for the little star lady. Our haircut will encourage the chickweed to branch many times and provide that many more tender shoots for our next cutting.

And our cutting keeps the leaves large. Well, large for chickweed. I see your point, but, look, some of these are nearly as big as your thumbnail. In a harsher habitat, the leaves don't get any bigger than your tiny toenail.

But large or small, all the leaves are an even, bright, clear green, absolutely smooth, and growing in opposed pairs. See how the leaf stalks get longer and longer as they get farther and farther from the growing tip?

Old chickweed is mostly stalk and not as edible as the tender leafy parts. Snip the growing leafy tops off, like this. And leave behind the soiled, stalky stuff. Lay it in the basket in a neat bundle, with all the stalks parallel. That makes it easier to chop for salad when we get back to the kitchen. No fuss, no mess, no dirt, no tedious washing.

Look at this line of hairs that runs up the stem. Just one tiny line of hairs on an otherwise totally smooth plant. That's not a second line of hairs; this one merely jumped to the other side there at the leaf node. It goes around to each of the four directions, as in a prayer to the four elements: fire, water, earth, and air.

You almost need a magnifying glass to see the hairs, unless you hold the stem to catch the light, just so, making the hairs visible.

Take another look at the stem. See how it barely rises from the ground? Not that it exactly creeps or lies on the ground, but chickweed can be said to grow out instead of up. There are so many branches to the stalk, and more here than usual, since my cutting increases the branching, that a single plant seems to grow like a super-nova, radiating out and up.

Pick one and feel the slightly swollen joints. Crush it, and note the juiciness. This is such a great plant to use as a poultice. Nothing like it for juicing things up and cooling off heat at the same time!

An inconspicuous plant, say most writers: smooth, green, small, low, no strong taste, and not very active medicinally. Inconspicuous, if you mean easily overlooked. Many a lawn owner is totally unaware of chickweed at play in the grass. What a feast of food and fun and fantasy they could have if the lawn mower didn't work.

Few town dwellers notice it either, though I've never been in a city yet, except in the tropics, that wasn't graced with chickweed. I was picking and eating chickweed off a curbside in West Berlin just a few months ago, much to the dismay of my German companions. At first, that is. A few salads later, they wanted to help me gather some more!

Most gardeners notice it. Small stature seems only to encourage our little star lady to a glorious abandon of abundance in vegetable or flower bed, thus bringing many an unladylike gardener's curse to the little star lady's ears. As any annual does, chickweed focuses her energy on producing as many viable seeds as possible.

Here's a seed capsule. Not much more visible than the rest of the plant. Maybe that's why wise women love the little star lady so: she's as invisible as they are.

The seeds in here will ripen even if you cut the plant or uproot it. If I pick a lot of chickweed and leave it in the refrigerator (it's one wild green that keeps well), within a few days the bottom of my storage bag is covered in a layer of tiny yellow-orange seeds that have ripened and fallen loose.

With your magnifying lens you'll see the teeth on the seed capsule. When the seed capsule gets wet, these teeth swell, and keep the capsule tightly shut. When the sun and wind dry the capsule, the teeth loosen and allow the wind to shake the seeds free.

These patches of chickweed seem almost perennial, they self-sow so readily and constantly. But we don't curse the chickweed; we bless it, and accept its blessing of abundant green.

Few patches of chickweed can outproduce my appetite for it! Last year I served chickweed salad to thirty women on spring equinox from this very patch. When I don't have that much help, I can eat quarts of chickweed a day all by myself.

Sometimes the chickweed is already flowering by spring equinox. Wouldn't you be surprised if this plain little plant had flashy flowers? Don't worry, it doesn't. Unless you use a magnifying lens.

Magnified, the pattern of delicate deeply-divided petals, each set off by a pointed green sepal, becomes a whirling mandala, a glittering star. The symmetry of the flower vibrates and the five white, cleft petals become ten slivers of light in your eye. The sepals' five-pointed under-star of shimmering green adds to the effect.

There you are peering through a magnifying glass at a tiny flower, and suddenly you're having an experience of cosmic proportions. That's the little star lady for you!

This patch of chickweed is out in the sun, so it dies early, as soon as the days lengthen and the heat builds. But there's a patch back at the house, under the roses. That patch doesn't give many greens in winter, but it stays so shady and moist that stars bloom there almost all year.

The little star lady prefers cool, rich, moist soil. Along misty coasts, deep in mountain valleys, and even in cities, she has no shortage of likely habitats.

She thrives here, along my quiet strand, though not as lushly as I once saw her growing.

I was in northern California, along the coast. The wind was fierce, so my walk that day wasn't far. Just far enough to find a little stream that ran down to the sea, spreading herself out and out as she came, and smoothing the way for acres of nearly knee-high chickweed (with a healthy bit of miner's lettuce mixed in to add to the bounty).

I would have lain down on the ground and eaten my way to bliss, but it was too wet. With my outer shirt as a makeshift carrying basket, and my ever-handy pocket knife, I cut enough to feast on for days to come, and plenty for sharing the earth's bountiful gifts with my chickweed-loving friends, too.

And why don't we do the same? Though we have a proper basket and won't have to undress to hold onto our chickweed! The days are short. Let's cut our salad and go have a cup of hot cider by the wood stove.

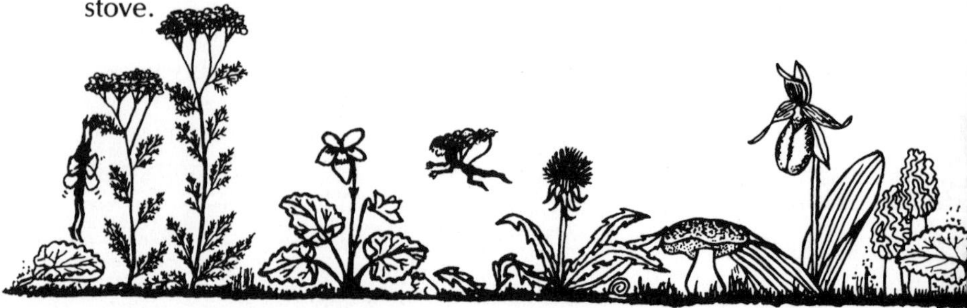

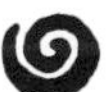

Chickweed Herb Properties and Uses

- **nutritive**, restorative, antiscorbutic, male tonic
- **cooling**, anti-pyretic, absorbent, alterative, refrigerant, carminative
- **demulcent**, emollient, vulnerary, pectoral

Chickweed is readily available and delicious **optimum nutrition.** Her ability to cool off those with fevers and infections is unsurpassed. In addition, chickweed contains **steroidal saponins**.

Saponins are soap-like; they emulsify and increase the permeability of all membranes. By creating permeability chickweed encourages the shifting of boundaries at all levels, from cellular to cosmic. Chickweed saponins increase the absorption of nutrients, especially minerals, from the digestive mucosa. Her saponins also gently **dissolve** thickened lung and throat membranes, emulsify and thus **neutralize toxins**, and weaken bacterial cell walls, making them vulnerable to disruption of their activities.

Fresh chickweed juice is so rich in saponins that it is used to **dissolve warts** and other growths. Chickweed tincture, taken faithfully for extended periods, **dissolves cysts**, especially ovarian ones.

Think of chickweed as increasing your permeability to solar, lunar, universal, and cosmic energies. What incredible nourishment awaits you.

Use chickweed, the whole fresh herb before or during flowering, as a nourishing, strengthening food, a cool helper when the situation is hot, a nourishing healer of wounds, an eye opener, an herbal diet pill, and a joint oiler.

- Dose of *fresh chickweed tincture* is 20-90 drops a day, in water.
- Dose of *dried chickweed infusion* is 2-4 cups/500-1000ml a day.

"The elixir of life. . . ." Paracelsus (1530)

Chickweed is a Nourishing Strengthening Food

(Numbers indicate milligrams per hundred grams chickweed herb)

Chickweed is bio-available optimum nutrition replete with minerals, proteins, carotenes, and vital life energy. Chickweed, the little star lady, thins the cellular membranes so nutrients are absorbed and utilized to their maximum.

Convalescents, weak children, anyone recovering from surgery or trauma will thrive on frequent salads of chickweed. Those in debilitated conditions, anemic, malnourished, with rickets or scurvy, gain strength quickly when allowed to eat freely of chickweed. A deep, rich sense of well-being and starbursts of spontaneous ecstasy arise from continued alliance with the lovely little star lady.

Chickweed is very high in aluminum (196), copper, iron (253), magnesium (529), manganese (15.3), silicon (15.7), and zinc (5.2).

She is high in calcium (1210), chlorophyll, cobalt (12.1), phosphorus (448), potassium (1840), protein (15-24%), carotenes, expressed as vitamin A (7229-32,500 IU), and fat (5).

She is a good source of vitamin C complex, expressed as ascorbic acid (375), chromium, molybdenum, riboflavin (0.14), niacin (0.51), thiamine (0.02), fiber, and naturally diuretic and heart-helping plant sodium. (More about sodium and the heart can be found in **Seaweed/ Ally with Lots of Heart**.)

The little star lady chickweed is a powerful nourisher to the glandular and lymphatic systems. Poultices externally, as needed, and twice daily doses of 40 drops fresh tincture are used with other Wise Woman ways for those with thyroid irregularities, reproductive cysts, swollen glands, ovarian cancers, and testicular troubles such as cancers, swelling, burning, or itching. Even persistent ovarian cysts dissolve with continual use of chickweed, though it may take up to a year.

Chickweed is a Cool Helper When the Situation is Hot

Those with fevers, infections, inflammations, all sorts of "hot" diseases are relieved, tempered, and chilled by the little star lady, chickweed. The way she retreats and vanishes in the sun's glare clearly indicates her ability to bring the crystal cool of evening stars to aid us.

Lungs love her moistening expectorant qualities. Lung infections respond promptly to her ability to dissolve bacteria membranes and nourish bronchial tissue. Try chickweed as your ally along with your other Wise Woman nourishments when healing yourself or others troubled with any heated chest congestion such as croup, asthma, smoker's cough, bronchitis, whooping cough, pleurisy, chest colds, flu, sore throat, lungs that are weak, bleeding, or inflamed, pneumonia, emphysema, pollen reactions, allergies, or tuberculosis. Drink chickweed broth daily or use tincture consistently for three or more months.

Bladders and kidneys relax at her cool touch. Include daily use of chickweed with your other Wise Woman ways when healing yourself or others bothered by chronic bladder infections/cystitis, bladder or kidney weakness, and low back pain from urinary system distress. Chickweed soothes and eases bladder discomfort in new mothers and those recovering from abdominal surgery, as well.

Livers become calm and the temper is soothed when the little star lady has her happy way. Chickweed, used freely, is reputed to restore superb hepatic circulation and revitalize the hepatic veins.

It is said that even the blood itself refuses to grow hot if chickweed is eaten or drunk in quantity! Some systems of health care maintain that hot blood is acidic, and associate acidic blood with chronic conditions. Alkalinizers neutralize the acidity. Whether through alkalinizing, cooling, or some mysterious means of her own, chickweed, as part of the daily diet, definitely helps change tendencies, habitual or hereditary, toward cancer, diabetes, and arthritis.

Those with digestive system problems crave plates of chickweed salad, for mineral-rich bulk and soothing, cooling energies to nourish their weak stomachs and bowels. Chickweed eases and helps those with yeast overgrowth, constipation, hard stools, hemorrhoids, stomach ulcers, intestinal ulcers, colitis, internal inflammation, stomach cancer, and those healing after treatment for appendicitis, peritonitis, or the like.

Those with hot, sore throats, dry coughs, or hoarseness enjoy frequent sips of chickweed tincture, 40-50 drops diluted in a glass of water.

"It grows all over the world and is so hardy that green leaves, and even flowers, may be seen underneath the snow." E. E. Pfeiffer (1951)

Chickweed is usually eaten by the handful, chopped and raw in salad, once or twice a day, throughout the growing season (though I often eat four or five times that much for weeks on end). Use of the tincture, 20-30 drops at a time, up to three times a day can be continued for years if desired. The infusion is the least effective form; try at least half a liter/two cups daily for six or more weeks.

Chickweed is a Nourishing Healer of Wounds

Chickweed, used as a fresh poultice, draws out infection; she has rich accepting resonance and energy. Chickweed heals all wounds; she has deep mending skills and wisdom.

Internal wounds, external wounds, visible wounds, invisible wounds: with chickweed, all are relieved of irritation, cleared of infection, and protected from further damage. In addition, chickweed nourishes rapid and thorough restructuring of damaged tissue by providing bio-available vitamin complexes, most notably A and C, and accessible mineral richness directly to the cell. Chickweed weakens, dissolves, and consumes bacteria.

Fresh chickweed poultices rapidly draw out splinters, venom, and infection, while reducing inflammation and swelling. Chickweed's remarkable extracting powers enable her to absorb and safely eliminate large quantities of unneeded materials from skin cells and all soft tissue.

Let the little star lady bring her cool hands in a poultice to ease and heal those with ulcers, erysipelas, splinters, pimples, boils, abscesses, infected cuts, blood poisoning, stubborn rashes and sores, cancerous testes, and gall bladder pain. She's good with trauma, too.

Chickweed oil or salve is more convenient than a poultice, and nearly as effective for helping to heal those with minor injuries, mosquito bites, rashes, chickenpox, measles, itches, sore spots, cold sores, fever blisters, herpes sores, mouth sores, hot spots, diaper rash, genital itches, bruises, hives, weals, scabs, blisters.

Baths and soaks of chickweed infusion are the easiest application if the irritated, erupted, inflamed area is extensive. Soak or bathe at least twice a day, and cover with ointment or oil overnight.

Think of chickweed as being as soft as slippery elm, as soothing as marshmallow, and as protective and strengthening as comfrey root. Turkish gypsies praise it lavishly.

"I have seen the fresh leaves [of chickweed] bruised and applied as a poultice to indolent, intractable ulcers on the leg, of many years' standing, with the most decided and immediately beneficial results; to be changed, two or three times a day." HW Felter, MD & JU Lloyd (1898)

Chickweed is an Eye Opener

The little star lady chickweed is used as a poultice to heal those with infected, injured eyes, often within a few days. She is a staunch ally to help those with eye infections, conjunctivitis, pinkeye, sties, ulcerated eyelids, ophthalmia (several clinical reports), inflamed eyes, and eyes sore and irritated from contact lenses.

After removing contact lenses, refresh eyes with chickweed lotion or a chickweed poultice. Helps clear the eyes and prevent squint lines.

Deborah writes: "When my little boy had his first experience with pinkeye I tried everything to help him, finally resorting to a medication prescribed by my doctor. Nothing helped his red, itchy, crusty-oozy eyes. And the prescription drops made him scream in pain. In the midst of this, I came upon a bountiful patch of chickweed glowing lush and green. And it was December! I picked some, went home, and made a poultice, which I applied directly to my son's closed eyes. He loved it! He laid his head on my lap as the chickweed gently embraced him with her healing strength. After only one poultice all the redness was gone. After two more (later that day and the next morning), the infection was completely cleared. No more calls in the middle of the night when he woke in panic with his eyes stuck together. Now, when his eyes get red and itchy, he's the one who finds the chickweed."

Chickweed is an Herbal Diet Pill

"Chickweed water is an old wives' remedy for obesity," says Maude Grieves. Since I trust old wives deeply, I asked the little star lady for more information about her alleged ability to remove excess fat cells from the body.

I've always assumed that the dried chickweed found in herbal weight-loss formulas was little more than a mild, mineral-rich diuretic. Not worth much, in other words, since weight lost through water loss is easily regained.

But chickweed reminded me of her soapy saponins, and that soap dissolves fat. I also know from experience that chickweed is a superb metabolic balancer and her regulatory effect on the thyroid seems to help women whose weight grows no matter what.

"I do take excess moisture from cells, sparing the kidneys," she reprimanded, "and spread my soothing cool touch to the urinary tract. But I do far more. I nourish the moistness of each cell and loosen the membrane so the cell relaxes. Then I grab the extra fat and run." She giggled, and high chimes sounded at the edges of my hearing. "It's not just fat I take with me when I leave, but any kind of excess baggage. And that's weight loss where it counts!"

Chickweed is a Joint Oiler

Those experiencing burning, hot, searing pain from arthtitis, rheumatism, stiff neck, sore back, sore legs, gout, backache, and bursitis find relief, often in a few hours, with hot chickweed baths, soaks, and poultices.

Those with chronic rheumatic pain can use Wise Woman ways and 20-30 drops of the fresh plant tincture (taken in water several times a day for several months) to restore joint mobility and ease pain.

To heal, stretch, and restore elasticity and strength to your tendons and ligaments, eat chickweed freely, and treat with poultices or hot chickweed oil packs.

Chickweed Pharmacy

Chickweed Poultice

- Apply the fresh herb, washed, directly onto sores, closed eyes, wounds.

or

- Cook the greens and stalks, especially when using older plants or treating deeply; cool somewhat before applying.

or

- Simmer chickweed in half water, half vinegar for about five minutes, cool and apply.

Then

Cover chickweed with a cotton towel or a thin layer of clay, and poultice for five minutes to three hours. Replace when poultice feels hot to the touch and oozes. (Yes, hot! Though most poultices are applied warm and removed when they cool, chickweed poultices actually heat up as they draw out infection and heat.)

Relief often begins within a few hours of the initial application, with pain and swelling diminishing steadily as treatments continue.

Poultices used on infections, such as pinkeye, must be thrown away after use. Poultices used on clean wounds and unbroken skin can be reused several times if chickweed is in short supply.

Chickweed Eye Lotion

4 oz/125ml distilled water 4 oz/125ml witch hazel 1 Tbs/15ml chickwd tincture	Combine all ingredients in a clean plastic dispenser-top bottle. Use prepared witch hazel from drugstore. Shake well.

To use: Wet a cloth or cotton ball with lotion and apply to closed eyes for 3 minutes. Discontinue if eyes are sensitive.

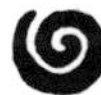

Chickweed Kitchen

Cooked Chickweed Greens

Don't do it! Ignore all recipes or suggestions to cook chickweed. It is at its buoyant best raw. Use chickweed like parsley: as a bland but salty, herby garnish. And try her in omelets, stuffed eggs, potato salad, pasta salad, and such.

Think Spring Salad

serves 8

4 c/1 liter fresh chickweed 2 c/500ml fresh watercress 1 c/250ml fresh flowers (e.g., violets, columbines) 2 tablespoons/30ml chives	Be careful when you harvest the greens. Leave roots and dirt in the stream and garden; then greens won't need to be washed. Don't wash flowers under any circumstances. Snip chives finely; mix all together. Serve immediately.

Preparation time: 3 hours: 1 hour to walk to the stream and pick watercress; 1 hour to visit with the fairies and pick flowers; 15 minutes to harvest chickweed; 15 minutes to mince chives and fix salad dressing; 15 minutes to tear greens and decorate salad.

Chickweed Tabouli

serves 13

2 ounces/60g dried mint
8 cups/2 liters water
2 quart/liter jars
5 cups/1250ml bulgur
2 c/500ml infused mint
dressing:
1 cup/250ml olive oil
1 cup/250ml lemon juice
1 tsp/5ml garlic powder
6 tsp/30ml tamari

plus:
6 ripe tomatoes
4 baby summer squash
3 c/750ml fresh chickweed
1 c/250ml fresh d'lion leaf
4 oz/125ml chives, scallions
1 c/250ml salty black olives

Prepare mint infusions: put half of mint in each jar and fill to the top with boiling water. Cap and steep overnight. To prepare bulgur, heat partially-strained infusions to boil and pour over bulgur in a large bowl. Cover and let sit while you make the dressing (combine all ingredients and shake), and harvest and chop greens and vegetables. Stir bulgur if you like, to insure even absorption of the mint. When all the liquid is gone, stir dressing to taste into the now "cooked" bulgur. Refrigerate at this point if storage is desired. Just before serving, stir in the chopped "plus" list and add more dressing if needed. Decorate with chickweed greens and calendula blossoms.

Preparation time: 90-120 minutes, but spread out over a few days. 10 minutes to put up the mint infusions. 10 minutes to reheat the infusions, measure the bulgur and put them together in a coverable bowl. 30 minutes in the garden and another 30 minutes in the kitchen with greens and vegetables. 15 minutes to put it all together and decorate it, too.

Chickweed Pesto

1 c/250ml fresh chickweed
1 cup/250ml fresh basil
2 cloves garlic
½ cup/125ml olive oil
optional:
3-4 oz/100g hard cheese
3-4 oz/100g pine nuts

Put all ingredients into your blender or food processor and pray for a smooth mélange. If your blender balks, stir and add more oil. If you elect to add nuts and cheese, they may be smushed in the machine at the same time. Great on dandelion noodles.

Preparation time: 15 minutes, unless I hang out to talk with the little star lady. This freezes well. To keep without freezing, put pesto in a jar and pour a good layer of oil right on top; keep cool.

Mild Curried Chickweed

serves 4

3 tablespoons/45ml olive oil
1 tsp/5ml cumin seeds
2 tsp/10ml mustard seeds
1 teaspoon/5ml turmeric
4 c/1 liter fresh chickweed
1 Tbs/15ml lemon juice
1 tablespoon/15ml tamari

Heat oil in cast iron pan. Add seeds, stir and cook two minutes. Stir in turmeric and cook another minute. Turn off heat. Add chopped chickweed, lemon juice and tamari. Stir well and serve immediately.

Preparation time: 20 minutes: 5 to pick chickweed, 5 to assemble spices, and 10 to cook. Great with basmati rice and yogurt soup on a warm spring evening.

Bacon, Chickweed, and Tomato Sandwich

serves 2

4 slices wholemeal toast
1 Tbs/15ml mayonnaise
1 Tbs/15ml yogurt
1 ripe tomato
3 slices fried bacon
1 c/250ml fresh chickweed

Combine mayo and yogurt so you won't worry so much about the bacon. Put thick slices of tomato on the mayogurt-spread bread. Add a handful of chopped chickweed, then the bacon. And the last piece of bread. Grin, and bite!

Preparation time: 20-30 minutes, depending on whether or not you can fry bacon, toast bread, and pick chickweed all at the same time. A well-deserved treat on fine fall days.

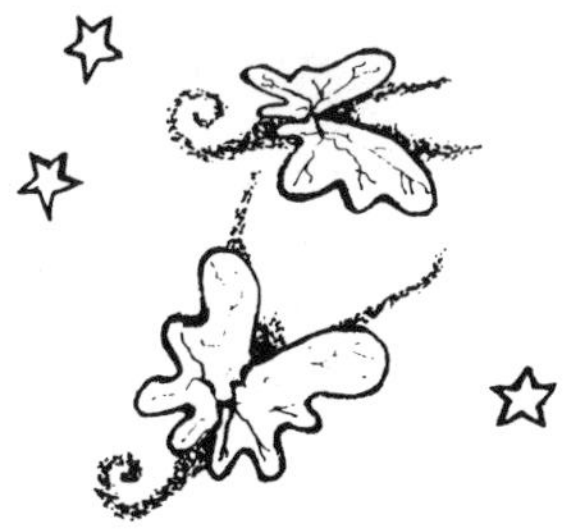

"Although chickweed is detested by farmers and gardeners, I love this little plant and can hardly bear myself to hoe it out. . . ."

Euell Gibbons (1966)

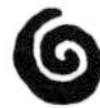

Chickweed Fun and Facts

• Henrietta Rau, in *Healing with Herbs*, treats chickweed with more respect and understanding than any other writer I've come across.

• Audrey Hatfield, writing nearly a hundred years ago in her *Weed Herbal*, clearly loves and enjoys our little star lady.

• *Wildflowers on the Windowsill* by Susan Hitchcock is a must read for all city dwelling weed-eaters. *". . . chickweed was one of the plants that got me started in this adventure of growing wildflowers on the windowsill."* (She's too polite to call it a weed.)

• For those with a scientific curiosity about chickweed, read: "Plant substances active against mycobacterium tuberculosis," F.K. Fitzpatrick, *Antibiotics and Chemotherapy*, 4(5), 528-536, 1954.

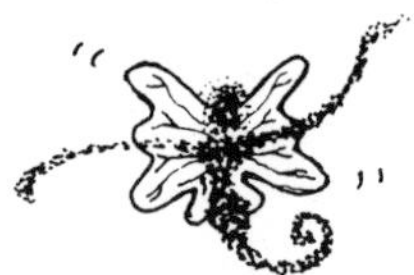

"Therefore, the fact that chickweed fossils have been found in the Lea Valley Arctic Bed and in the soil stratum of Britain's late-glacial period should not surprise us." Audrey Wynne Hatfield (1898)

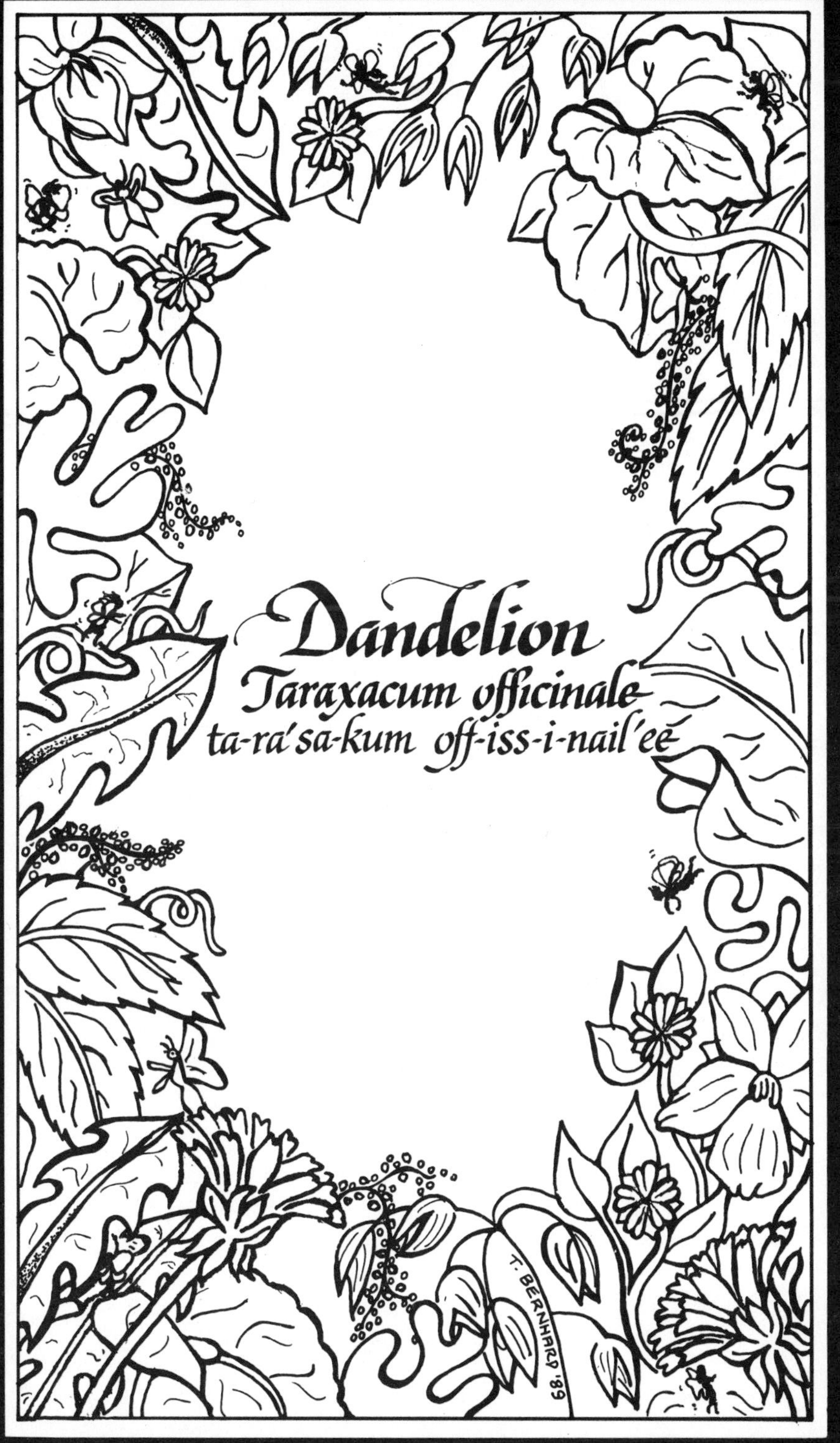
Dandelion
Taraxacum officinale
ta-ra'sa-kum off-iss-i-nail'ee
T. BERNHARD '89

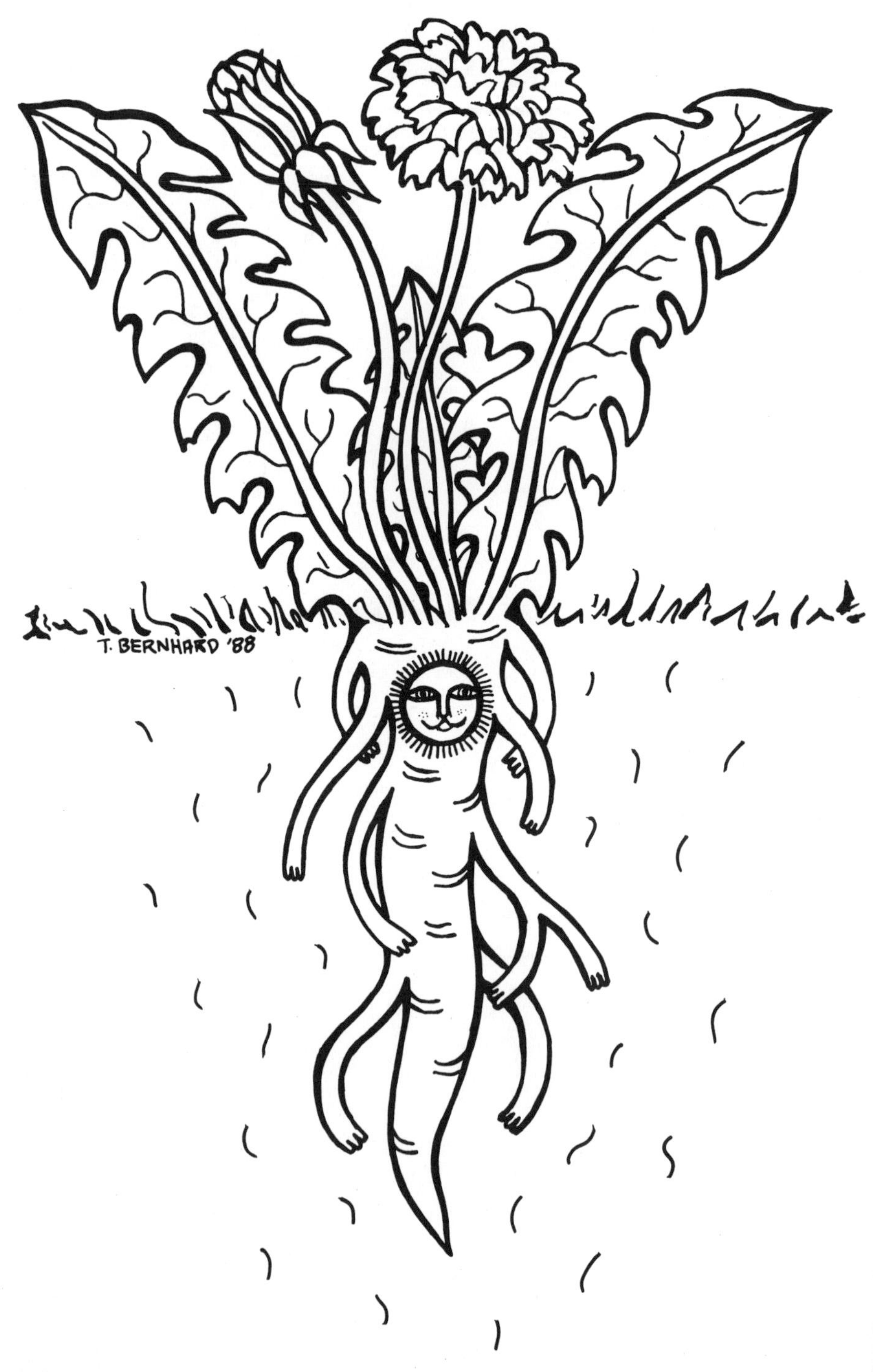
T. BERNHARD '88

Dandelion Speaks

Bon jour, ma chere!* Is it not a day magnifique? Beautiful! I am so full of delight zat you have come to play with me, amie.

See how full zis day is with sunshine and singing birds and golden bees. Does it not make you want to sing and buzz and glow as well, eh?

Non, non. Why are you looking up, eh? Look down. (Silly humans, whenever zey hear a voice and do not see a person zey look up. What do zey expect, eh? An angel? Mon Dieu?)

Look down . . . down here at your feet . . . down . . . oui, down! I speak to you from ze earth. Oui! It is I, tooth of ze lion, dent-de-leon, dandelion, who speaks to you of ze day magnifique. Doctor dandelion, s'il vous plaît.

Ah! Allô. What is zat? Am I a medical doctor? An MD? I guess you could say so, but I have no degrees, eh? So maybe we'd better say I am an SD, spirit doctor, or SD: self-healing doctor, or SD: spirit dancer. I am a doctor who prescribes ecstasy and unity and self love, eh? Joy can heal, eh?

I say joy makes ze spirit whole, and zen ze whole person can heal, eh? Some people, zey consider me a very powerful doctor. Ozers, zey say I am an aggressive foreigner. Please do excuse my accent. It is true zat I am not from your beautiful country, zough I am very much at home here, merci.

But what to say of myself, eh? Even I sometimes do not understand myself perfectly well, eh? I am so full of dramatic opposites. And I love all my opposites. To me zis is not contradiction, but vast variety. Always it is my task to expand to encompass fully ze dualities of my existence. A large undertaking, eh, chère?

You see me here, golden, in ze sunlight, full of myself, bold, and brazen. Erupting with fountains of bright spring yellow. Crowning myself with twenty, fifty, a hundred golden headdresses. Ze queen of life. Unbounded life! Delirious with joie de vivre! Buzzed over wildly by ze bees and ze fairies, all ze petite zings avec wings, eh? Zey love to come to me.

Zey are all attracted to me. Are you not attracted to me, chère?

See* **Doctor D's Appendix, *page 162*.

Do you not find yourself compelled to me, eh? Have you tasted my nectar? Put your probing tongue to my pollen? Non?

Are you in awe of my intensity? You zink maybe I have an overzealous personality, eh? Maybe you are a bit embarrassed zat I show off and strut my stuff, eh? You zink a doctor should be more reserved.

Perhaps you are even afraid of me, eh? Am I not ze leon? Do you see me as a créature splendide? Great yellow gold lioness, in touch wiz all of existence, eh? And zat includes death . . . Do not worry . . . I play nice. . . .

But what of ze cool, hidden part of me? What of my melancholy? What of ze part of me zat sinks into ze earth as far as I can reach, to be alone, alone in silence? What of ze part of me zat closes up so fast when ze storm threatens? When ze sky grows dim, I do not shine in ze gloom. I hide away. And what of ze part of me zat blows off my seeds? Zat sends them like tears, flying on ze winds of time? Alors, stranger even to my own children!

Take off your shoes . . . oui . . . and now your socks . . . put your bare feet on ze earth here . . . are you surprised at ze cool? I keep my toes down in ze cool deep moist earth, chère, so I keep my cool, even when I get hot. I am so full of ze opposites, eh? Oui, oui, I am all zere is, all that there is.

What you zink? You zink you will have a good time playing with doctor dent-de-leon, eh? Sometimes together we will be dark and quiet, sometimes we will shine as brightly as we can, sometimes we'll be rooted for years and years and years in one spot, and sometimes we will go on endless flights. I am all ways, all zings. Zis, I zink makes me good doctor. I am whole in my many ways, eh? You play wiz me, and you feel more whole in your many ways, eh? Is zis not what a self-love doctor must do?

What is zis you are saying? I am a weed? Not a doctor? Eh? Who tells you zees tings? You say doctors do not take off shoes and put feet in earth? You say doctors do not make sexy jokes? You say doctors especially do not go where zey are not wanted, invading neighborhoods, and disturbing ze residents. Well! Something wrong with your idea of doctors, I zink.

I tell you again. I am a doctor of life, of spirit. I exist to help you live your life to ze fullest, to experience all ze parts of yourself, to enjoy yourself, your food, and your sex, and your work. I am here to open you to life! Your life! Your whole life! How can I do zis if I do not live where you live, eh? How could I do zis if I did not follow you everywhere? I must be under your very feet to call out to you, eh?

You are asleep, ma chère, mon amie. Someone must be ze alarm clock, eh?

Wake up! Wake up! Enjoy your life. Enjoy yourself. Zis is doctor dent-de-leon, SD, speaking.

You have more problems wiz me? Old fashioned? Doctor dent-de-leon is old fashioned? Of ze old country? Not modern? Of ze old country; oui, chère. Old fashioned; non. I am ze great wholeness which contains all opposites, eh? Ze great lioness of unity. I am modern, contemporary, fresh, young, and still I have ze ancient knowing, eh? Still I have ze ways of ze ancient times inside me, eh?

First woman and I were friends way back zen. She, whole, me, whole, no speaking did we need. We played glad games of creation. Her every thought, fantasy, and dream took form, became dolphins in ze sea, lions stalking antelope, snakes warming living spirals on rock altars, honeybees singing joy.

Ah, here was first woman's first problem . . . honeybees hungry. So first woman asks for my help, eh? She sees how many flowers I make, and how much the bees love my largesse of pollen, how zey suck my nectar. She says to me: "Make more."

"How do I make more?" I wonder. I wonder and I ponder. I ponder very deep, very long. I brood on zis request. I pull my sepals up around my flower so I can zink.

And as I ponder "How?" a wondrous zing occurs: inside my closed flower, under my sepals curling and green, are seeds. And each one holds a gossamer parachute. I am so astonished by zis zat I open my sepals. Whoosh! Ze wind blows and away fly my seeds on zer silky puffs. My little bébés, ze seeds, gone!

Away flew my dreamseeds. And though today my seeds make only more dandelions and fly no further zan you could walk in an hour, zat day zey flew to every place on ze planet earth. And each seed became ze seed of a différente new jolie fleur of ze green nation. So all ze flowers were born, and all ze bees became so happy zey began to buzz! And zey still do!

Such a happy story, eh? But I do miss my seeds, chère. Are zey not naughty children to fly so far from me?

Zat was a long time ago. But ancient memories do not make one out of date, or old fashioned, eh? Doctor dent-de-leon has had a punk hairstyle for a long time. Is zis not modern?

C'est bon zat we talk; c'est bon; good, good. What else bother you? Make you not want to play wiz doctor dandelion, eh? Make you not trust doctor dent-de-leon? You tell me; we talk, eh?

Bitter? You have been told zat I am bitter? Ah, well, ma chère . . . ze bitter comes with ze sweet of life, eh? But I do not zink I lay so heavy on ze tongue as all zat!

I like to zink of myself as sharp, not bitter. Salty and sharp. Do I not dress sharp, eh? Quite a looker, eh? I like to be sharp, quick, on ze alert. I like to be on ze edges, ze cutting edges of new thought, new fashion. Doctor dandelion cuts a sharp image, eh?

I like to be in ze public eye. I like to show off, eh? I like to be in ze middle of things. I like to hear all ze gossip. I like to be in ze know. And I like to shine. And when I am in ze spotlight, I am not sweet, eh? When I shine it is best to be a little bitter. But come to me, chère, after ze show, and believe me, I serve you some tasty dishes!

Now what? I zink you are going to stay and play, and now it seems you go? What is zis? You say you are going to study dandelion wiz some woman named "Weed"? How silly! Quelle absurdité! Stay here. Study wiz dent-de-leon. Believe me, you don't need zat woman Weed, whoever she is. *I* tell you ze facts and take you on ze weed walk and tell you all about how to find or buy and use dandelion, eh? Who knows better, eh? You get it right from ze doctor's mouth, eh? You play with me and we learn lots of zings, eh?

Bon! Get your notebook and pen, s'il vous plaît. Doctor dent-de-leon is going to give to you all ze facts:

Dandelion Facts

Botanical name: *Taraxacum officinale*; taraxos (Greek) means disorder; achos (Greek) means remedy; taraxacum means I am ze remedy for disorders; officinale means I am indeed an official medicinal plant, eh? **Other useful species:** *T. mongolicum, T. magellanicum, Leontodon taraxacum*; approximately one hundred species, all useful. ***Natural order:*** Asteraceae/Sunflower family. ***English names:*** Piss-in-bed, lion's tooth, blow ball, fortune-teller, red-seeded dandelion, arctic dandelion, doonheadclock, tell-time, clock flower, bitterwort, yellow gowan, swine snort, Irish daisy, wet-a-bed, priest's crown, cankerwort, puffball, wild endive. (Zey give me some wild names, eh, chère?) ***Chinese names:*** Huang-hua ti-ting, ju-chi ts'ao, ai-chiao p'u-kung-ying, kung-yin, pu-kung-yin. ***French names:*** Dent-de-lion, pissenlit. ***German names:*** Löwenzahn, Kuhblume, Pfaffenrohrlein. ***Greek names:*** Radiki: "radiating from the center like the sun's rays or the spokes of a wheel." ***Indian names:*** Dudhal, baran, kinphul. ***Italian names:*** Diente di lieone, Radicchiallar, Tarassaco, Soffione. ***Persian names:*** Trakhasnkun. ***Russian names:*** Oduvanchik, pushki. ***Spanish names:*** Chicoria, diente de leon, consuelda. ***Turkish names:*** Kara hindiba otu, yabani, aci marul. ***Dye uses:*** From my flowers comes a light yellow color for your wool; from my roots, a rich magenta. ***Food uses:*** My greens are gathered and eaten wherever I grow; my roasted root is a common coffee substitute; my fleurs make a vin excellent. ***Medicinal uses:*** You will find me for sale in many places, prepared in many ways; keep your eyes open for me, chère. ***Soil uses:*** Note carefully; regardez! I create drainage channels in compacted soils, restore mineral health to abused soils, aerate and attract earthworms in all soils; not so bad, eh? Maybe you let me hang out in your garden, eh? ***Animal uses:*** My seeds are eaten by many wild birds, including ze Canada geese; my leaves are relished by animals from chipmunks to bears, especially rabbits; and I am a most important all-season bee food. ***Habitat:*** Wherever you go, I will follow, chère; just give me some open ground, eh? a field, pasture, lawn, or wayside will do, if you've no garden room. ***Natural range:*** Greece, Arabia, Asia Minor; I lived in all ze first cities, eh? ***Current range:*** Worldwide; especially throughout ze north temperate zone of China, Europe, New Zealand, Australia, and North America. ***Toxicity:*** Chère, enjoy! Zere are no reasonable limits to ze amount of dandelion zat you may consume, zough ze cooked greens can be laxative at first, ooh, la, la. Watch out! I loosen you up! Even ze tincture can be taken by ze glassful without harm, eh? Then you get very loose! I tell you, we have a good time; enjoy life! ***Best identified by:*** Know me as dandelion, none other, by my bright yellow flowers in your lawns and field; my leaves of dark green which are absolutely hairless (check the back of the mid-rib, chère) and grow stalkless from a center point; and, of course, my seed heads enchantés which you so enjoy blowing upon.

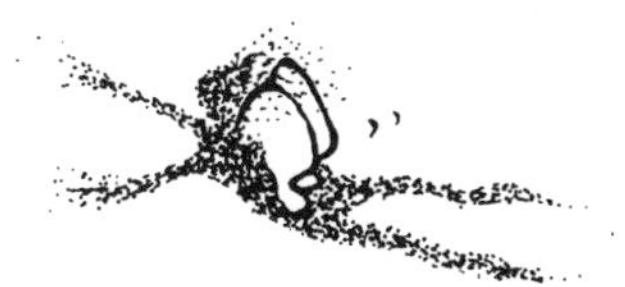

"It is a pleasant sight of spring days to see these new-fledged Americans dotting the fields and waste lots near our big cities, armed with knives, snipping and transferring to sack or basket the tender new leaves of the well-beloved plant, which, like themselves, is a translated European."

C. Saunders (1920)

Dandelion Weed Walk

Now, alors! Time for ze weed walk. I cannot walk. And I do not want you to pick me at the moment, s'il vous plaît. You go for a petite promenade, eh? Find dandelion, zen come back. . . .

In the sun the bees hum about the sweet flowers of dandelion.

Bien . . . bien . . . let me see. What have you brought back? Teeth, teeth, handfuls of teeth. See? Zer are big teeth on ze leaf, eh? And ze petite pointy teeth on ze fleur. And zis broken tooth of a root. See how ze white sap leaks out here . . . where you broke ze root, and here . . . where you broke ze hollow flower stalk, eh?

You be careful now when you see zis white sap, eh? Milky sap is very, very powerful. Not to mess around wiz, eh? Zis is part of why I am ze family doctor. It is because I am of ze white sap family, so I have ze power, power I can use to help or hurt. I help you, eh, chère?

I choose to help people, eh? To help especially ze ones who are sick in ze liver: les maladies de foie—my spécialité. Without the happy foie, zer is no joie! What you zink, eh? I find a way to make ze poisons in your liver so slippery zey slide right out of you, eh? I make your liver very energetic, very powerful, so poisons cannot affect you, eh?

Alors, OK! OK! Zis is ze weed walk . . . I talk about my properties later, right? Eh, chère? We go in ze proper order. Oui. Oui.

What is first? We examine first ze fleur. Zis is what you notice first, eh? My flowers. Mes fleurs: le sacre du printemps. Ze first song of spring. Ze crowning of spring. Ze first gold, eh?

Notice: one stalk, one fleur. Very important. Some imposters (quacks, I say) try to look like doctor dandelion. But zey don't have ze power to have a hollow, unbranched stalk, eh? One stalk, one flower. Remember, eh?

Très amusant. Here is a funny joke. I tell ze little lie. Zis is not one fleur. Zis is many flowers, not one. Take a look, eh? Pull one "petal" off and you can see all ze flower parts in zat one petal.

Ze petal is actually a flower and ze flower is but a petal of ze larger pattern. So one is many, yet ze many become one. You see here zat to make ze bigger picture beautiful and bright, you must be as much yourself as you can, eh? Ze whole blossom must be from ze cooperation and fulfillment of each individual, eh chère?

Unité. Individualité. Another of ze opposites I encompass, chère. My single blossom's brilliance is ze life force of not one but hundreds of individuals, eh? Each one independently alive and each one integrated into ze larger pattern.

Look into zis fleur, now. Very deep into zis fleur. Let ze color come in through your eyes and your nose and let it flow to your stomach. Put your hand on your stomach. Non, non . . . your stomach, not your belly. Put your hands near ze bottom of ze rib cage. Oui, très bien. In ze middle: ze stomach. On your right: ze liver. On your left: ze spleen and pancreas.

Alors. Hands on ze stomach. Attention on ze fleur . . . fleur d'or . . . golden flower . . . let ze luminous honey-colored light flow up to your lips. Lick it off. Swallow ze taste. Feed yourself on ze essence of dandelion. Now breath in ze bright/deep, sweet/itchy, familiar/strange scent. Zen open your eyes, very wide, breathe deeply and let your vision get very large. Do you see ze air full of fragile flickering rainbowed glittering wings, eh? Oh, chère . . . I love it when you look at me zat way! We could make lovely wine together!

We look next at ze leaves, eh? What is zat? Seeds? Seeds . . . ah, that is my melancholy. My sadness. Ma joie, oui. My pride, oui. But such a price, eh? All my dears, my bébés, gone, gone before I get to know zem.

Let us go on to the leaves, eh? I shall not burden you wiz my great longing and suffering. All my wishing for ze children I have given to the winds, sent out into ze world alone, alas.

So, ze leaves. Ze leaves are very important: good food, good médecine. OK, OK, I leave zat for later. Ze leaves are important to identify ze dandelion, because you use ze root and ze leaves when ze dent-de-leon is not flowering, eh? So if you can only identify dandelion by ze flower, you're, how you say, "Out of luck, Charlie."

Let us see if you can identify ze leaf of dandelion, eh? Look now at ze leaves you brought back. Do zey all look ze same? Non, non, non! See, some have deep sharp teeth, some have shallow jags, some teeth point down, some point out. Zis leaf has a whole mouthful of teeth. Zis leaf does not have a single one, eh? Maybe it is from a baby lion? All are different.

Are zees leaves all dandelion? Non. Not all leaves of dandelion. Some are of chicory. But it is not because of ze teeth. You cannot tell ze difference by ze teeth. Here is how to tell. Turn ze leaf over; look on ze back, along ze midrib. If she is smooth and hairless, is dandelion. If she is hairy, is chicory (she Italian, eh?).

Non, size is not ze good way to tell. Chicory leaves can be bigger, smaller, or same size as dandelion. Hair on ze midrib is ze only positive way to tell. Doctor dandelion is a smooth talker, eh? And a smooth mover, eh? You will not confuse me wiz ze hairy doctors, eh? Just take my smooth leaves home and put them in your salad, or cook yourself up a mess of greens, eh?

Oui, and remember you need to find ze leaves without ze fleur, eh? Ze leaves are only tasty when I am finished playing blossom games with ze fairies and butterflies and bees. So you come pick leaves in ze early spring and late fall, eh? Ze frost she does not hurt us, eh? Eat my leaves, maybe cook and freeze if too many, but don't bother drying zem, zey won't stay useful long zat way, eh?

We have left ze grandest for last: ze grand dent-de-lion, the big tooth, my root. Here, too, you see I'm made up of opposites: dark-skinned without and light-fleshed within.

Zis grand root tooth is fastened securely in ze gums of ze earth's mouth, eh? And zere I grow year after year, reaching down two of your handspans in loose soil, and looking like a slender carrot. In rocky soils, I divide into many roots and stay small, even in advanced age. But everywhere, rich soil or rocky, I search out ze earth's mineral richness wiz my roots.

To dig zis root, you must take special care, eh? Ze juice is ze goods! We don't want to break ze root and lose any of ze juice, eh? So we must be digging very slowly. Maybe chant or sing while loosening the dirt ever so carefully. Oui, oui. Très bien. I like zis chant you sing, chère.

I give my root to you, eh? My melancholy is eased by your song, chère. I will go home wiz you, eh? You will sing to me, eh, chère? It is time, chère. Ze frost is in ze air but not in ze ground. Time for doctor dent-de-leon to find a warm home full of song to spend ze winter in, eh? Time for you to dig my fat, rich autumn roots, full of stored food and energy, ready to nourish you all winter long.

Do not delay. Soon ze ground will too hard, too frozen, to dig into, and you will have to wait until spring softens it to lift me out. And in the spring I can only give you sharp, mean roots: concentrated in tonic bitters, my sweet sugar used to sustain me in the cold and to fire my fast spring growth after winter's long nights are past. And, if you wish to dig my roots in spring, you must take zem only in zat brief spell between ze warm loosening of ze earth and when my buds begin to swell. Once you see my fat green fleur buds you must leave my root alone, eh?

I give my root to you because you put your own life and love into your hands when you touch me, when you touch ze earth. I tell you to take me, chère, but gently, s'il vous plaît. Pull me very gently free, so I will only break off a finger or toe to leave behind, not an entire limb, eh? Though you know zat each bit of me will grow into a new me in time, eh?

I give you my deep connection to ze whole of life and all of life's parts. I give you my ability to include ze most extreme opposites in yourself without settling for ze ordinaire, ze average, eh?

You wish some more dandelion roots, eh? Oui. Oui. My kin here are well pleased to share your warmth and songs. Take not ze oldest plant you see. Remember her as first woman. Take not ze younger plants. Zey have need of more growth. Look for ze wiser, older plants. You get roots as big as your finger or bigger, eh?

Wash me tenderly. Sit me in a bit of water, eh? Or let ze running stream wash my muddy root and play wiz me, heh, heh, while you dig an ozer root, eh? Très bien.

Soft sounds of water and chanting join in chorus with the bees' hum.

Très bien. OK. Here is doctor dandelion, all cleaned up and at home wiz you. It is nice and warm inside, and we are still singing, eh?

Take me to your kitchen, eh? We make some dandy brews. You know, zis makes me so happy to come home with you. So happy to be singing wiz you. Zat's why I cry, eh?

So, take hold of me, chère. Tie a string around my middle, and hang me up to dry. Like zis, eh? Do not take off my leaves, s'il vous plaît. And don't cut! Remember ze juice is ze goods, and it leaks out through ze cut, even through ze cut leaves.

Non, it is not worth drying any others, chère, for you will never keep me around for long zat way. Dried dandelion root is so nutritious (high in sugar, protein, and minerals) zat mold, maggots, and all manner of beetles will eagerly eat all ze dandelion you dry if you do not use it first, fast.

But I want you to dry me, and watch ze emergence of my spiral wrinkles, for I sense zat you will learn much about me zat is beyond words in zis way, eh? Yet I am not beyond words, here, eh? Even hanging from ze ceiling!

Très bien! Très bien. What a grand panorama I have from here where you have hung me.

Now zen . . . alors! Where do I begin? I want to teach you so much, chère. Let us begin wiz an elixir of long life. You will make zis from zes grand roots wiz zer glistening green leaves. Chop ze plants, if you wish, or just coil zem into a jar to fit. We like a tight fit, eh, chère? Oui.

You can use roots only in your elixir, but is better to use all of me, eh? Ze whole thing: leaves and roots. Do keep a tight fit in mind here and fill up ze jar, eh? Zen pour over all some nice vodka, eh? Oui, or some very organic vinegar from ze apple cider. Zen we leave our elixir alone for a moon cycle and a half. After zat, is ready, eh? Put ze date on ze jar, now, so we can remember when to use, eh?

Alors! Again, I go out of order. Excusez-moi. I will leave ze recipes for last and we go right into my powers, eh? (Save some of zees roots and leaves to cook with, eh? I give you *lots* of recipes!)

Now we talk about ze root, ze heart of ze dandelion, eh? Now we talk about some real power, eh? You take zis elixir of long life (maybe you call it dandelion root tincture) and . . .

What? Can you make zis elixir, zis tincture out of dried dandelion? Non, non, absolument non. And do not buy zis unless guaranteed from fresh dandelion, eh?

Your fresh root tincture (made from fall-dug roots), zis elixir of long life, it is full of starch and sugar. You can see ze white sediment in ze bottom of your jar in a few weeks. Part of zis is *inulin,* and in ze fall I am full of it, up to a quarter of my weight in fact. In spring I have none left, alors. (1.7% in March-dug roots.)

Zis starchy sugar is soluble in water and alcohol (like vodka) when you have ze fresh root. But in ze dried root, inulin is only soluble in hot water, eh? So, that dried root is no good for our elixir of long life. It's not soluble in alcohol, and how can it share life wiz you when most of its life is dried up and gone?

Now, when your tincture of fresh dandelion root is ready to take, in six weeks, shake it before you take it. Shake it so you get all zat white stuff at ze bottom, eh?

Zis inulin is ze goods, eh? Oui. And *taraxacin* is ze goods, too, eh? Zis taraxacin, unlike the inulin, is soluble from ze dried roots, and is highest in ze spring-dug roots. Is very bitter, very medicinal. But only good if you soak it in ze cold water, not hot. Oui. Oui. I am full of contradictions.

But not to worry, chère. Just use me fresh, eh? I say my fresh live energy is very complex, very whole. I show you how to be healthy/whole/holy, like me, eh? I am both more simple and much more complex than any alkaloid your scientists may discover, and my complexité, chère, being contrary as I am, is in my simplicité, eh?

Now pay close attention, eh?

"An irritable condition of the stomach and bowels and the existence of acute inflammation contraindicate its use." Henrietta Rau (1968)

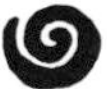

Dandelion Root Properties and Uses

- ***hepatic,*** cholagogue, lithotriptic
- ***tonic,*** nutritive, galactagogue
- ***digestive stimulant,*** stomachic, aperient, laxative, diuretic
- ***deobstruent,*** bactericide, fungicide, astringent
- ***hypnotic,*** sedative

What's wiz all zees big words, eh? Zey break your mind! I tell you in plain English (well, I *try* in English). I, doctor dandelion, affect ze **liver** most profoundly, encouraging its juices, strengthening and nourishing its ability to help you live. I help you function better, eh? I make you strong, and sure of yourself. You leave it to doctor dandelion. I improve your **breasts,** and your **stomach,** and even your guts, eh? I get rid of stuff in ze way, no matter what: any kind of blockage, resistance, doubt. And if you need, I put you to **sleep.** For the hard jobs, you get burdock to work with me, eh? We all have a good time, chère!

Use dandelion root as a supreme liver ally, a tonic (what else?), a trouble shooter, a lover of ze ladies, and a real pisser.

- Dose of *fresh dandelion root tincture* is 10-100 drops a day, in water.
- Dose of *dried dandelion root infusion* is ½-2 cups/125-500ml a day.
- Dose of *fresh dandelion root juice* is 3-6 tablespoons/45-90ml a day.

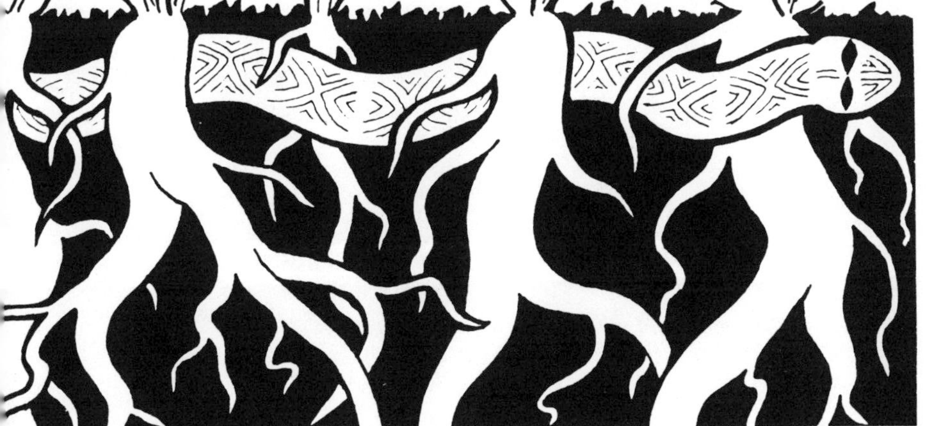

Dandelion Root is a Supreme Liver Ally

Do you realize how much of your life is in ze hands, so to speak, of your live-er?

Every minute of every day fifteen hundred milliliters (zat's three pints) of your blood circulate through your liver. On one hand, your liver takes away: filtering chemical contamination, unneeded hormones, metabolic breakdown by-products (referred to as toxins in some circles), some infectious organisms, and ammonia from your blood. And on ze other hand she adds: bile, glucose, lipoproteins, urea, cholesterols, phospholipids, and plasma proteins, to mention a few.

Sorry, chère. Not to worry, chère. You don't need to remember any fancy words, just remember your liver does more than five hundred functions and deserves a lot of love and cherishing (wiz ze help of doctor dandelion) if you want to live a long and happy life, eh?

Oui, happy. Ze one whose liver is not right cannot enjoy life, n'est-ce pas? Is zis one not full of bitterness? And does zis not disturb ze sleep? and ze appetite? and ze sex life? Ah . . . how can such a one be joyeuse?

What qualifies doctor dandelion to be your liver ally, eh? Chère, I love life, I am a liver of life. And I am full to the brim of zings your liver loves, eh? Choline. Carotenes. Mineral salts. I am ze stuff, chère. I am ze hot stuff for your liver.

I will activate, charge, shine into, rev up, energize, and strongly nourish your solar plexus, eh? I will stimulate ze production and flow of bile from both your gallbladder and liver, eh? If you eat meat, chère, you need me. If you live in ze city, chère, you need me. Let's get going!

I can be your ally, along with your Wise Woman wisdom, when you're healing yourself or others of liver distress: swelling, tenderness, torpidity, or congestion; stress from pregnancy, rich food, chemotherapy, and other chemical exposure; damage from alcohol or drug abuse, jaundice (even in bébés), and hepatitis.

Doctor dandelion is on ze job when you have bile duct swelling and blockage, cholesterol-based gall stones (biliary calculi), indigestion, dyspepsia, and chronic constipation (especially of ze elders, who do not get out of bed, eh?).

"A broth of dandelion roots, sliced and stewed in boiling water with some leaves of sorrel and the yolk of an egg, taken daily for some months, has been known to cure seemingly intractable cases of chronic liver congestion." Maude Grieves (1931)

And do ask me to help when you have poisoned yourself, eh? I am especially good at restoring life to those suffering from botulism and mushroom mistakes (with activated charcoal or slippery elm to help neutralize ze poison and relieve ze liver).

Alors, I can even help you when you have ze beginning stages of cirrhosis. But don't wait zat long to get to know me, eh, chère?

Eighty percent of ze patients treated with dandelion root preparations in Chinese hospitals recovered from appendicitis without surgery, according to Adele Dawson.

Dandelion Root is a Tonic, What Else?

(Numbers indicate milligrams per hundred grams dandelion root)

Have I not been used for hundreds of years, all over ze world, from ze Mediterranean to China as a bitter tonic?

Doctor dandelion is strong enough, gutsy enough, and toothy enough to get your innards in gear. Ally yourself wiz me, and we'll tone up your liver (we already talked about that, eh?), your spleen, your stomach, your pancreas, your kidneys, your skin, and your nervous, glandular, digestive, urinary, circulatory, immune, and lymphatic systems. I tell you, I am one powerful doctor, n'est-ce pas?

You know I am full of extremes, eh? But in my constituents, I am exceptionally well balanced, eh? Tonifying everyzing with a skillful blend of earth mineral salts and improving your nutritional bases at a cellular level, eh? No wonder zey zink of me as an appetite stimulant. I make you crave ze fullness of life itself! And I increase your vitality, eh?

My root has high amounts of iron (96), manganese (6.8), phosphorus (362), protein (16.5%), aluminum (65.6), and carotenes expressed as vitamin A (14000 IU).

And I give you average amounts of calcium (614), chromium (0.9), cobalt (8), magnesium (157), niacin (3.3), potassium (1200), riboflavin (.21), silicon (4.7), sodium (113), tin (1.3), zinc (1.3), and ze vitamin C complex expressed as ascorbic acid (38).

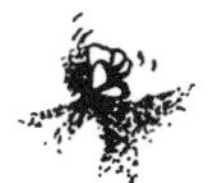

> *"[Dandelion] leaves can be picked young or blanched to use fresh in salads, or picked a bit older and steamed or boiled like spinach, the flowers form the basis of a very good golden wine; the seeds can be sprouted and the roots can be chopped and used like parsnips or roasted and ground to make a very nice coffee substitute."* Gai Stern (1986)

Dandelion Root is a Trouble Shooter

My tonic effect is not just for maintaining your health, eh? I can help you wiz some troubles. Oui. I help you wiz troubles like cancer, heart and lung problems, digestive woes, and painful joints. I tell you, I am ze hot stuff, doctor dandelion, the family doctor supreme!

I can create a potassium-rich anti-cancer environment for you, chère. I can help eliminate free radicals, those gangsters and hoodlums. And I have a special way with viruses, heh, heh.

Let me be your ally, along with your other Wise Woman ways, when you are healing yourself and others with cancer, swollen lymph glands/nodes, EBV, or mononucleosis. Ask for my help when confronted with infections and fevers.

I am a trusty friend, chère, for your chest (later I tell you about breasts, ooh, la, la). Try me in any form for helping yourself or others when you want to nourish, soothe, and heal those with chronic chest pain, bronchitis, pneumonia, and tuberculosis. Try me as well for eliminating, or at least reducing, high blood pressure, arteriosclerosis, and elevated cholesterol levels.

Because I am so good for ze liver, ze whole digestive system is strengthened when you ally yourself wiz me: stomach, pancreas, gall bladder, even ze intestines.

Of course I am ze greatest for restorative therapy after liver illness. But did you know that I stabilize ze blood sugar, help ze pancreas, reduce hypoglycemia, and can even help prevent middle-age-onset diabetes, eh? Try me to increase ze appetite of zose who are convalescing, enfeebled, or anorexic. In addition, I help to relieve chronic constipation; for zis, ze fresh root must be used, eh?

What else? I have so many abilities, eh? A soothing warm cup of root infusion, maybe wiz lait (zat's milk) to help your insomnia; sips of infusion or frequent ten-drop doses of tincture to improve acute skin eruptions in a day or two; three tablespoons of my fresh juice (oui, you must put into ze juicer machine for zis) diluted in water and drunk once or twice a day for eight weeks to loosen and oil your rheumatic, arthritic, stiff joints.

Wiz me, and your Wise Woman ways, everyzing gets healthy/whole/holy, eh?

"The constituents of dandelion are taraxasterol, taraxerol (both water insoluble), fructose, inulin, choline, pectin, and, in the early spring, mannite. The leaves also contain inositol." M. Moore (1979)

Dandelion Root is a Lover of ze Ladies

Oui, oui, chère. I do love ze ladies. Tincture or infusion of my fresh root, or even my juice, taken conscientiously, is well known by wise women as a specific for nourishing and helping heal ze ladies' breasts, ooh, la, la, and ze uterus and ovaries.

Try me wiz your Wise Woman ways to help you with menstrual cramps, premenstrual breast swelling and tenderness, premenstrual digestive variances.

Frequent sips of my fresh tea after delivery of ze bébé encourages prompt expulsion of ze placenta.

Native American women used me in a cold infusion with thistle root to prevent conception, but the precise dosage and species of thistle is not known. (Well, maybe I know, but maybe is not so good to tell, eh?)

As well as ingesting me, use my fresh and grated roots when you are healing/wholing ze woman whose breasts have sores, tumors, cancers, cysts, or impacted milk glands.

You want to be in good shape, ladies? You stick wiz me, eh?

Dandelion Root is a Real Pisser

Is not for nothing, chère, zat my name is pissenlit, piss in bed. I can be a real pisser, for sure, eh? But for zis, you use ze spring roots, OK? You can make an infusion or tincture, either one.

Try me as a wise woman's ally when helping yourself or others heal kidney and urinary problems, including all kidney and bladder diseases (oui, even cancer), kidney stones, diabetic kidney problems, gout, dropsy, edema, renosis, urinary stones and gravel, and ulcers in the ureters, urethra, or bladder.

I am well endowed, zis you know. My root is especially well endowed with sodium and potassium, electrolytes needed in plentiful supply when a strong diuretic effect is to be accomplished without stress to the kidneys. I tell you before, I play gentle, eh?

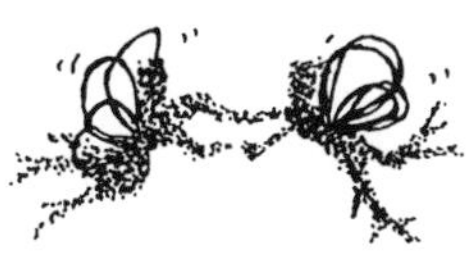

"This is one of the most esteemed plants of the herbalist, a favorite of the great Arabian herbalist Avicenna. . . . A diet of the greens improves the enamel of the teeth." Juliette Levy (1966)

Dandelion Leaf Properties and Uses

- ***nutritive,*** alkalinizer, tonic, galactagogue
- ***stomachic,*** cholagogue, aperient
- ***diuretic,*** depurative, mild detergent
- ***vulnerary,*** anodyne, slight narcotic

Alors, chère, here are ze big words again. Zey say my leaves of glorious green are one of ze best **foods** you ever eat, eh? Zey help you stay alkaline (not a sourpuss) and active. Ze **breast milk** is made rich (I tell you I like ze ladies!), ze **stomach** and **liver** is made strong, and ze **wounds** are healed when doctor dandelion is your ally. And don't forget my effect on your **kidneys.** You don't want to wet ze bed, eh?

Use dandelion leaves, especially fresh, as a nutritious free food, a digestive bitter, and a real mover in your blood and lymph.

- Dose of *fresh dandelion leaf tincture* is 10-45 drops a day, in water.
- Dose of *dried dandelion leaf infusion* is ½-2 cups/125-500ml a day.
- Dose of *fresh dandelion leaf juice* is 1-6 tablespoons/15-90ml a day.

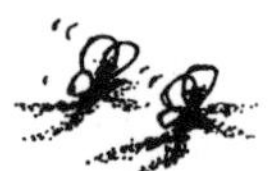

"The leaves are eaten raw or cooked by the Digger and Apache Indians, who value them so highly that they scour the country for many days' journeys in search of sufficient to appease their appetites. So great is their love for the plant, that the quantity consumed by a single individual exceeds belief."

Dodge (1870)

Dandelion Leaves are a Nutritious Free Food

(Numbers indicate milligrams per hundred grams of dandelion leaves)

You have a nice stack of dandelion leaves, chère? Wash zem very well. Dry half and put them in a folded towel in a cool place. Oui, icebox is good. Zis other half, we chop. Zen we look up a recipe in **Dandelion Kitchen** and cook zem, eh?

I know you like ze numbers, so I give you ze numbers, zen we talk some more about ze leaves, eh?

Dandelion leaves have very high amounts of carotenes expressed as vitamin A (21,060-58,335 IU), ze vitamin C complex expressed as ascorbic acid (33-652), potassium (397-2757), and calcium (252-4223).

Ze fresh or cooked leaves have also high amounts of iron (3-29), phosphorus (59-526), and the B-vitamin complex including riboflavin (0.29-1.8), thiamine (0.23-1.70), niacin (.80), and choline (essential for liver function).

Also you get manganese, sulphur, magnesium, silica, very low sodium (76-79), potash, and vitamin D. And don't forget ze taraxacin, and taraxacerin, eh? Zey are not only in my roots; I like to spread my goodness around to my leaves, eh?

Ze half we put in ze icebox, eh, we make a salad wiz tomorrow. Or a nice dip? A big bowlful, in fact a whole liter (oops, quart) of dandelion leaves contains only 44 calories, eh? You can eat a lot of zis salad. Try lemon or orange juice, with ginger and tamari for ze dressing. Keeps ze figure slim, eh? And my leaves are 19-32% protein; zat's high, so you feel full, not starved.

Because my leaves are so nutritious, I suggest you eat zem whenever you can. But if you need excuses to eat them, I suggest ze last two months of pregnancy, and throughout ze nursing year, eh? And for ze anemic, especially around zat certain time of ze month, eh? Ze ones who don't want to eat, ze anorexic teens, ze bored elders, zey will find zer appetites returning when doctor dandelion is ze ally, eh? And ze liver will be happy.

Dandelion Leaves are a Digestive Bitter

Doctor dandelion is ready to orchestrate great happenings in your digestive tract, eh? First, I will increase ze hydrochloric acid in your stomach, that will help you digest better, get more calcium out of your food, and avoid nasty tummy aches.

Then I'll get to work on lowering your cholesterol levels (I have phytosterols, chère, which don't give ze wrong fats a chance), and rebuilding your liver. I don't want you to have any difficulty in digesting fat, chère, we have a lot of parties to go to together, n'est-ce pas? No sluggish liver, no run down feeling for us, eh chère? No constipation, eh?

Here is what you do. You make yourself a dandelion apéritif.

On ze way home from work, you find a place to pick a few dandelion leaves. I cannot tell you where; but dandelion is everywhere. I know you can find some, eh? You will be careful for dog doo and chemicals, eh? Sometimes sidewalk is safer zan ze lawn!

Zen you buy some nice vin, vin blanc, nice French white wine, eh? And go on home . . . wash off zose dandelion leaves, chop zem up, put zem in a glass, and pour ze wine right over zem.

Go away for an hour, or better yet, make dinner, which you'll accompany wiz your dandelion apéritif.

You don't like wine? You just use water, eh? Pour boiling water, not wine, on ze leaves, and let sit for an hour.

OK. Now you have dandelion apéritif. Drink. Every evening. Big zings in store for you. Doctor dandelion likes to keep zings moving, chère!

Dandelion Leaves are a Real Mover in Your Blood and Lymph

I get zings going in your fluid circulation, eh? I get your blood going, chère! I make those cells take notice, eh? Ze leaves of dandelion are a very safe means of increasing ze amount of water and blood waste eliminated through ze kidneys and urine. Zey act specifically to eliminate congestion and fluid swelling.

Sounds good, non? How we do zis, eh? It's easy. Just eat dandelion, and drink dandelion, infusion or tincture, as much as you want. But for a while, eh? I like a long affair, eh?

Once I get to know you, zen doctor dandelion will be your ally (I know you use your Wise Woman ways, too) to heal yourselves or others with low blood pressure, poor circulation, diabetic edema, rheumatic swelling, arthritic congestion, recurrent mastitis, premenstrual water retention, and cancer of the breast, liver, and urinary organs.

Oui, I am willing to help in some emergencies. Make a strong tea, or infusion from fresh or dried dandelion leaves, chère. After you strain it, drink ze liquid and poultice with ze plant material. Try zis with your Wise Woman ways for healing zose with fevers, swelling from broken bones and sprains, bruises, mastitis, and chronic skin problems, especially swollen and weepy rashes, eczema, and acne.

"A veritable army of weed killers and tools has been employed to get rid of this lawn 'spoiler,' but have you ever seen a field made a glorious sheet of gold by millions of dandelions?" Adrienne Crowhurst (1972)

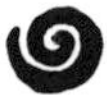

Dandelion Flower Properties and Uses

- ***emollient,*** anodyne, vulnerary
- ***hepatic,*** calmative, cardio-tonic

Use dandelion flowers as a beautifier, a pain reliever, and a friend to your heart.

- Dose of *fresh dandelion flower tea* is ½-3 cups/125-750ml a day.
- Dose of *dandelion flower wine* is ¼-1 cup (2-8 ounces)/60-250ml a day.

Dandelion Flowers are a Beautifier

Chère, why suffer from unsightly freckles, large pores, oily skin, rough chapped skin, windburn, sunburn, insect bites, age spots, tired, red eyes and other untidy evidences of your human frailty? Doctor dandelion will be so kind as to help you, eh?

Steep fresh dandelion blossoms in a covered container for at least an hour in water freshly boiled. Strain, reserving both flowers and liquid. Put ze warm wet fleurs on your face and lie down for ten minutes. Zen wash it all off wiz ze liquid. Do not rinse. Also splash zis infusion on your skin before you go to sleep. Leave on overnight for best results. I make you so jolie, chère.

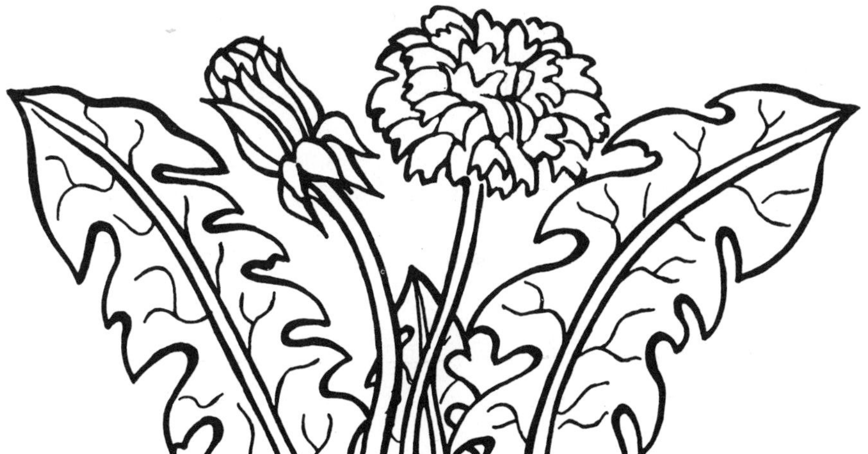

Dandelion Flowers are a Pain Reliever

Chère, how can you be beautiful when you are frowning? Let me help you erase zose frowns.

Go out on a sunny spring day and pick ze fully open dandelion fleurs. Listen to ze bees; zey tell you which fleurs are best, eh? Put some in your salad; zat's good for a smile.

Use my golden blossoms to make vin de dent-de-leon (see recipe, page 151). Zis is so good for ze heart zat maybe you fall in love, eh?

Steep a handful of ze fresh blossoms in a teacup of boiling water. Add honey and drink to relieve and heal yourself and others with headaches, menstrual cramps, backaches, stomach aches, even depression, eh? Jolie et joyeuse!

Make a dandelion flower oil and use it wiz your Wise Woman touch to ease the pain and help heal those wiz stiff necks, arthritic joints, sinus headaches, back tension, and weepy, swollen skin sores.

Ze société fleur essence (zat's Flower Essence Society, eh?) recognizes ze ability of my huile de fleur (zat's flower oil) to promote deep relaxation and facilitate release of emotions locked in ze muscles.

I insist you loosen up and enjoy life!

Dandelion Sap Properties and Uses

• ***discutient,*** anodyne, keratolytic, fungistatic, bacteriostatic

Use dandelion sap as an eraser—externally.

Dandelion Sap Is an Eraser

Oui. I will erase zings for you. Just daub on ze sap and see what happens to warts, corns, calluses, hard pimples, bee stings, old sores, and blisters. No need to wait, I tell you what happens: zey dissolve and disappear!

My sap is ze most potent part of me, eh? Zer is much sap in ze flower stalks, and in ze fresh root or leaf, eh? Zat's right: just break me anywhere and I will bleed a healing white sap for you.

Hey! Doctor dandelion. This is Susun Weed. How 'bout if you take a break and let me do the recipes for the pharmacy and the kitchen? You can come back and finish up with fun and facts, OK? OK!

Dandelion Pharmacy

Dandelion Wine à la Laughing Rock

Our year's supply for rituals and medicine

2 gal/8 liter crock
3-5 qts/3-5 liters blossoms
5 qts/5 liters water
***

3 pounds/1.5 kg sugar
1 organic orange
1 organic lemon
***

1 pkg/8 grams live yeast
wholewheat bread toast
***

Find a field of dandelions in bloom on a glorious shining day. Follow the honey bees to the finest flowers. Pick them with a sweeping motion of your parted fingers, like a comb. I leave the green sepals on, but get rid of all stalks. Back home, put blossoms immediately into a large ceramic, glass, or plastic vessel. Boil water; pour over flowers. Cover your crock with cheese cloth. Stir daily for three days. On the fourth day, strain blossoms from liquid. Cook liquid with sugar and rind of citrus (omit rind if not organic) for 30-60 minutes. Return to crock. Add citrus juice. When liquid has cooled to blood temperature, soften yeast, spread on toast, and float toast in crock. Cover and let work two days. Strain. Return liquid to crock for one more day to settle. Filter into very clean bottles and cork lightly. Don't drink until winter solstice.

Preparation time: A week's worth of effort yields a drink not only delightful but good for your liver, as well.

Dandelion Apéritif

several months' supply

2-3 cups/500-750ml fresh dandelion blossoms
⅔ cup/160ml sugar
rind of half a lemon
1 quart/1 liter vodka

Do not wash flowers. Cut off green. Mix all ingredients into jar; cap. Shake daily. Resist for at least two weeks, then strain and enjoy! Enjoy with ice and lemon. Enjoy with hot water and honey. Enjoy it by itself, before or after meals.

Preparation time: Not much more than half an hour. Any edible flower or herb can take the place of dandelion blossoms, in case you want to experiment with this easy effective way of making your medicines.

Doctor Dandelion's Homebrew

15 bottles of beer

1 lb/475g sugar
1 oz/30g cream of tartar
½ oz/15 grams ginger
½ lb/235 grams dandelion
5 quarts/5 liters water
1 cake or 1 Tbs/15ml yeast

Wash well a large non-metal fermentation vessel. Put sugar and cream of tartar into vessel. Wash dandelion (use any mix of roots and leaves) and chop coarsely. Boil 10 minutes with grated ginger and water. Strain through cloth into fermenting vessel. Stir well until sugar is completely dissolved. When cooled to blood temperature brew is ready for yeast. Dissolve yeast in water and add to vessel. Cover the lot with a clean cloth and let it ferment for 3 days. Siphon off into sterile bottles and cap. Store bottles on their sides for a week before opening. Tastes best well chilled.

Preparation time: 10 days is not very long to wait for bottled cheer. You can make up lots of batches of beer while you're still waiting to open the first bottle of your dandelion wine. Thanks to Audrey Hatfield for preserving the way of this delightful beer.

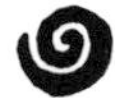

Dandelion Kitchen

Very Fancy (but easy) Dandelion Salad

serves 4-6

4 c/1 liter dandelion greens
4 c/1 liter lettuce leaves
1 hard boiled egg
croutons:
2 slices stale bread
2 tablespoons/30ml olive oil
garlic powder & salt to taste
dressing:
¼ c/60ml olive oil
1 tablespoon/15ml tamari
2 tsp/10ml lemon juice

Wash and dry greens; tear into bite-sized pieces in a blue or red bowl. Slice egg and add. Cut bread into small cubes and fry in oil until crisp. Sprinkle with garlic powder and salt. Make dressing in a small jar. Toss into salad just before serving; garnish with croutons and edible flowers.

Preparation time: 15-20 minutes in the kitchen; ten minutes or so in the garden. Remember to make the hard-boiled egg ahead of time!

Dandelion Egg Noodles

serves 6

2 c/500ml minced d'lion leaf
1 c/250ml boiling water
1¾ c/440ml wh. wheat flour
1 egg, well beaten
2-4 Tbs/30-60ml broth
***
3 quarts/3 liters water

Cook finely minced leaves in water until mushy, 15-20 minutes. Drain, reserving broth. Combine with flour, egg, and enough broth to make a very stiff dough. Roll out, on a floured surface, thinly. Let dry 2-4 hours. Cut into noodles. Cook in boiling, salted water about 30 minutes. Serve with sauté of garden vegetables.

Preparation time: 3-5 hours, but only 15-20 minutes of that is active. The color of these noodles is incredibly green, and what a flavor!

Dandelion Blossom Syrup

tastes like honey

1 qt/1l dandelion flowers
1 quart/1 liter water
2 pounds/1kg sugar
½ lemon, organic if poss.

Put blossoms and water in an enamel pot. Bring just to a boil, turn off heat, cover, and let sit overnight. Strain and press liquid out of spent flowers. Add sugar and sliced citrus (peel and all, if organic) and heat slowly, stirring now and again, for several hours or until reduced to a thick, honey-like syrup.

Preparation time: Two days of gathering and steeping, squeezing and slowly simmering give you lots of time to feel the Wise Woman wisdom in this brew. It is a treasure passed from wise woman to wise woman. I first tried it many years ago. Maria Treben says she learned it from her mother, who learned it from a woman she saw carrying dandelion blossoms. Who will receive it from you?

Dandelion Coffee

serves 8

8 Tbs/120ml roasted dandelion root
6 cups/1.5 liters water

Dig dandelion roots in autumn. Cut leaves off a short distance from root crown. Eat greens; dry roots whole. When roots are crisply dry, in about two weeks, roast them in a very slow oven. Check frequently and remove from heat as soon as dark. Grind whole roots as need arises. Brew in a percolator if at all possible.

Preparation time: From dried root to coffee cup in not that much longer than getting in a car and driving to the store, all in all. This drink is stimulating to the digestion, like coffee, but not to the nerves, so it helps you get a move on without getting stressed out.

Dandelion Bud Breakfast

serves 4

2 cups/500ml dandelion buds
½ cup/125ml water or butter
***
½ onion, minced
2 tablespoons/30ml olive oil
3 Tbs/45ml wholewheat flour
1 cup/250ml milk or water
1 cup/250g cheese
***
4 slices wholemeal bread
4 poached eggs

Steam buds 3-5 minutes and drain. Or cook in foaming butter. They may burst into bloom! Set aside. Make sauce: sauté onion in oil until tender; add flour; cook and stir a minute or two; slowly stir in water or milk, then cheese, and salt to taste; cook until thick, stirring. Sauce may be stored overnight if desired. Add cooked buds to warm sauce before serving. To serve, top toast with egg and sauce. Garnish with violets and columbine.

Preparation time: This rather elaborate breakfast takes 45 minutes to prepare, but what a great excuse to be outside early, barefoot, in the dew! Any extra buds are great in omelets and spectacular in stir-fry.

Fast Flower Fritters

serves 2 generously

1 c/250ml wholewheat flour
2 tsp/10ml baking powder
pinch salt
1 egg
½ c /125ml milk or water
2 tablespoons/30ml olive oil
1 c/250ml yellow parts of dandelion flowers

Mix dry ingredients. Beat egg; add liquid and oil. Stir into dry mix. Stir in yellow florets. Cook like pancakes. Serve very hot with jam, syrup, or butter.

Preparation time: When the dandelion is in full bloom I can pick a cup of blossoms in five minutes. Then it's another 15-25 minutes until the first fritters are hot off the griddle. For a super heart-healthy variation, leave out the egg and cook without any oil. The help of several children adds great joy to the preparation of this recipe.

Stir-Fry Dandelion Roots

serves 4

- 1 lb/475g young d'lion roots
- 6 ounces/170g mushrooms
- 1 cup/250ml sliced onion
- 4 cloves garlic, minced
- 3 tablespoons/45ml olive oil
- 3 tablespoons/45ml tamari
- 1 Tbs/15ml dark sesame oil

Wash and chop young dandelion roots and leaves harvested from the early spring garden. Drain. Sauté onion and sliced mushrooms in oil until soft and a little brown. Add garlic and drained dandelion; cover and cook 5-10 minutes, until tender, stirring occasionally. Turn off heat; add tamari and dark sesame oil. Let sit a minute or two before serving.

Preparation time: 25-30 minutes in the kitchen, plus harvesting time in the garden. I usually make this at the same time I'm putting up spring-dug dandelion tincture.

Dandy Pumpkin Soup

serves 3-6

- 2 c/500ml pumpkin cubed
- 4 cups/1 liter water
- 2 c/500ml dandelion leaf
- 1 large onion, chopped
- 3 tablespoons/45ml olive oil
- 2 c/500ml milk or water
- salt to taste

Combine pumpkin pieces with water and finely chopped dandelion leaf in a large pot and simmer, covered, until tender. Meanwhile, sauté onion, and garlic if you like, just a little. *For a smooth soup:* put everything in a blender and blend, using liquid as needed. *For chunky soup:* blend most of pumpkin and dandelion, pour back in pot with remaining chunks. Add sauté and milk. Garnish with chrysanthemum petals.

Preparation time: 25-35 minutes. A surprisingly sweet soup which I sometimes spice up with fresh grated nutmeg. A delicious way to get ready for cold weather.

Dandelion Dip

serves 2 for dinner, 6 for a party

¼ cup/60ml yogurt
½ c/125ml cottage cheese
1 c/250ml dandelion greens
garlic powder
salt to taste

Mix cottage cheese and yogurt. Mince greens well, then add. (Or combine all ingredients in blender.) Season with garlic and salt. Serve with oatcakes (recipe, p. 209) or corn chips.

Preparation time: Not much more than 10-15 minutes unless there's a particulary marvelous sunset that detains me whilst picking the greens.

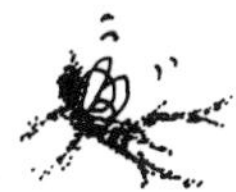

"When splendid salads were appreciated, dandelion's bitter leaves, shredded or chopped roots, and sweet, tangy flowers were all highly prized ingredients." *Audrey Wynne Hatfield (1898)*

Standard Greens

with international variations

per person:
1 c/250ml dandelion greens
¼ cup/60ml water in pot

Wash greens well. Chop coarsely without drying. Add to pot with water. Bring to a boil. Reduce heat and cook to your taste: some like 'em firm and some like 'em mushy.

French style: Add sliced raw garlic two minutes before greens are done. Serve with olive oil, salt and fresh pepper.

English style: Add up to 1 tablespoon/5ml vinegar and dash of salt to the cooked greens.

Russian style: Serve greens topped with sour cream and thin slices of raw onion.

German style: Add a lump of butter and slices of hard-boiled egg before serving.

Southern style: Depending on your means (that's Southern for how rich you are) add a piece of salt pork, or fat back, or even ham to the greens, and boil 'em up real good.

New York style: Fry one piece bacon per person. Crumble over hot greens.

Oriental Dandelion Soup

serves 4-6

8 c/2 liters water
5 oz/175g soba noodles
8 c/2 l dandelion greens
1 c/250ml onion, chopped
1 Tbs/15ml olive oil
2 Tbs/30ml dried kelp
1 Tbs/15ml grated ginger
½ c/125ml scallion tops
3 Tbs/45ml miso
(diluted in ½ c/125ml water)

Bring water to a boil. Add noodles; cook ten minutes. Add chopped greens and reduce heat to very low. Sauté onion in oil until clear. Add to soup along with all other ingredients except miso. Cook 5-10 minutes. Turn off heat. Dilute miso and add to soup. Garnish each bowl with a a single calendula blossom or a carrot swirl.

Preparation time: 35-45 minutes in the kitchen; plus 15-30 minutes in the garden to enjoy the sun and the birds and, oh yes, to cut onion tops and gather dandelion leaves.

Worthy Winter Soup

serves 3-6

1 cup/250ml dried beans
4 cups/1 liter water
2 cups/500ml onion, diced
2 tablespoons/30ml olive oil
1 c/250ml fresh d'lion root
or ¼ c/60ml dried d'lion rt.
1 c/250ml wild/garden carrot
½ c/125ml dried seaweed
8 cups/2 liters water
salt to taste
1 tablespoon/15ml miso

Soak beans in warm water overnight. Drain (water your houseplants with the soaking water). Sauté onion in oil in a soup pot until brown. Add soaked beans, chopped roots, seaweed and water, but no salt. Cover and cook slowly for several hours. Just before serving, dilute miso in some of the broth and add to soup.

Preparation time: 5 minutes (and a forethought the evening before) to soak the beans and then maybe 15 minutes cutting and cooking. While you wait the 2 hours for the soup to cook, why not put a bread in the oven?

Dandy Autumn Dish

serves 4

- 4 c/1 liter dandelion leaves
- 4 potatoes, cubed
- 1 large onion, chopped
- 2 tablespoons/30ml olive oil
- 1 c/250ml chopped tomatoes
- 1 c/250ml cheese

Wash dandelion leaves and chop. Put in saucepan with potatoes and water to cover. Bring to a boil and simmer for 15 minutes. Meanwhile sauté onion (and up to 1 c/250ml wild mushrooms if available) until soft. Drain saucepan; reserve water for future soup or bread. Stir in sautéed stuff, tomatoes, and salt to taste. Crumble cheese on top and bake at 350 F/80 C until cheese melts.

Preparation time: A slow and easy 30-40 minutes will take you to dinner, if potatoes and tomatoes are already harvested and close at hand, and a bag of dandelion greens is in the fridge.

Love of the Earth

serves 4-6

- 1 c/250ml dandelion roots
- 4 c/1 liter cubed potatoes
- 2 c/500ml dandelion leaves
- 2 c/500ml onion, diced
- 2 or more cloves garlic
- 2 tablespoons/30ml olive oil
- 2 tablespoons/30ml vinegar
- salt to taste

Clean and chop dandelion roots and cook with potatoes in water to cover. Meanwhile, sauté onion 5 minutes, add chopped dandelion leaves, cover and cook over low heat until potatoes in other pot are done. Drain roots and spuds, reserving water for future soup or bread, and put in serving bowl. Mix everything else together and add to bowl. Serve hot or cold.

Preparation time: 30-45 minutes once in the kitchen. Coming in from the garden with a bucket of dandelion and potato, onion and salad greens, I turn on the oven and mix up a cornbread. While it cooks, I make "Love of the Earth" and a salad. Dinner's on the table in an hour.

Hot Stuff Dandelion

serves 6-8

1 lb/500g dandelion root
2 tablespoons/30ml olive oil
4 or more cloves garlic
¼ cup/60ml sesame seed
1 Tbs/15ml hot sesame oil

Wash roots (fine to use leaves too) and slice thinly on a diagonal. Cook in water to cover until tender, 15 minutes. Drain and sauté in oil for 5 minutes alone, then for 5 minutes with sesame and garlic. Add hot oil and serve.

Preparation time: 40-45 minutes, or just long enough for a pot of brown rice to cook (start it first) and for you to put together a salad. How long it will take you to actually dig the roots beforehand depends . . . most days, most places, a good hour at least.

Dandelion Fun and Facts

And now ze part I've been waiting for, where I get to be catty (I am a lion, eh?) and say what I zink about what zey say about me! And where I get to really strut out my stuff. Ooh, la, la, chère. Here goes.

• Bradford Angier is a real gentlemen, oui. He describes me most poetically in his exceedingly useful *Field Guide to Edible Wild Plants.*

• And I love Monsieur Moore. He has a real good grasp on me in *Medicinal Plants of the Mountain West.* And I do like men with a good grasp.

• Maria Treben is a dear friend of mine and she has her own Wise Woman ways wiz me. She suggests using a tea made from ten of my fresh flower stalks every day for half a moon cycle (two weeks) to heal those with liver pain, metabolic disturbances, diabetes, and spleen, stomach, and skin problems.

• Don't you just adore how tasty I am? Thanks to Connie and Arnold Krochmal for "Dandelion Noodles" and "Dandy Pumpkin Soup" recipes. Their petit livre *Cooking with Wild Plants* has lots more, including amazing pancakes. Invite me for breakfast, eh, chère?

• Ze prize for ze most dandelion recipes goes to Gai Stern in *Australian Weeds.* She has eleven ways to intoxicate yourself wiz my deliciousness.

• John Evelyn, in *Acetaria,* says of my leaves: *"With this homely salley, Hecate entertained Theseus."* (Salley is a salad, eh?)

• Maida Silverman is a true friend to ze weeds and she has nice words, nice stories, and nice recipes for dandelion in *A City Herbal.* Une bonne fille, eh? I hear her book is out of print and zink someone should do somezing about it.

• My root is official medicine all over ze world. In America, you find me in ze United States Pharmacopoeia (1831-1926) and in ze National Formulary (1888-1965).

• One of ze many studies showing my power is reported in "Pharmacology of inulin drugs and their theraputic use. II. Chicorium intybus; taraxacum offinale," by L. Kroeber in *Pharmazie,* 5, 122-127; 1950.

• Ze société fleur essence sells a dandelion gift pack, of all zings! You get a bottle of dandelion flower essence, a bottle of dandelion flower oil, and a pin-up photo of moi! Très jolie! Ze address is: FES, POBox 1769, Nevada City, CA, 95959.

• Now a little brag. Is OK, because zis is ze time to brag, and how will you know zes zings if I don't tell you, eh? In addition to being an important source of food for bees, dandelion pollen is used by more than 90 different insects. Impressive, eh?

• Ze whole dandelion plant is one of the six herbal activators in biodynamic compost starter. I tell you, I am ze hot stuff, eh?

• Do you recall, s'il vous plaît, that I am one of the five bitter herbs of the Bible, book of Exodus?

• While I am actively growing, I exhale ethylene gas. While zis gas does slow ze growth of nearby plants, and so makes me an unwelcome guest near many prize specimens, it is ever so useful in ze orchard making ze fruit ripen evenly and early. (And do not forget how attractive I am to ze bees which pollinate ze fruit blossoms, chère.)

• Messages, messages . . . my seed parachutes are ze original overnight express mail. Send a message to your love zis way: hold a single stalk gone to seed in both hands, focus your mind on your message, and blow! Any leftover seeds are parts of the message zat aren't sent.

• Some of my flying seeds have been found over ten kilometers, zat's more than five miles, from me!

• Children, alors, ze children. Mine fly away, so I call to ze human children to play wiz me. And zey do! I love ze delight and joy zey exude while weaving crowns of my glorious fleurs. Ah, chère, children they fly. I have no more to say today. Perhaps another day you sing to me some more, eh? Zen we talk. Au revoir.

Doctor D's Appendix

alors: so, then
apéritif: before-dinner drink
bébé: baby
bonjour: good day
chère: dear (to a woman)
  ma chère: my dear
complexité: complexity
créature splendide: splendid creature
différente: different
enchantés: enchanted
excusez-moi: excuse me
fleur: flower
individualité: individuality
joie: joy
joie de vivre: joy of living
joyeuse: cheerful
le sacre du printemp: the rites of spring
les maladies de foie: liver disease
magnifique: magnificent
merci: thank you
moi: me
n'est-ce pas?: isn't it so? right?
non: no
oui: yes
petite livre: little book
petite promenade: little walk
petite zing avec wings: little winged things
quelle absurdité: what a joke!
regardez: regard, look
s'il vous plaît: if you please
spécialité: speciality
très amusant: very funny
très bien: very good
très jolie: very pretty
une bonne fille: a good girl
unité: unity

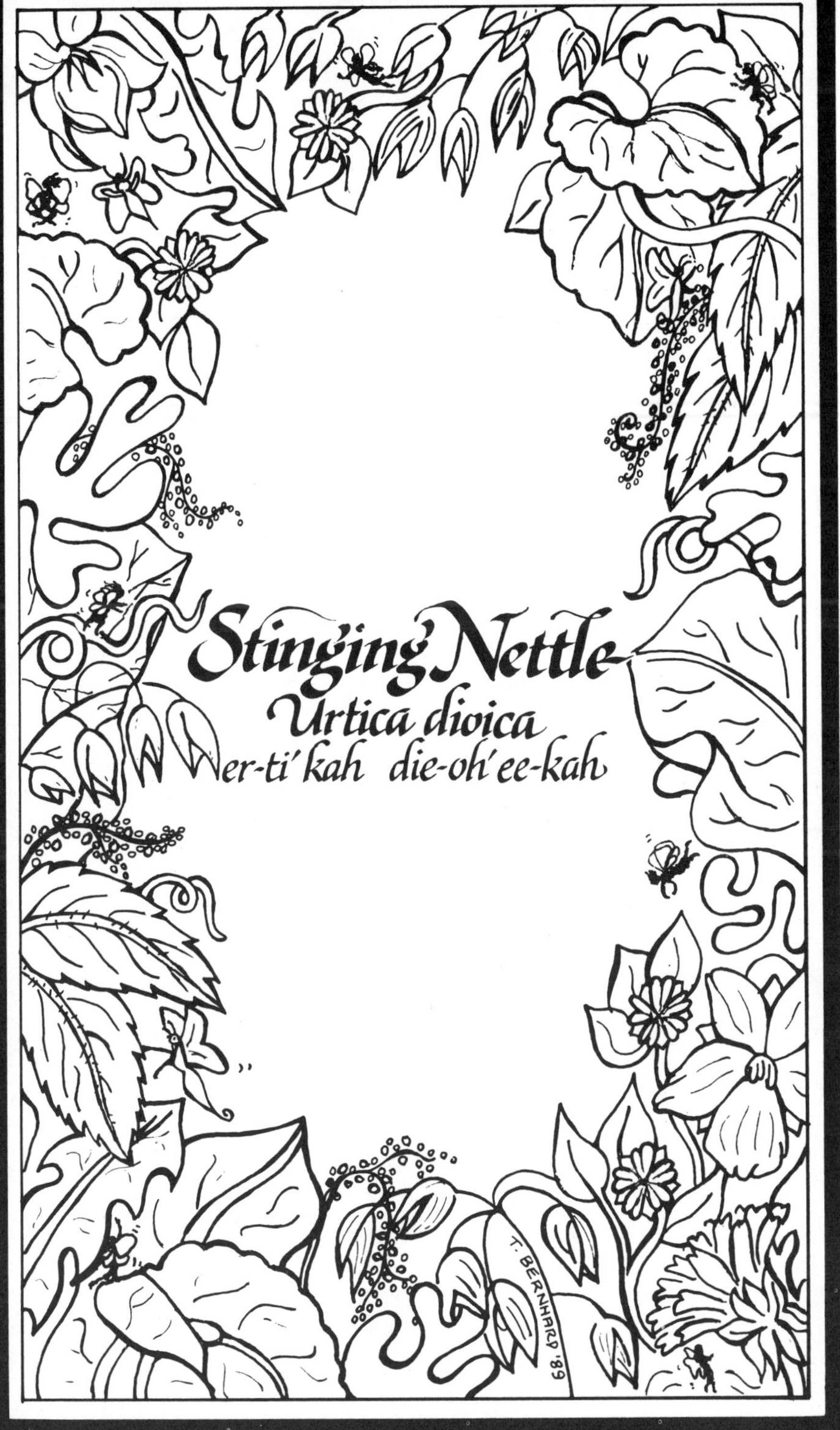
Stinging Nettle
Urtica dioica
er-ti'kah die-oh'ee-kah
T. BERNHARD '89

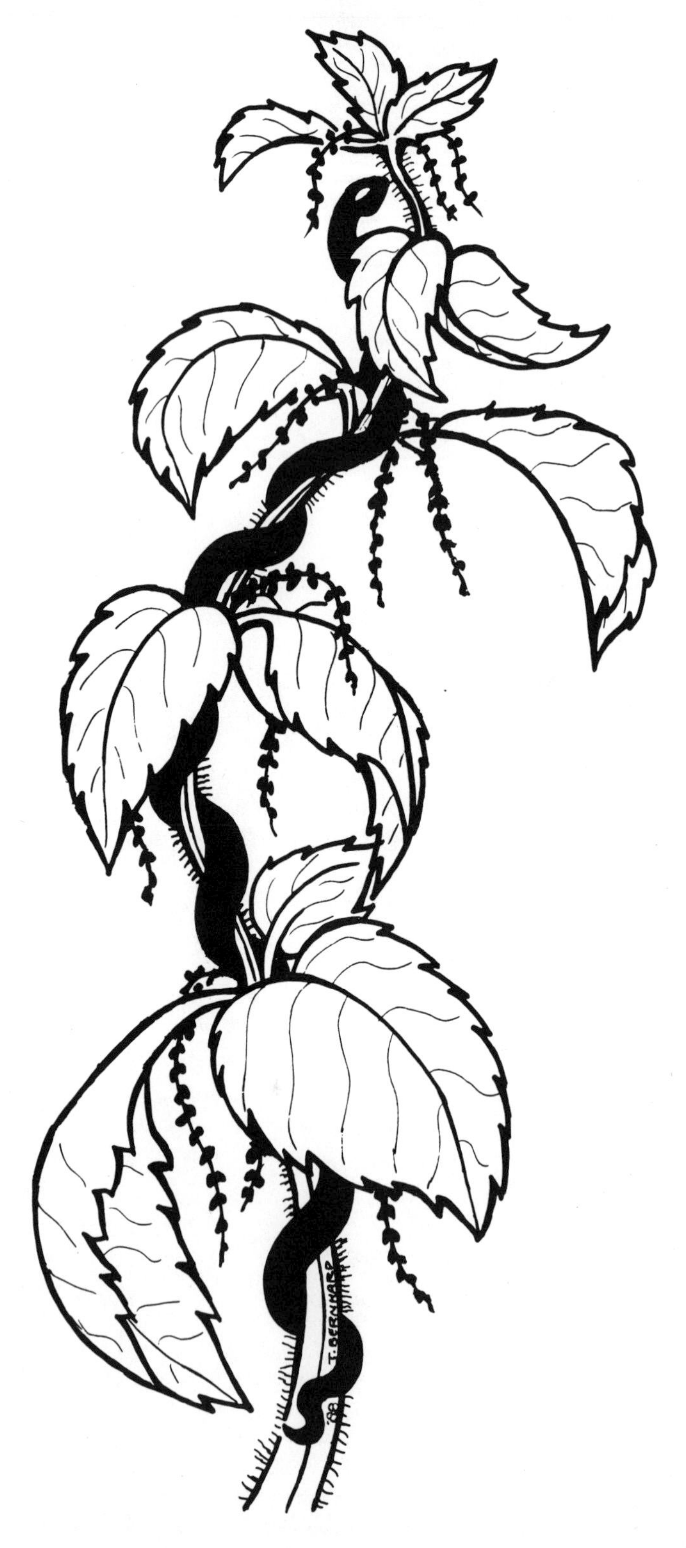
T. BERNHARD
'88

Stinging Nettle Speaks

Now pay attention. Do pay attention so I don't have to repeat myself. You humans do not seem to pay much attention. Do you think you can quiet yourself enough to pay attention to me? I am stinging nettle, though you may call me sister spinster, if you like. I have some things of import to impart to you, if you will just pay attention.

How can I help you pay attention? Let's try this: close your eyes and become aware of the sun on your skin, and the breeze tickling your temples, and the rich scent of the earth, and the chuckle of the stream. Feel the complex and satisfying nourishment available to you here where I live. And know that this is what I am: this complex nourishment of sun, wind, soil, and water, transformed by my attention and my care, transformed into food for you, into milk for you.

Green milk for you. Are you finding it easier to pay attention? Keep your eyes closed now; and continue to feel the warm sun, the gentle zephyrs, the deep earth, the sensitive waters. Feel all the rich and varied sensations available to you here in my home.

Let my voice move into your awareness, as I spin my sister story, as I tell you of my ability to feed you fully: I can nourish your energy, your being, your sense of self worth, and every cell in your body. Sister spinster, great green nettle, will nourish you with the care and joy that a mother brings to her task. I transform the very elements into green milk for you, green milk vibrantly alive with chlorophyll, calcium, iron, trace minerals, vitamins, proteins, and my own zest and love for life. I become, I am, the milk of your mother, the earth. I am the full breast of the earth, ripe for you to thrive on. I am the sweetness and richness that sustains you and heals you at your mother's breast.

Now, pay attention to the green as you slowly open your eyes. Continue to pay attention to the sounds, fragrances, tastes, and energies around you, and pay special attention to the green. Pay special attention to my green. My green is my love for you. What a delicious, dark, deep spinning green I am. What a lovely lilting green I am. Luxuriant green! Creative green! Sister green. Eat my green. Drink my green glow, my green that makes your blood so red, and your movements so flexible. My green that makes your mothers' milk so abundant, so rich. My green that makes your skin, your hair, so gleaming, so glowing.

Pay attention to my green. Pay attention to my words. Pay attention to the life that surrounds you, that moves you in its rhythms. Attention holds the image; attention snares the thought; attention pierces to the heart of the matter.

Pay attention to sister spinster stinging nettle. I feed you. I heal you. I teach you. I offer you the best of the earth. I guide you to walk in beauty. I inspire you to honor the earth and her green give-aways to you. And I sting you to attention!

Close your eyes, once more, dear sister. And remember with me the days of sisters spinning and weaving. As you spin and knot my nettle fibers into nets, know that I help you catch the many fishes: fish of the ocean, and fish of the mind, swift spirit fish, too. As you twine and weave my fibrous strength into carrying bags, remember to let me help you grasp the totality of life, to help you contain securely all that you have gathered. As you twist my resiliant inner fibers, fashioning me into rope, let yourself be spun as one with me. Let me tie it all together for you. String along with me. Spin sister, spin with me, the great green spinster.

Come spinning to me in the spring. Cut and eat my greens for two moons after they begin to grow, no more. And I will spin greenly into you. I will nourish your vital energy, increase your chi force, fertilize the ground of your garden and the ground of your being, and strengthen your kidneys and adrenals, so you may enjoy long life. What a delicious delight of spring green is the taste of your sister spinster.

Come as sister to cut my stalks at maturity and I'll supply you with thread, cloth, and cord. Come whenever you can, spinning or still, sister or nameless one, come, learn my ways, and I will guide you in the ways of attention. I will guide you along the spiraling beauty way.

It's all in the quality of one's attention.

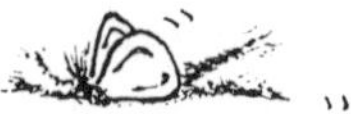

"Nettles are so well known that they need no description. They may be found, by feeling, in the darkest night." Culpeper (1561)

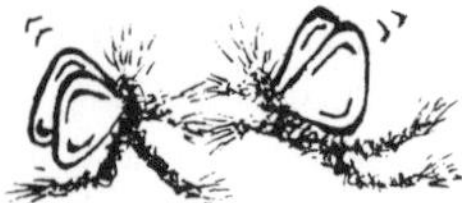

"I have eaten nettles, I have slept in nettle sheets, and I have dined off a nettle tablecloth. . . . I have heard my mother say that she thought nettle cloth more durable than any other . . . linen." Thomas Campbell (1803)

Nettle Facts

Botanical name: *Urtica dioica*; uro (Greek) means urine (nettle strengthens the kidneys); di-oikos (Greek) means in two houses (male and female flowers are separate). ***Other useful species:*** *U. gracilis, U. urens, U. procera, U. canadensis, U. pilulifera*, and related species, including *Laportea canadensis*/wood nettle. ***Natural order:*** Urticaceae/ Nettle family. ***English names:*** Stinging nettle, stingers, wild spinach, plaything, devil leaf (and no doubt more colorful names as well, to suit the moment). ***Chinese names:*** Hsieh-tzu-ts'ao. ***French names:*** Ortie, grande ortie. ***German names:*** Brennesselkraut, Kleine Brennessel. ***Huron (Native American) names:*** Anonhasquara. ***Pakistani names:*** Bichu, chicru. ***Russian names:*** Krapiva. ***Fiber uses:*** Nettle may have been cultivated in Mexico as early as 8,000 years ago; her fiber is used as paper pulp and is spun and woven into strong thread (fifty times stronger than cotton, almost as strong as silk), durable cloth, and long-wearing cordage. ***Dye uses:*** Various shades of green from the stalk and leaves, quite permanent; yellow from the root decocted with alum. ***Food uses:*** This spring potherb is avidly sought by old wives in the know. ***Medicinal uses:*** Commonly available in European, American, and Australian specialty shops as dried cut herb or in prepared hair lotions. ***Soil uses:*** Incredible soil enricher: add to compost heap; brew into plant food; grow in your garden as a boon companion to tomatoes and aromatic herbs. ***Animal uses:*** Favorite farmyard fodder and food supplement, dried, for dairy animals and poultry; good disinfectant wash for stalls. ***Habitat:*** Rich, wet soil; often near people; barnyards, gardens, streamsides. ***Natural range:*** Temperate Eurasia. ***Current range:*** From the Yukon of N. America, through Mexico, and Central America to S. America, even in the Andes; Sweden, Russia, Europe, Australia, New Zealand. ***Toxicity:*** *Externally,* nettle sting is intense, but short-lasting, except in some tropical species where the pain may be felt for years. The common nettle sting itches and burns for a few minutes to several hours, turns the skin red temporarily, and raises an occasional small blister. *Internally,* there is a small chance of adverse reactions such as nausea, a burning sensation in the digestive system, or hives from fresh nettle preparations. Use of plants that are, or were, flowering increases the risk of adverse effects. *Urtica ferox*, a native of New Zealand called *ongaonga* or tree nettle, is so toxic that the extract of five hairs can kill a guinea pig, and a fatal human poisoning has been reported. ***Best identified by:*** Deeply grooved stem; transparent short hairs on stalks and leaf undersides; blue-green, opposed, serrated leaves, like a giant mint.

Nettle Weed Walk

Come out into the richness of spring, the moist richness of spring to search with me for stinging nettles. We won't have much of a search, actually, since this dependable perennial shoots up her dark blue-green growth in the same places every year.

Come down here, where the water wells and seeps. Here's nettle. Come over here, in the corner where the barn meets the garden. Here's nettle. Look here, in the black soil spilled up by the river. Here's nettle.

So close to May Day we shall find plenty of big tender nettle leaves and stalks for our supper. See how the pointed and serrated leaves grow in pairs up the unbranched stalk, making her look like some huge, lush mint? And how deeply grooved the stalk is? When I cut through the stalk with my fingernail or knife, we can see inside the stalk, where it is hollow, and threaded through with pink. What a beautiful surprise!

The stinging hairs are also a hidden surprise. They stay discreetly underneath the leaves and scatter themselves down the stalk. They aren't sharp at all, just delicate. Lightly touch them or accidentally brush by them and drops of stinging acid are flipped at you. Touch them with attention and the acid stays put, where it can't sting you.

Ah! Look, in the sunnier spots the nettles are knee-high and taller. By the time this year's wheel has turned to harvest fest, some of these will be as tall as your head. They're so beautiful now, aren't they? Luscious revved up green energy . . . in the flush of growth . . . spring in her wildness!

Nettle is playful in the summer. She's grown so tall, and sports two kinds of flowers dancing, nodding, and frolicking in the breezes. No, you can't see the flowers now. May is too early in upstate New York.

You can hardly even see them when they're there, truth. But if you wait three moons, then come back, and look right here and here, at these places where the leaves grow from the stalks (those are her armpits, axils to the botanist), why, there you'll see lots of little strings of tiny light green pearls, the female flowers, arching out and down. And look here, at this plant, when you come back in the summer, look nearer the top and you'll see the tiny male flowers in dense tufts, pointing up.

I'll return here in autumn to harvest seed. Meanwhile, I'll keep a sharp eye on those female flowers. They set their seed and drop it to the ground in rapid succession once they bloom. So I have to time my seed collecting very precisely and ask the weather deva to give me a sunny day. Nettle is so lovely in autumn sun and autumn winds, about to bend to winter and return to her underground roots.

Have you ever seen the root? No, let's not dig one up today. I'll tell you what it looks like. It is small and white and skinny, and called not a root but a rhizome. I declare she can sting. This nettle, she likes to keep her roots, or rhizomes, to herself, I guess. Though if you can endure the sting, the roots can be transplanted easily enough. And what's more, they make a superb hair lotion.

Strange though it may seem, I've found that I won't get stung by nettle leaves or stalks if I pay careful attention and grasp firmly. Hmmm . . . maybe I've never paid enough attention to the nettle roots. Let's gently uncover these.

See how the nettle rhizomes cross over each other and weave a net in the earth? Do you know they talk to each other through this neural net? I found the truth of this last spring.

Contrary to my usual encounters with nettle (I am known for picking nettle bare-handed and for occasionally eating it raw) every time I went to pick nettles last spring, I got stung and stung. Some of the welts blistered and made my joints tingle, then feel numb. I couldn't figure out what was wrong; I was paying lots of attention to my beloved nettle. Why was she stinging me so?

Then I found the answer. I noticed some blue-green tips struggling out from under some unused garden pots I'd hastily piled in a corner of the greenhouse. Nettle! What a surprise. She'd never grown inside the greenhouse before. I cleared the pots away so she could grow up straight and apologized for not paying attention.

Next day (with the moon in Pisces, and still some weeks before the nettle would flower) I began my main harvest of tender nettle tops. Some we cooked for lunch, some we cooked and froze, but most I quickly hung in small bunches in a shady place to dry until crisp.

And I wasn't stung to attention by my sister spinster—though I admit that after a full day of handling nettle barehanded, my arms did tingle from fingertips to shoulder blades well into the night. I enjoy the sensation; it is intense, but not painful, like the pins-and-needles you get when circulation returns to a part that has "fallen asleep." Other people could feel the buzz in my hands whenever I touched them that evening. The next morning only a lingering warm glow reminded me of my reunion with sister nettle.

The harvest won't be for another few weeks this year, so you have plenty of time to get ready for it. Come here every day. Really pay attention to the nettle. Sing to her; talk to her; focus your full attention on the nettle. So long as you give her your full attention, she won't have to sting you to get it.

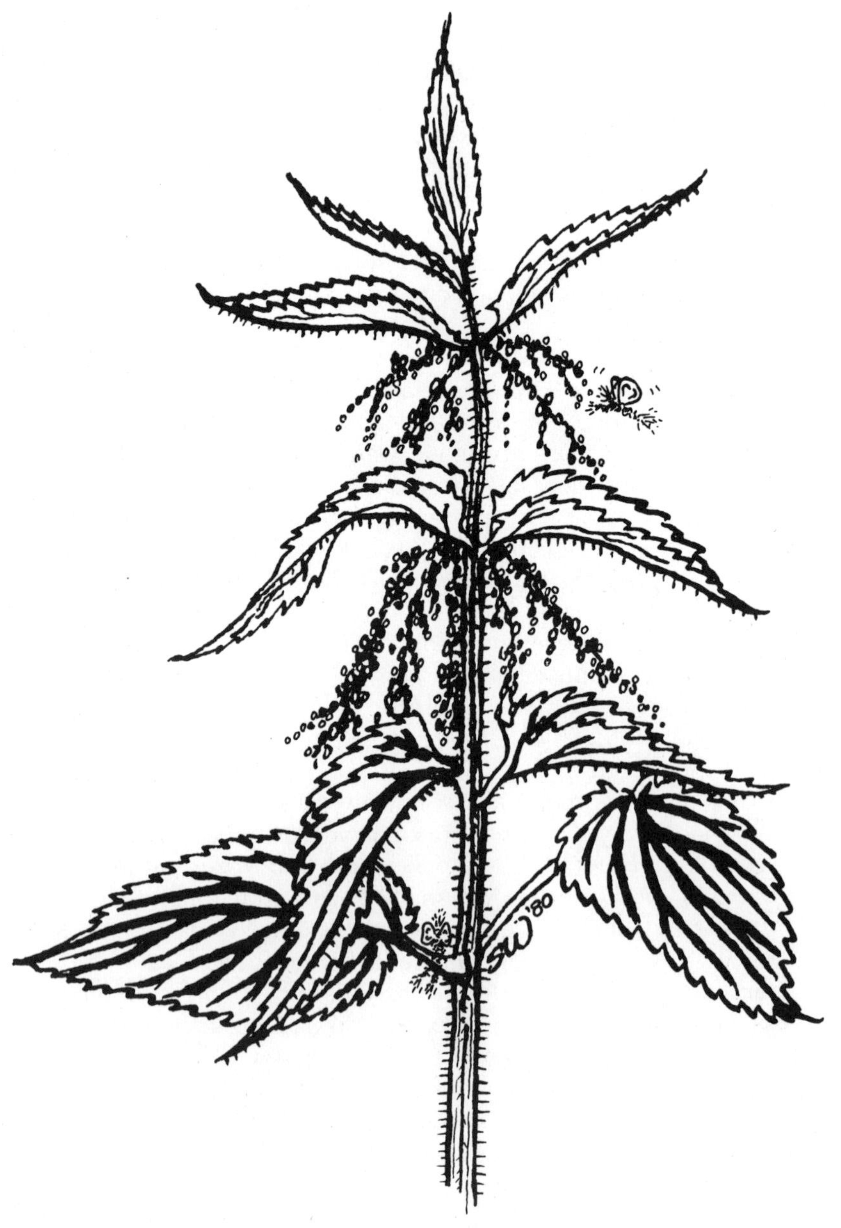

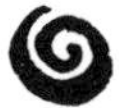

Stinging Nettle Leaf/Stalk Properties and Uses

- ***nutritive,*** tonic, galactogogue, anti-anaemic, anti-scorbutic
- ***kidney ally,*** diuretic, laxative, lithotriptic, anti-purine, chi strengthener
- ***alterative,*** antiseptic, depurative, anti-diabetic, anti-rheumatic
- ***pectoral,*** astringent, anti-asthmatic, expectorant, epispastic
- fresh nettle juice is ***hemostatic,*** styptic, anti-hemorrhagic

Stinging nettle leaves and stalks are gentle enough for an everyday **nourishing** brew and powerful enough to **heal** damaged tissue. **Kidneys, lungs, intestines,** and **arteries** are **tonified, strengthened,** and gradually **altered** toward optimum functioning with consistent use of nettle, freshly cooked or infused. Women love this rich green plant during **pregnancy, childbirth,** and **lactation** for its safe **diuretic** effect, its gentle restorative **laxative** effect, its assured **anti-hemorrhagic** power, and its contribution to their over all well-being. **Antiseptic** when fresh juice is used as a wash for skin, kitchen, or stable, nettle also clears **auras** and energetic pathways. **Hair** gleams, grows, thickens, and darkens when nourished and rinsed with nettle infusions. In my long-time alliance with sister spinster, I have also found nettle a powerful ally in restoring and maintaining the vibrancy of my **adrenals,** my hormonal and circulatory systems, my energetic, bio-chemical, and magnetic fields, and my emotional, sexual sensitivity. A friend well worth knowing, I say. Worth bringing home to dinner, in fact!

Use nettle leaves and stalks as an everyday nourisher, an energetic changer, a marvelous kidney/adrenal ally, a digestive restorative, a respiratory strengthener, an ally for women, a hair and skin nourisher, and a prompt hemostatic.

- Dose of *fresh nettle leaf tincture* is 5-100 drops a day, in water.
- Dose of *dried nettle leaf infusion* is 1-2 cups/250-500ml a day.
- Dose of *fresh nettle juice* is 1-3 teaspoons/5-15ml a day, in water.

Nettle Leaves and Stalks are an Everyday Nourisher

(Numbers indicate milligrams per hundred grams nettle herb)

Fresh young nettle is an excellent source of minerals, vitamins, and amino acids, protein building blocks. (Recent Russian research shows less amino acids in dried nettle.) Her superb, bio-active nourishment is readily absorbed by all soft tissue and working fluids: blood, lymph, hormones, and neurotransmitters. This results in increased ease and energy in the operation of the circulatory, immune, endocrine, nervous, and urinary systems. Sister spinster stinging nettle is highly recommended for pregnant and lactating women.

Sister spinster is very high in calcium (2900), magnesium (860), trace minerals, and chlorophyll (6 grams are extractable from a kilo of dried leaves).

Stinging nettle is high in chromiun (3.9), cobalt (13.2), iron (41.8), phosphorus (447), potassium (1750), zinc (4.7), copper, and sulphur, as well as the B complex of vitamins, especially thiamine (0.54) and riboflavin (0.43), and the carotenes, measured as vitamin A (15,700 IU).

Nettle leaves and stalks also supply niacin (5.2), protein (10.2%), manganese (7.8), selenium (2.2), silicon (10.3), tin (2.7), vitamin C complex, measured as ascorbic acid (83), and vitamins D and K.

Sodium levels (4.9) in nettle are quite low.

Frequent use of nourishing sister stinging nettle (as infusion or cooked green) along with Wise Woman ways is recommended for those wanting to stabilize blood sugar, reset metabolic circuits to normalize weight, reduce fatigue and exhaustion, restore adrenal potency to lessen allergic and menopausal problems, and eliminate chronic headaches. Nettle is also a powerful preventive for those with hereditary susceptibility to rheumatic complaints.

"If they would eat nettles in March, and drink mugwort in May, So many fine maidens would not go to the clay." Funeral song of a Scottish mermaid

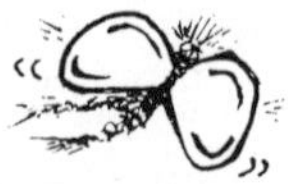

". . . cows fed on it give much milk and yellow butter. Makes horses smart and frisky. Stimulates fowls to lay many eggs." Rafinesque (1830)

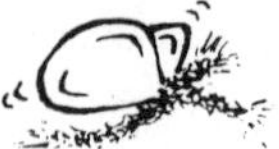

"I use lots of Urtica for all kinds of things. It is my favorite herb and I use it as a base in many formulas. I'm especially drawn to it for pale, pasty types." Cascade Anderson-Geller (1989)

Nettle Leaves and Stalks are an Energetic Changer

Nettle not only changes energy with her stings, she gives an herbal treatment to the entire energetic system: nerves, neurons, chakras, and subtle bodies. Nettle's sharp energy cuts loose old patterns and reweaves connections. Her glowing green nourishment strengthens reception of planetary and galactic pulse patterns, thus allowing natural strengthening of individual energy, and consequent strengthening of the immune system.

Nettle is a ally which—combined with Wise Woman ways—can help the gradual healing of a person with a chronic condition such as Epstein-Barr virus (EBV), hay fever, allergies, lymphatic swellings, ARC/AIDS, nerve inflammations (including lumbago and sciatica), persistent headaches, high blood pressure, inexplicable lethargy and exhaustion, repeated bouts of flu and colds, hardened arteries, weakened veins, infertility, rheumatism, joint aches, continuous skin eruptions, and loss of nerve sensitivity. With the help of sister spinster stinging nettle, and our Wise Woman ways, we are abundantly nourished and so grow to encompass more and more of ourselves along the spiral way of transformation.

Try a cup/250ml of nettle infusion, or a half cup/125ml cooked fresh greens and pot liquor, or a teaspoonful/5ml of the juice every nice spring day for at least a month.

Nettle Leaves and Stalks are a Marvelous Kidney/Adrenal Ally

Nettle infusions heal kidney cells like nothing else I've ever seen. The usual curative dose is one or two cups of infusion daily for ten to twelve weeks, or longer. Used in conjunction with Wise Woman ways, I have seen stinging nettle forstall the necessity of proposed dialysis.

As a tonic for adrenals and kidneys, try a cup daily for six weeks and then three or four cups a week for as long as you like.

Ask nettle to be your ally in healing those with gravel or stones in the kidneys or bladder, bloody urine, kidney pains, chronic urinary tract infections (UTI), diabetic water retention and kidney stress from insulin, chronic cystitis, dialysis and kidney surgery, stress, allergies, childbirth trauma.

Sister spinster's water energy (most potent in wild nettles) reestablishes chi/energy flow in the urinary, nervous, and subtle body systems.

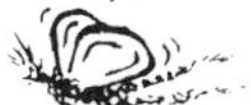

"The whole plant is powerfully medicinal, from the roots to the seeds."

Juliette Levy (1966)

Nettle Leaves and Stalks are a Digestive Restorative

Invite sister spinster stinging nettle to dinner. If she arrives dried, serve her as an after dinner tea or infusion. If she arrives freshly picked, use her as a fresh juice or eat the cooked greens (see **Nettle Kitchen**).

Do it often, for at least three weeks, and she'll help improve your digestion and prevent stomach aches by: tonifying your liver, gall bladder, and spleen; healing stomach and intestinal ulcers; nourishing the mucus membrane of the intestinal tract; relieving constipation; eliminating or reducing diarrhea; restoring tone to digestive system veins so hemorrhoids shrink; and clearing some intestinal infections. (Nettle extract inhibited Shigella strains and Staph. aureus in Russian tests. E. coli and Pseudomonas were unaffected.)

Those with hemorrhoids respond strongly to nettle sitz baths, as well as regular daily tonic use of the infusion to strengthen veins. Use two quarts/liters of nettle leaf infusion. Soak your sitzer in the warm infusion for ten minutes two or three times a day. Also, daub on fresh juice when available. An 1833 hemorrhoid cure calls for boiling nettle juice with "a little sugar," and instructs: "Take two ounces of it; it seldom needs repeating."

Another old book suggests that humans or beasts with roundworms or threadworms (pin worms) may be treated by steeping fresh nettle leaves in whey and drinking this exclusively for three days or longer until worms are gone. My experiences with worms have led me to believe that, while many cures will reduce worm infestations, chronic problems are best treated with drugs to debilitate the worms and herbs to prevent reinfection at high levels. Tonification of the digestive mucosa, circulation, and energy fields with nettle infusions after chemical deworming will go a long way to reducing chronic worm problems.

Nettle Leaves and Stalks are a Respiratory Strengthener

Breathe deeply. Make some fresh nettle juice. Blend a small amount of water, then an abundant amount of honey into the juice. This can be your ally, taken by the teaspoonful/5 ml, to help heal bronchial and respiratory tissues, stop internal bleeding, and curb excess mucus.

Try this nettle honey and some Wise Woman wiles when healing those with colds, flu, asthma, bloody coughs, bronchitis, pleurisy, lung or chest wall sores, pneumonia, AIDS-related respiratory diseases, even tuberculosis.

Old wives' stories circulate of people who cured themselves of severe lung diseases with daily use of nettle. Try a half-cup serving of nettle greens several times a week for up to three months, repeated for several years, or drink up to two cups of nettle infusion daily for the same length of time. And ask yourself these Wise Woman questions: *How is this problem my ally? What gifts does this problem bring? How can this make me, and the world, more whole?*

Boiled with barley and eaten as porridge several times a day, the fresh or dried leaves of sister spinster stinging nettle loosen and bring up deep congestion without irritating sensitive respiratory tissues.

Considered a specific for adults with asthmatic allergies, nettle tincture is used for acute care, and the infusion for restorative and healing care.

The fumes of nettle, inhaled in a sweat bath or from the steam rising off a reheated infusion, are an effective ally when healing yourself or others during and after pneumonia, bronchitis, or other (especially watery) chest complaints.

Nettle Leaves and Stalks are an Ally for Women

Sister spinster stinging nettle is the cherished friend of the tired teenage woman, the ever-hungry new mother, the crampy executive, wise woman midwives, and the emerging crone. Two cups/half liter of nettle infusion daily nourish and stabilize energy in the reproductive/hormonal systems, build nutrient-rich blood and expand the cells' capacity to metabolize nutrients.

Nettle is a wonderful ally for women with night sweats, exhaustion, anemia, chronic profuse menstrual flow, menstrual cramps, and those who have had a large blood loss during childbirth, surgery, or accident.

Many midwives suggest regular use of nettle infusions during the last trimester of pregnancy to add a plentiful supply of vitamin K and iron to the blood. They affirm sister spinster stinging nettle's reputation in reducing both the likelihood of hemorrhage and serious effects from postpartum hemorrhage. Should you hemorrhage, postpartum or otherwise, fresh nettle juice sipped frequently is your ally to help stop it. And to nourish yourself afterward, nettle infusion, of course; drink it regularly for several months.

Two weeks of two cups of nettle infusion daily will noticeably improve the quantity and quality of many women's breast milk. Three or more cups of the infusion weekly will provide optimum bio-active minerals, especially calcium, vitamins, and proteins to nourish you and ensure nutrient-rich milk. If I had acres of it, I'd make nettle hay for my milking goats!

Nettle Leaves are a Hair and Skin Nourisher

Glossy, thick, vibrant hair, healthy, hard nails and clear, lustrous, smooth skin are yours when sister spinster stinging nettle becomes your ally. So say the gypsies, myself, Czech researchers, and every friend who's tried it. Use a half cup/125ml of cooked nettle or drink up to one cup/250ml of infusion three or four times weekly, in addition to using nettle hair rinse at least once a week.

The simplest rinse is made by combining a cup/250ml of rainwater and a spoonful (any size spoon) of nettle vinegar. See **Nettle Pharmacy** for fancier potions.

Recommended especially to balance over-oily skins and scalps, nettle treatments nourish new growth, check falling hair, encourage supple strength, and remove fungal and bacterial infections of scalp, nails, and skin, including acne. Try nettle infusion, from fresh or dried plants, as a facial, hair rinse, bath, and dentifrice (great for gums).

When your skin is a chronic problem, try Wise Woman ways and nettle. For healing yourself or others with problems such as acne, eczema, fungal infections, eat at least half a cup/125ml of cooked nettle daily, or drink up to two cups of infusion daily, for six to ten weeks.

Tincture of fresh nettle, fresh nettle juice, or homeopathic Urtica is preferred for easing pain, nourishing the immune system, and helping heal those with acute skin rashes, such as hives, measles, or chicken pox. Try 1/4 teaspoon/1ml fresh juice or 5-25 drops tincture in water. This may be repeated up to six times in a day, but only for a few days. Thereafter, use only one or two doses a day.

Russian herbalists use the fresh juice as a toothache cure.

Fresh nettle leaves bruised, or pounded with salt, applied at least three times daily, help heal those with external ulcers, boils, foul sores, abscesses, and infected splinters.

A wash or soak of nettle infusion (or the fresh juice) is your antiseptic healing first-aid for those with cuts, minor wounds, heat rash, burns, corns, diabetic foot problems, and sore feet.

Try nettle lotion or ointment to relieve those with swelling and stinging from insect stings and bites, rashes, burns, hives, fungus infections, and pityriasis (a mild, self-limiting rash known also as "Christmas tree rash.")

"Most people know Nettle by experience or reputation, but rather fewer by appearance." M. Moore (1979)

Nettle Leaves and Stalks are a Prompt Hemostatic

The juice of fresh nettle, the broth from her cooked greens, and full strength nettle infusions are all reliable ways to use one of sister spinster's most notable properties: stopping bleeding. Sip frequently, during and after hemorrhage.

Nettle is an excellent ally along with your other Wise Woman ways when you're healing yourself or others with profuse menses, nose bleeds (epistaxis), bloody urine, hemorrhage from lungs, bloody coughs, bleeding hemorrhoids, bloody stools (check for possible cancer), bloody vomit, and childbirth hemorrhages.

Jamaicans put fresh juice into open wounds.

Finely powdered nettle leaves make a fine styptic to stop bleeding from razor and glass cuts, nosebleeds, and other minor wounds.

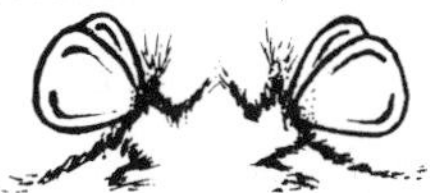

"For hemorrhages, the expressed juice of the fresh leaves is regarded as more effective than the decoction, given in teaspoonful doses every hour or as often as the nature of the case requires."

GP Wood, MD & EH Ruddock, MD (1925)

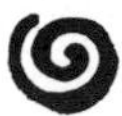

Nettle Seed Properties and Uses

- ***antiseptic,*** rejuvenative
- ***vermifuge,*** anthelmintic, laxative
- hypnotic

Nettle seed nourishes the **endocrine glands,** antidotes poisons internally and externally, and provides a curative, unique wine. **Hair** and **skin** are strongly influenced by nettle seeds.

Use nettle seeds as a thyroid helper, a poison antidote, a skin and scalp tonic, and a curative wine.

- Dose of *fresh* or *dried nettle seeds* is ¼ teaspoon/1ml daily.

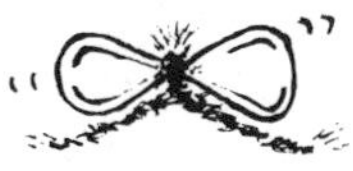

"The seed of nettle stirreth up lust. . . ." Gerarde-Johnson (1633)

Nettle Seeds are a Thyroid Helper

"A sovereign remedy for big neck," says Gunn in 1859. A century and a half later, herbalists still agree that nettle seed can help nourish the thyroid and reduce both excess weight and goiter. Thirteen seeds taken three times a day is the ritual dose.

Nettle Seeds are a Poison Antidote

Eating nettle seeds is a reputed antidote to poisoning from hemlock, henbane, nightshade, spider bites, bee stings, snake bites, and dog bites. The immune system is alerted and energized rapidly by use of any nettle preparation, so that may justify this use. I've not had occasion to try it. Nettle's ability to strengthen the kidneys and liver (organs responsible for eliminating poisons) is also noteworthy when considering the validity of this poison antidote assertion.

Nettle Seeds are a Skin and Scalp Tonic

To revitalize and remove infection from human scalp and hair, as well as the skin and fur of animals, use nettle seeds internally and externally. Soak one teaspoon/5ml seeds in hot water for twenty minutes. Strain, then sponge liquid onto scalp or skin, leaving on overnight. Or use as a final rinse after shampooing.

Alternately, try powdering seeds and mixing with honey to form a sticky ointment; especially recommended if the scalp/skin irritation is exceptionally dry, flaky, or hot. Cover and leave overnight. Wash out next morning.

Nettle seed oil may be used as a daily hair dressing, or applied to smaller, local sores for healing help.

Nettle Seeds Make a Curative Wine

A tablespoon/15ml of nettle seeds soaked in a glass of wine overnight, the whole lot warmed and sweetened, and taken throughout the day, is part of a Wise Woman way for healing those with fevers, flus, impotence, testicular irritations, and diarrhea (if acute, seeds may be cooked in wine for five minutes and taken immediately). This also helps return tone and capillary strength to respiratory tissues stressed by bronchitis, pneumonia, whooping cough, and such. Increase consumption to three wineglassfuls a day if needed.

Nettle Root Properties and Uses

(especially of *Laportea canadensis*/wood nettle)

- ***tonic,*** diuretic
- ***astringent,*** antidiarrheal

Use nettle root as a hair and scalp tonic, a urinary strengthener and stimulant, an immune system/lymphatic strengthener, and for a bit of first aid.

- Dose of *fresh nettle root tincture* is 5-90 drops a day, in water.
- Dose of *dried nettle root infusion* is 4-8 ounces/125-250ml a day.

Nettle Root is a Hair and Scalp Tonic

Those with thinning hair, dandruff, scalp infections, and hair loss after chemotherapy or giving birth, can try rubbing the scalp every morning and night with nettle root decoction or tincture. The mild hormonal effect of nettle leaf or seed taken internally strengthens the effect of the external applications. See **Nettle Pharmacy** for some hair tonic recipes.

Nettle Root is a Urinary System Strengthener/Stimulant

Frequent sips of nettle root infusion or decoction ease those with urinary discomfort and initiate strong kidney action. Ask sister spinster stinging nettle to give you her roots to help reduce water retention, stop bleeding and encourage the passage of kidney stones and gravel from the urinary tract, relieve dropsy symptoms (as well as helping to prevent incipient dropsy), reduce urethral swelling/urethritis and prostate swelling/prostatitis, and help eliminate chronic cystitis.

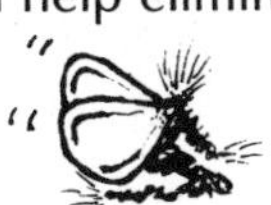

"I myself rub this tincture [of Nettle root] into the scalp daily; I even take it with me on trips. It is worth the effort; no dandruff, and the hair is thick and soft with a beautiful sheen. . . ." Maria Treben (1982)

Nettle Root is an Immune System/Lymphatic Strengthener

When immune system stress is severe, as in people dealing with AIDS/ARC, EBV, genetic tendencies to cancer (including DES children), intermittent fevers such as malaria, and constant exposure to chemicals, try daily use of nettle root tincture (5-30 drops, up to three times a day) along with your other Wise Woman wiles. *Note: Overuse or excessive doses are reported to cause hallucinations.* Sips of the root decoction are used if the tincture is unavailable or inappropriate.

Nettle Root is a Bit of First Aid

Sipping nettle root decoction helps stop dysentery, loose bowels, and diarrhea.

Speakers and actors ward off hoarseness by mixing the dried, powdered root with an equal amount of molasses, forming lozenges, and sucking them.

Using the root vinegar as a salad dressing is excellent for the spleen.

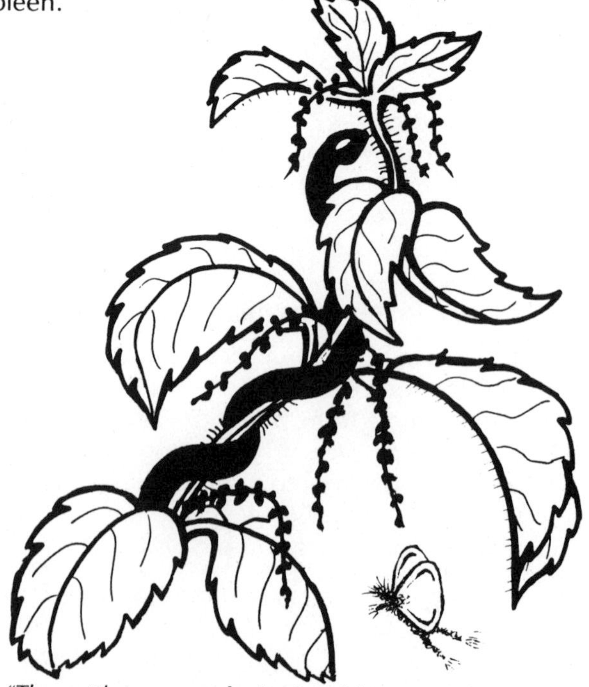

"The nettle, or ***wergulu****, in the old Wessex dialect of the tenth century, was one of the nine sacred herbs along with mugwort, plantain, watercress, chamomile, crab apple, chervil, and fennel."* Adele Dawson (1980)

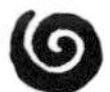

Nettle Sting Properties and Uses

• ***stimulant,*** rubefacient, antiseptic

Nettle Sting is No Joke

Being stung by nettles accidentally is frightening, painful. Why would anyone do it on purpose? (Must be a masochist.)

Counter-irritation, as in hitting yourself on the toe to cure a headache, is the usual explanation given for the effect of urtication, the technical term given to lashing the skin and joints with fresh nettles, a supposedly out-moded technique.

Earth-honoring peoples in Australia, Eurasia, and the Americas have long recognized the unique value of being stung by sister spinster stinging nettle.

A few writers make the connection between reported cures of arthritis from bee and ant stings and some of the acidic compounds in nettle. But the story is much larger.

Urtication creates an intense physical and energetic stimulus to capillaries/circulation, nerves/meridians, muscle fibers, lymphatic flow, and cellular metabolism, combined with multiple surface injections (like a vaccination) of a fluid containing, among other things, histamines, acetylcholine, and formic acid. No wonder modern herbalists still note that nettle stings "bring dormant energies into action."

My initial experiences were from unintentional urtication, but the results led me to pursue it purposely. Injuries from glass cuts, old but still occasionally painful, and an arthritic pain in a knuckle or two completely disappeared after three springs of attention from my sister stinging nettle.

Nettle is traditionally used (with Wise Woman ways) for healing those with palsy, paralysis, chronic headaches, muscle tightness and congestion, rheumatism, arthritis, neuritis, sciatica, cold feet, gout, and other chronic congestions.

Fresh stinging nettle oil (or ointment) is said to make you sweat when applied. Sounds great for a chilly night! This oil is an honored ally, one of the best, some writers exhort, for those with hives (technically known as urticaria, by the way), allergic reactions, stress reactions, itchy rashes, and itchy bites. Combine with daily use of nettle leaf infusion if the condition is chronic.

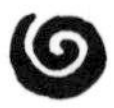

Nettle Pharmacy

Nettle Juice

Rinse fresh nettle leaves and stalks in clean water. Juice immediately in a mechanical juicer, or wrap wet nettles in a cloth and heat gently for thirty minutes. Wring out and collect juice. Use at once or keep refrigerated no more than a day. To preserve longer, combine one part juice with four parts vodka. This can be stored at room temperature and will keep for up to a week.

Stinging Nettle Hair Tonic

½ ounce/15g dried nettle*
2 cups/500ml boiling water
1 Tbs/15ml nettle root tinc.

*leaf, stalk, and/or seed

Pour boiling water over nettle in jar, cover tightly and let sit overnight. Next morning, strain into a plastic bottle, and add tincture (optional). Keeps only a day or two. Use as a final rinse after shampoo and conditioner, leaving it in hair.

Thickens hair texture, helps eliminate dandruff, aids in preventing hair loss during chemotherapy and in restoring hair growth afterwards.

Nettle Hair Lotion

Mild enough for everyday use

4 oz/120g fresh nettle *or*
1 oz/29g dried nettle
4 cups/1 liter water
¼ cup/60ml vinegar
3 drops rosemary *or* lavender oil

Prepare infusion (see p. 261) of nettle. Strain out plant material. Add oil and vinegar to infusion. Keep in refrigerator between uses.

To use: Pour a handful of nettle lotion on wet hair after shampooing. Rub in well. For best results, don't rinse.

Nettle Hair Rescue

1 entire nettle plant:
leaves, stalk, seeds, root
2 c/500ml olive/almond oil

Wash roots only of freshly harvested nettle. Snip entire plant into small pieces with scissors. Fill a jar with the pieces. Pour as much oil as possible into the nettle jar, poking and shaking to dislodge air bubbles. Steep in the closed jar for an entire moon cycle. Remove plant material.

To use: Warm a teaspoon/5ml oil and massage into scalp. Leave on overnight; wash out in the morning. Finish with nettle hair lotion or tonic. Repeat weekly or as needed.

Nettle Face Saver

2 c/500ml fresh nettle leaves
1 cup/250ml water
1 lemon
½ cup/125ml water

Simmer leaves in water in closely covered pan for ten minutes. Cool a bit. Chop or mash leaves and spread evenly on a thin cloth. Steam face and then apply warm nettle pack. Leave on 10-15 minutes. Finish by washing face with lemon water.

Weekly use helps prevent blemishes, oily build-up, loss of skin elasticity, and sun damage.

Nettle Rennet

Enough to curdle four gallons of milk

1 quart/1 liter fresh nettle
1 quart/1 liter water
1 teaspoon/5 ml salt

Cook nettle in simmering salted water in well-covered pan for ten minutes. Strain and add to warm milk. (Each cup/250ml of this will curdle 4 quarts/liters of milk.)

Green Goddess Plant Food and Sister Spinster's All-Purpose Insecticide

1 ounce/30g dried nettle or
¼ pound/125g fresh nettles
4 cups/1 liter water

Pour boiling water over nettle in quart/liter jar and let steep overnight. This recipe may be increased at will. We keep a 55 gallon drum near the greenhouse and gardens filled with water, nettle leaves, comfrey leaves and other weedy inspirations. And tightly lidded to contain the smell.

- ***Foliar Feed:*** Strain nettle infusion through cloth; add three tablespoons/50ml to 2 cups/500ml water. Spray on plants.
- ***Root Feed:*** Pour 1 cup/250ml cooled, unstrained (leaves and all) infusion on ground under tree or shrub. Water in.
- ***Insecticide:*** For mildew, white flies, aphids, and other plant pests: dilute 4 ounces/60ml strained nettle infusion with 1 quart/1 liter water; add one teaspoon of liquid soap. Use immediately as a spray. Again, this may be made in very large batches.

"While growing, they [nettles] stimulate the growth of other plants nearby and make them more resistant to disease . . . nettle humus [compost] quickens life in otherwise sterile peat [soil]." Audrey Wynne Hatfield (1898)

Herbal Compost Activator

A boon for rickety or lazy gardeners

1 oz/30g dried nettle
1 oz/30g dried yarrow
1 oz/30g dried dandelion
1 oz/30g dried chamomile
1 oz/30g dried valerian
1 oz/30g dried oak bark
1 gallon/4 liters water

Combine dried herbs and pour into water, mixing very well. Let stand at least 24 hours. To use: make a heap of layers of soil, manure, weeds, and kitchen waste roughly 4x2 feet/2 square meters. Let mellow for 3 days, then make holes in the heap about 1 foot (300mm) apart with a fat (diameter of two inches/50mm) stick. Put three inches/75mm of liquid activator in each hole. Cover well with soil. Compost will be ready to use, with no turning (!), in one month.

Nettle Kitchen

Pick only the tender tops too young to flower. Stored in a plastic bag in the refrigerator or other cool spot, your fresh nettle greens will last for up to a month uncooked. Once cooked, the nettle spoils rapidly, so eat promptly or freeze.

Nettle Sesame Salt

A delicious low-salt seasoning

1 cup/250ml sesame seeds
¼ cup/60ml dried nettle

Roast sesame in heavy pan over medium heat. Stir constantly to prevent scorching. When browned to your liking, pour into blender or mortar with a pinch of salt and nettle leaves. Grind fairly fine.

Preparation time: 10 minutes. This disappears as fast as I can make it. Superb on salads and cooked grains.

Rich Russian Nettle Tonic

serves 4-6

4 cups/1 liter nettle tops
1 cup/250ml water
2 cloves garlic
½ cup/125ml sour cream
salt to taste

Cook fresh nettles in water, well covered, 10-15 minutes, until tender. *For sauce:* Drain well, then blend, or run through a food processor with garlic and sour cream (or yogurt). Serve immediately over rice, noodles, toast, or vegetables. *For soup:* Blend nettles, cooking water, garlic and sour cream. Reheat gently.

Preparation time: This is a quick dish, taking only 20-25 minutes, so you can spend your time in the nettle patch instead of the kitchen. Though lush and rich, this tonic gives you get-up-and-go!

Spring Song Soup

serves 4

2 cups/500ml nettle tops
1 cup/250ml yellow dock lvs
½ cup/125ml dandelion lvs
2 cups/500ml water
1 large onion, minced
2 tablespoons/30ml olive oil
2 carrots, diced
2 turnips, diced
6 cups/1500ml water
3 Tbs/45ml brown miso

Wash greens; chop, and cook until tender in water in a large pot. Meanwhile, sauté onion in oil until golden. Add onion, carrots, and turnips to nettles. Add water and a pinch of salt and simmer for at least thirty minutes. Thin miso and add just before serving. Garnish with pansy blossoms.

Preparation time: 90 minutes counting picking, cleaning, and chopping greens and vegetables, unless, of course, the day is full of sunshine and birdsong and the greens picking just goes on and on and on.

Nettle Soufflé

serves 2-4

1½ c/375ml water
4 c/1 liter young nettle tops
2 tablespoons/30ml olive oil
1 onion, minced
2 tablespoons/30ml flour
1 c/250ml milk or nettle broth
1 or 2 egg yolks, beaten
2 egg whites, stiffly beaten

Cook nettle in boiling water for 5-10 minutes. Drain well; save broth. Purée nettle in blender, sieve, or processor; set aside. Sauté onion in oil until golden. Add wholewheat flour and cook, stirring, for two minutes. Slowly add a cup of nettle broth and cook, stirring often, for a few minutes, until thick. Add a little of this at a time to the beaten egg yolk, until they are well mixed. Now stir in nettle purée and salt to taste. Last, carefully fold in egg whites. Put in a souffle dish; bake at 350 F/80 C until firm, 30-40 minutes.

Preparation time: I figure on an hour: 35 minutes of cooking plus another half hour washing up the mess while the soufflé's in the oven.

Nettle Goat Cheese Casserole

serves 8-10

3 cups/750ml brown rice
6 cups/1500ml water
pinch salt
6 cups/1500ml nettle tops
2 cups/500ml water
4 cups/1 liter goat cheese

Cook rice in boiling water in very tightly covered pan for 40 minutes. Cook young nettles in water until tender. Lightly oil casserole dish. Layer rice, greens, cheese, rice, greens, cheese. Bake at 350 F/80 C until the cheese is melted and brown, about 15-20 minutes.

Preparation time: 60 minutes if you grease the casserole, pick and cook the nettles, and grate the cheese while the rice cooks. Otherwise an hour and a half.

Shitake-Nettle-Tofu Quiche

serves 8-12

1 ounce/30g dried shitake
1 cup/250ml warm water
2 baked pie shells
6 cups/750g nettle tops
1 pound/500g tofu
1 onion, cut in crescents
4 tablespoons/60ml olive oil
2 cups/500ml milk
3 eggs
1 tablespoon/15ml tamari

Soak shitake in warm water. Rinse nettles; cook in water to cover until tender; drain immediately. Sauté onion (and some garlic if you wish) in half of olive oil until partly soft. Slice the softened shitake and sauté with onion for 3 minutes. Cut tofu in small cubes; sauté with shitake, rest of oil, and onion for 4 minutes. Remove from heat; stir in cooked nettle; put in prebaked crusts. Beat eggs, milk, and tamari together and pour into piecrusts. Bake at 350 F/80 C for 40-50 minutes, until center is set. Decorate with sprigs of nettle and spring flowers and serve.

Preparation time: When I'm a kitchen witch, I whiz this out in two hours: 30 minutes for the crusts; 45 minutes of cooking; and 45 minutes of baking. I start soaking the shitake before I head out the door to collect the nettles.

Nettles Plain or Nettles Fancy

serves 4

1 cup/250ml water
1 pound/500g fresh nettle
***
4 tablespoons/60ml butter
4 cloves garlic, minced
½ cup/125ml pine nuts

Cook young nettle tops in water until tender; don't be afraid of overcooking. For nettles plain, serve as is, in the delicious broth. For nettles fancy, warm garlic in butter, add pine nuts, and serve over drained nettles. (Save that broth to use as soup base!)

Preparation time: 30 minutes. I cook nettle leaves and stalks until soft, usually 15 minutes. Melt in my mouth is what I want. Add another 10 minutes in the garden to snip nettle tops and sniff spring.

Nettle Porridge/Pudding

serves 6-8

1 cup/250ml barley
3 cups/750ml water
6 cups/1500ml nettle tops
1 cup/250ml dandelion leaves
1 cup/250ml watercress
½ cup/125ml sorrel leaves
½ cup/125ml black currant lvs
1 sprig mint
1 onion with top, minced
2 tablespoons/30ml olive oil
1 beaten egg
salt to taste

Cook barley in water until very soft. Wash greens. Chop finely. Stir into soft barley with onion, oil, egg, and seasonings. Put all into a tightly covered glass bowl or enamel pan, which is then placed on a rack in a large pot containing several inches of water. Cover both pans well; bring water to a boil; steam pudding for ninety minutes. Don't let steam get in the pudding. Serve with miso sauce.

miso sauce:
1 onion minced
2 tablespoons/30ml olive oil
4 tablespoons/60ml flour
3 tablespoons/45ml miso
1½ cups/375ml water

Sauté onion in oil until soft. Stir in wholewheat flour and cook for 2-3 minutes, stirring. Dissolve miso in water. Pour water into flour mix slowly, stirring. Cook until thick.

Preparation time: The whole affair spans 3 hours. I use the 30-40 minutes it takes to cook the barley to gather and wash the greens, and pray that I don't get distracted. The actual steaming requires very little attention. The miso sauce takes about 5 minutes.

Nettle Beer

One of the most delightful medicines for joint pain I've ever taken.

1 pound/500g raw sugar
2 lemons
1 ounce/30g cream of tartar
5 quarts/5 liters water
2 pounds/1 kilo nettle tops
1 ounce/30g live yeast

Place sugar, lemon peel (no white), lemon juice, and cream of tartar in a large crock. Cook nettles in water for 15 minutes. Strain into the crock and stir well. When this cools to blood warm, dissolve the yeast in a little water and add to your crock. Cover with several folds of cloth and let brew for three days. Strain out sediment and bottle. Ready to drink in eight days.

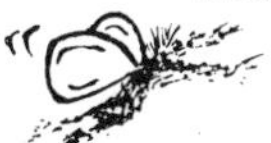

"Nettles were once tithed, they have so many uses: medicine, food, fodder, fertilizer, beer, dye, fiber for thread, nets, durable cloth, paper, hair restorer, aphrodisiac, and smoke!"

Nettle Fun and Facts

• *Weeds and What They Tell,* by E.E. Pfeiffer, is a dynamic little book which ends with inspiring tales of nettles in the garden.

• Audrey Hatfield obviously adores nettle and has filled her *Weed Herbal* (1898) with lots of wonderful nettle recipes, including nettle porridge and nettle beer recipes I've adapted to modern standards and included here. I love her description of nettle pollination: *"The stinging nettles have an enchanting early morning festival when the males gaily puff their pale golden pollen into the air to be caught by the females. And the plant fancier enthralled by novel plant habits will not be disappointed if [s]he drags [her]himself out of bed early enough to catch this graceful ritual."*

• Maria Treben quite thoroughly describes nettle's ability to help those with chronic problems in *Health through God's Pharmacy.* She suggests up to two liters/half gallon of infusion or tea daily for chronic headaches, eczema, allergies, leukemia, and cancers of the spleen and stomach.

• My newest nettle book is the hardest one for me to read: *Rund um die Brennessel: Kochen-Heilen-Zauberei,* by Marlene Haerkötter; 1987, Eichborn Verlag.

• *Discussing the chemical constituents of nettle, E. E. Shook, in Advanced Treatise in Herbology*, 1934, says, *"It is fairly well known that iron phosphate (organic) is nature's quickest and best remedy for all inflammation, that potassium phosphate is the basic food for the brain and nerves, and that potassium chloride is nature's masterpiece solvent of fibrin."*

• *Weaver's Garden* by Rita Buchanan, 1987, Interweave, discusses the fiber uses of sister spinster, but Rita has yet to learn to pay attention and honor this green ally.

• Noedl (Anglo-Saxon) is needle. Ne/net is related to Sanskrit nah (bind), German na-hen (sew), and Latin nere (spin).

• *Laportea canadensis*/wood nettle and *Boehmeria cylindrica*/stingless nettle and *Boehmeria nivea*/ramie are useful fiber plants closely related to nettle.

• Maude Grieves has an excellent discussion of the history and uses of nettle fiber in *A Modern Herbal.*

• The Algonquin have a myth about how the making of nets from nettle came to be: Sirakitehak, who created heaven and earth, invented nettle nets after watching the spider spin. She told the women to twist the fibers on their thighs. And so they do, to this day.

• Nettle flowers in England provide the nectar which is the sole nourishment of peacock butterflies and tortoiseshell butterflies.

• Nettles are mentioned in *Rob Roy,* by Sir Walter Scott, and in *Les Miserables* by Victor Hugo. Nettles are the star of *The Princess and the Eleven Swans,* retold by Hans C. Andersen.

• Samuel Pepys ate nettle porridge on 25 Feb. 1661 and noted it in his diary.

• Albrecht Dürer painted an angel flying to heaven and carrying nettles.

• The Tibetan Buddhist saint Milarepa, student of the great translator Marpa, lived exclusively on nettles in his retreat; and it is said that he became both green and enlightened.

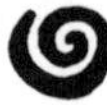

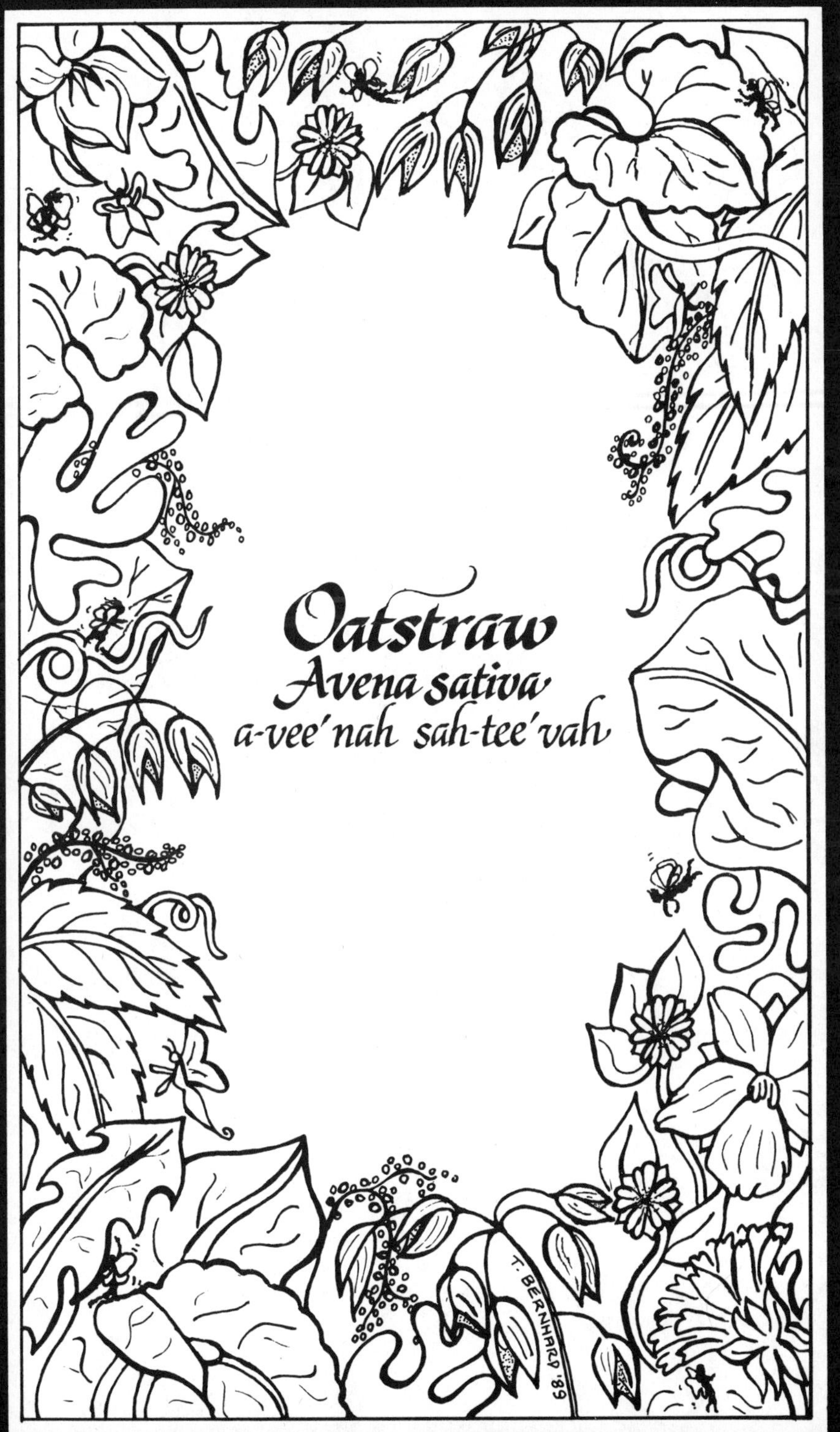
Oatstraw
Avena sativa
a-vee'nah sah-tee'vah
T. BERNHARD '89

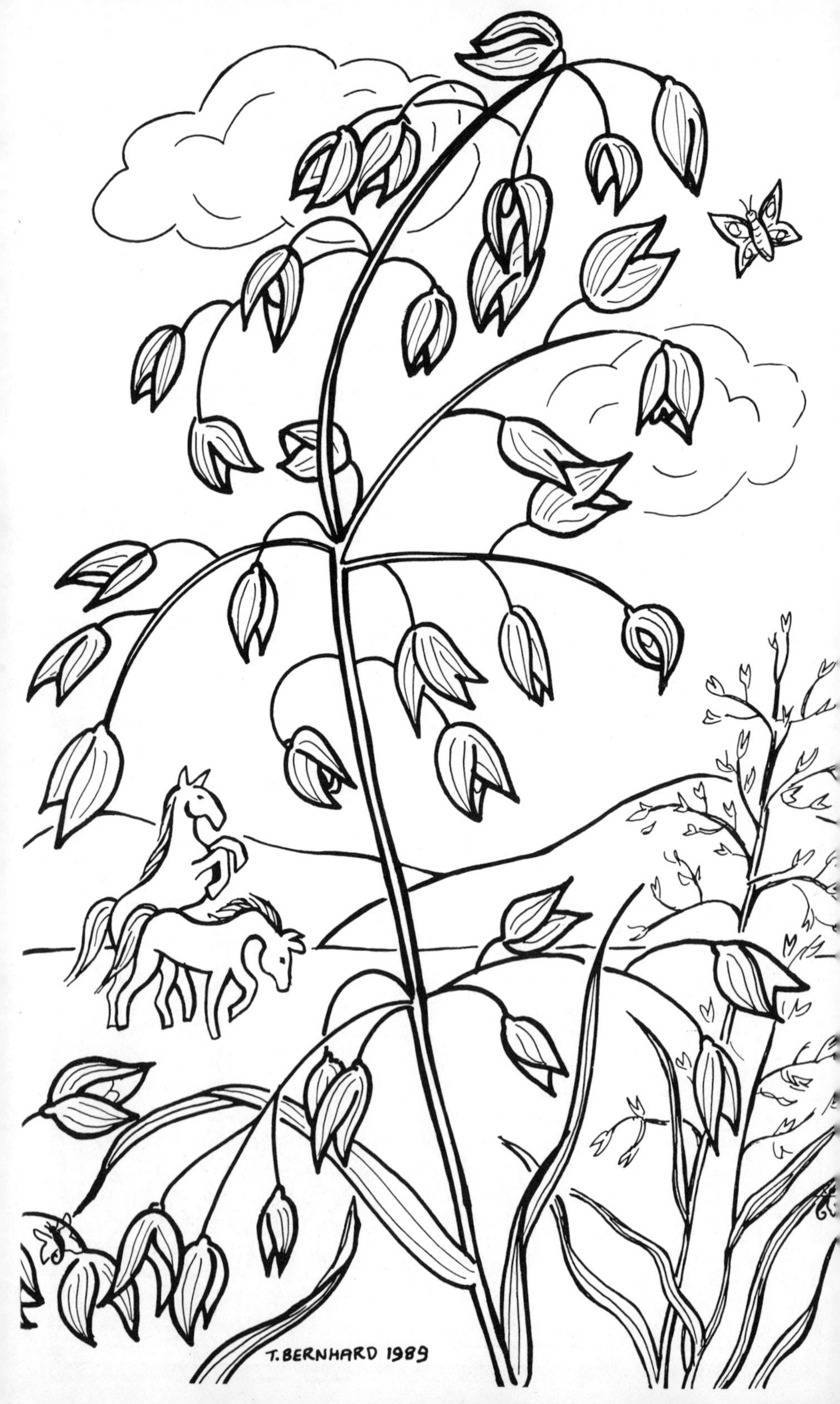
T. BERNHARD 1989

Oatstraw Speaks

Feeling your oats today? Whoa! Now do mind your manners. Don't stop . . . just be . . . discreet . . . I do love the way you stroke my blades and touch my kernels. My grain's milky ripeness is pleasing, is it not? Come and move with me. Let your heart ripple with me. Let your imagination soar with me a while, while the wind lifts my long green leaves, like feathers, flying.

My name is Oats. I am priestess of Ceres, great mother of grain. Yes, yes, do touch me there.

I am the archetype of fertility. I am the image of optimum nourishment. I am Corn Mother. I am the mother of many, many breasts. Welcome warm womb am I; seed filled with life am I; born of heaven and earth am I, I who nurture all. Yes, do suck there. Ummmm.

Those with four legs graze my green grass. Ummmm. The creeping, crawling ones find shelter and sustenance among my hollow stalks. Ohhh, that does feel so pleasant; do continue. The feathered flying ones, and you, the ones with hands, relish my seeds. My seed, my sweet grain, the milk of the earth's breast, is your first food after your own mother's milk.

You look so beautiful there in the dapple of my shade. Come, be more bold upon me. Imbibe me. Grasp me and harvest my sweet, short life to feed your own. Drink deeply of me. Take me into you. Open yourself to me. Do not hesitate. The fullness and richness of life is yours.

I know you see me as a simple woman, a country woman, with little wisdom, a woman easily taken. Yes, do lie down here with me. This ignorance is fortunately recent. In ages past, I was known as goddess. Further back, I was honored with art, dance, poetry, and love. Yes, yes, love. Do come lie down with me here in the hay.

I am the mother's gift of nourishment. I am the mother's gift of love. Love. Love! I am love in form. Love from your mother, my great granny Gaia. I bring contentment. I bring rich, full nourishment for spirit, hearth, community, earth wherever I am grown with honor, joy, and love.

It is true that I am young, and that my roots are shallow. Compared to yonder oak, I am of less note than the passing butterfly. But I carry, conscious, the memory of all my sisters: sisters of the sacred cycle. And so I know more than my youth suggests.

Yes, I am wise and sweet, far wiser yet and richer sweet than you may guess. We grasses have seen, year after year, the great play of life here on this sweet, green earth, we grasses who are the great green heart of the mother earth. I am life. Learn how to nourish yourself with me and you will find yourself steady, vital, sensitive, strong, at one with the mother of all.

I have grown here under stars, moon, and sun, and have concentrated the lights of heaven into myself. I have investigated the earth for minerals. I have found stability in storms and the mother's love. I have concentrated the power and subtlety of many transformations into my being.

Now, you eat me. All this comes to you, through me. You are gifted by the Goddess, whose priestess I am.

Fertility priestess. Your books say: "temple whore." Yes, do rub a little harder there. Ummmm. Come a little closer. Watch the graceful curve of my neck. Flare your nostrils and catch my enticing, soft, secure scent.

Breathe deeply; breathe evenly; be aware of your breath. Be aware of the stallion. Remember the stallion covering the mare. Remember the gleam of his dappled coat, here in the dappled shade as you breathe deeply, and fully, and remember.

Yes, remember.

Remember the stallion covering the mare: the fierce brightness of his eyes, the lightning energy of his moving muscles. Remember the stallion grazing here, eating me, becoming filled with me.

Breathe slowly, remember. I am the gleam in his dappled coat, shining bright. I am the gleam in his fierce eye, looking keen. I am the gleam of his muscles, lightning energy. Remember, remember me.

Remember.

I remember. She made me promise not to tell, but that was so long ago. Thousands of years ago. Thousands of years ago when it was the hot gossip. She swore me to secrecy then, but that was so long ago. Who cares now? Who even remembers ? Who wonders what really went on between Poseidon and my mother Demeter?

You want to know? Yes, let me brush your cheek here; I'll tell you. Though Demeter didn't tell me. We are close, very close for mother and daughter, but she would have us all believe the official stories, me included.

No, Mother never discussed with me her relationship with my father. "That is over and done with," she would tell me when I asked. But my great granny Gaia was kind of sweet on my dad, if you ask me. Yes, do turn this way. Anyway, Gaia made sure I got the real story. Well, the real story according to her.

It wasn't just a matter of Poseidon lusting after my mother, Gaia told me. Gaia said Demeter was just as avid for him as he was for her. But she wouldn't let on! I mean, even though she is a fertility goddess and all, mother is really stern and severe. She always leaves the erotic, sensual parts for Aphrodite.

No, it would not do at all, my mother must have thought, to consort with her own brother, Poseidon. Not at all. Nor, especially, to let on to anyone (except granny Gaia) how she lusted after his salty tang.

So, hoping to forget her eagerness for Poseidon's treasure, Demeter threw herself into her work. Early one misty morning, under granny Gaia's guidance, she shape-shifted. She shape-shifted into a roan mare.

As mare, Demeter lifted her head, breathed deeply, and quivered in ecstatic communion with the vital essences of grass, earth, sun, and wind. And riding that bliss was the image of Poseidon. The repressed, denied longing to merge with her brother came to her full force on the morning breeze. (Did she really tell great-granny this? Did she really share her desire? Or did Gaia just sense what must have happened?)

Her primal heat awoke and spread. Her skin felt boundless and deep; her eyes closed as sparks flared through her nerves. And in that instant, Poseidon appeared.

Poseidon appeared as a dappled stallion. Dappled stallion he, he knew the way was clear for him now. As mare, Demeter would receive him; she could not, as mare, deny her ardent wish to enfold him, to pull him into her, to fill herself bursting full of him. This wish, this truth, she could deny in human form. As mare, Demeter could not deny. She could only act the truth.

Great-granny Gaia never really told me what happened then. I mean, not the details! By the time I was born, he was back at sea, and nobody was the wiser, so far as Demeter was concerned. I loved the seaweed he would send from time to time. But no one would talk about my father. Remember, it's a secret.

But to get on with the story, I was born. And so was my dumb brother, Arion. Well, he isn't really dumb. In fact, he's very gifted. I mean he can actually speak. And that's really something for a horse, don't you think? A talking horse. Ha, ha. A talking horse for a brother.

Yes, we were both embarrassments to Demeter, I'm afraid. You can hardly hide the results of your lust, even if you're intent on making everyone believe you're demure. Not that anybody in Olympus ever cares if your lover is your brother or mother or whatever. But we did have a way of reminding her of a secret she would rather forget.

Arion's horse shape spoke to her every day of her inability to deny her desire, her primal heat. And you can bet she resented him for that. And maybe his gift of speech made it even worse for her. (Personally, I always wanted him to shut up.) And as for me . . .

As for me, well you know me now. I take after mother, and great-grandmother, too. I'm tall and slim, graceful, and hauntingly beautiful. I'm blond and breezy and ready for you. Demeter tried to hide me; and great-granny Gaia said I shouldn't tell my name to mortals. But I don't think anything will happen if I tell you my story and tell you my name.

I am Avena: daughter of earth and ocean pulsing together. I am Avena, nourished by mare's milk, brought up as human. Avena, avena, will you whisper it with me? Avena, avena, like silk skirts whispering in a breeze. Avena, avena.

Avena, that's me.

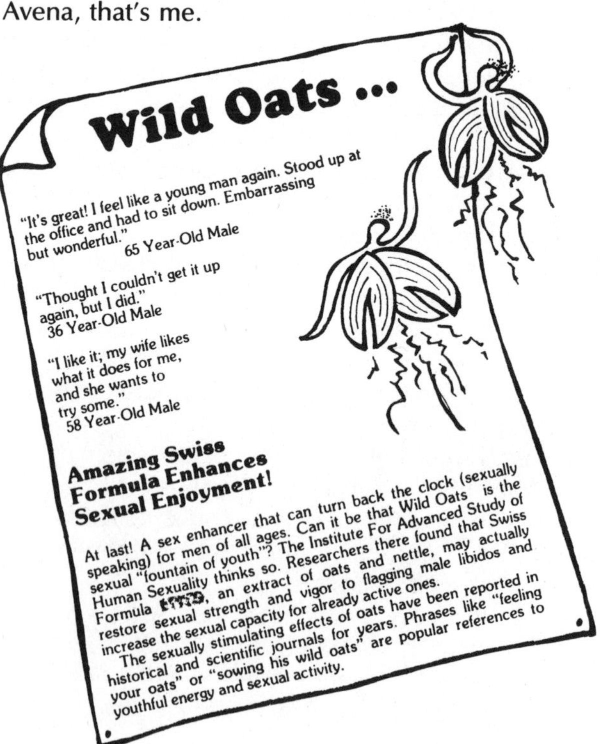

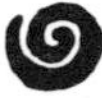

Oatstraw Facts

Botanical name: *Avena sativa*; avena (Latin) means oats; sativa (Latin) means cultivated. ***Other useful species:*** *A. fatua, A. barbara* are wild oat species; *A. orientalis, A. nuda*, and *A. stringose* are modern cultivars. ***Natural order:*** Graminaceae/ Grain family. ***English names:*** Oats, groats, wild oats, naked oats, tartarian oats, bristle-pointed oats. ***Chinese names:*** Yen-mai. ***French names:*** Avoine cultivée. ***German names:*** Hafer, Saathafer, Gruen Hafer. ***Russian names:*** Oves. ***Welch names:*** Ceirch llwyd, blewgeirch. ***Fiber uses:*** Husks are used to stuff bedding. ***Food uses:*** Rolled oats, steel-cut oats, and whole oats are readily available as people/animal feed; production world-wide for 1988 was 55 million metric tons. ***Medicinal uses:*** Still recommended by MDs for acute itchy dermatitis, like chicken pox. ***Soil uses:*** Helps prevent erosion, especially on marginal (acidic, depleted) soils. ***Animal uses:*** Oat hay and oats are important foodstuffs; widely used for horses. ***Habitat:*** Cultivated land, banksides, grainfields. ***Natural range:*** Mediterranean, Near East. ***Current range:*** Cultivated and growing as a weed on all the great plains of the world, especially China, Europe, North America, Australia, New Zealand, Asia, and South Africa. ***Toxicity:*** Unhazardous internally and externally; wind-blown pollen is allergen. ***Best identified by:*** Hanging, swaying seed heads; large milky grain; the sigh the wind makes in her hair.

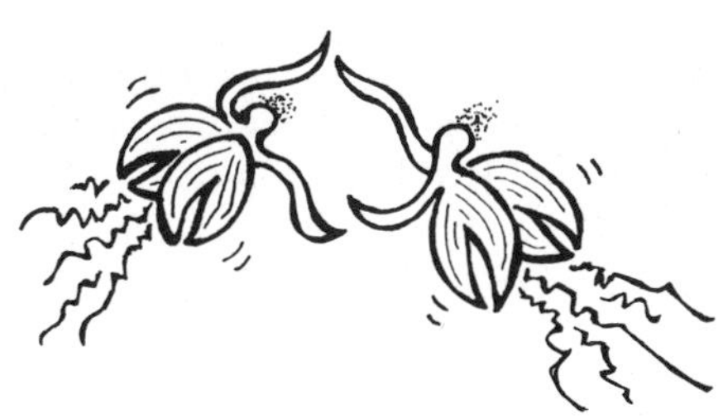

"It is the oats which grow so quickly after rains have come. It is the wild oats which ripen so rapidly. Their graceful open tassels shake in the wind . . . glisten in the sun . . . give the coastal breezes their distinctive sound . . . a rustle as of stiff silk petticoats. . . ." E. Anderson (1969)

Oatstraw Weed Walk

What a mellow September day, full of slanting sun and grasshopper wings in gaudy colors. We could be walking in an ancient grainfield in Mesopotamia as easily as here in the closing years of the twentieth century.

This field of oats is eternal, is it not? The blue sky doesn't have a date. The mouse scurrying there doesn't belong to any particular century. Who can say if the wind is old or young?

Does it make you feel peacefully free to see the oats rippling under the wind's caress? Does it ripple in your eyes and your mind and set you free? Free for even a short while of the constraints of your own time and your own place? Free . . . and relaxed . . . and just here, which could be any oat field . . . that's where we are.

Here, chew on this green, sweet stalk of oats as we stretch our legs for a long walk. See how it's hollow, like a straw. That's an oatstraw. Let the soft green sweet taste you suck from it help you remember your new friend: Avena.

We could imagine, but for the heat, that we're here in spring to see the delicate shoots of oatgrass come up out of this now-dusty earth. The earth then would be dark from rain and easily broached by the first green darts of oats. Yes, just one long, straight leaf at first, as befits a grass.

The root, at first one thin white tendril, becomes many. And the many thin fibers spread out in the earth, and down in the earth, finding what minerals are there, what water is available.

The stalk lengthens, unfurling other slender leaves, pushing upward to swing flowers and oat seeds in the breeze. That hollow, jointed stem . . . pulled away from gravity, yearning up toward the sky . . . that oatstraw . . . so graceful. Is it not the straw of connection between the earth and the sky? Let us sip and suck through it and remember our connections, and all our relations, as my Native American friends say.

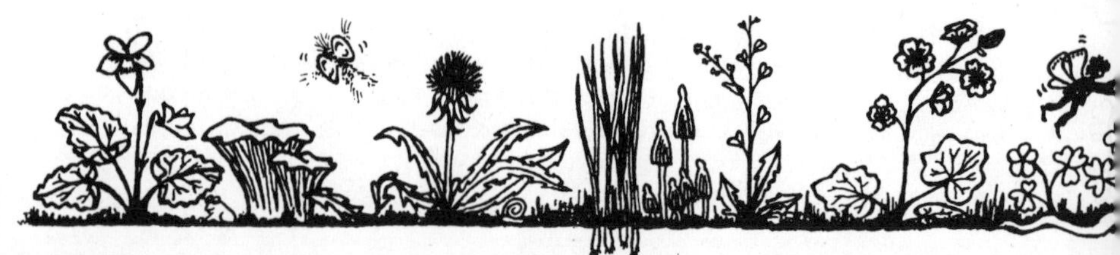

First the oatgrass is as high as your knees. Then, so fast you can almost see it grow, it's as tall as your armpits, and puffing flower pollen with every breeze. The leaves grow rougher, more narrow, and pale, as the first delicate flowers appear just a few moons after the seed has sprouted.

Dark flowers they are, pendulous spikelets, swaying magically and suggestively against the pale green leaves and straws. Each tiny perfect flower forms two seeds. Each flower, wind obliging, will ripen two seeds. Two awned seeds of green that will darken until golden ripe. Two seeds that will dance looking at the earth.

For though the oatstraw stretches to the sky, the oat herself, Avena, looks back down to the earth. Her flowers and seeds look ever back at their loving mother, and dance with their loving sisters.

This is a good spot to harvest some. We have permission to cut a bit from the edge of the field, but I feel more energy, more essence emanating from these wilder oats, the ones that aren't in the field. Maybe they really are wild oats, though most likely they're grown of some cultivated seed that the birds spread. I like the way it grows in the patterns of the earth's energy, not like the orderly rows in the field.

Come sit here with me a moment before we begin. Feel again the sunshine on your eyelids and hear the drone of the insects. Allow yourself to accept the blessing you are being given. Be blessed by each touch of the grass. Envision yourself harvesting this life-sustaining grass in a graceful way, in beauty. Ask Avena to be your ally, your friend. Wait a moment.

Yes, now we may begin. Cut an armful, no more. I only dry enough for a year, maybe two. And it's a long walk back to the car. We don't want to have too much to carry.

Back home, we'll spread this out to dry so it keeps the soft green color and a good bit of the green seeds. We don't want it to look like hay, so we won't dry it in the sun. When it's dry the stalks will snap easily. I store it, as unbroken as possible, in plain paper bags, ready to make my favorite company tea. Everyone loves the smooth taste of oatstraw. Umm . . . just thinking about it makes me want to get home and make some. How about you? Ready to go?

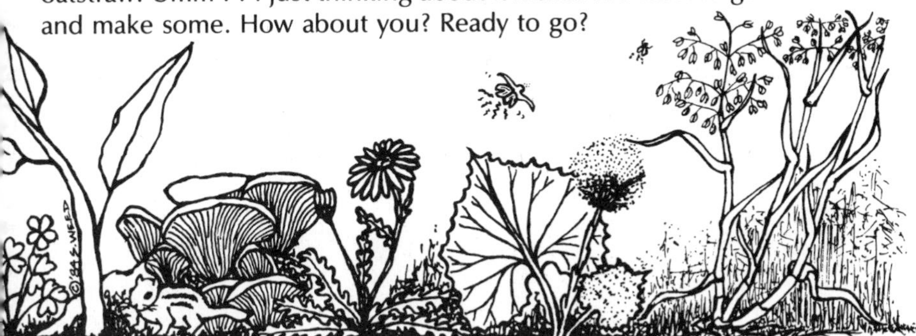

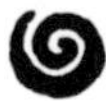

Oatstraw Properties and Uses

- ***nutritive,*** tonic, demulcent
- ***nervine,*** antispasmodic, antidepressant
- ***cooling,*** febrifuge, diuretic, diaphoretic, carminative

Oats and oatstraw are (for the purposes of this book) the same herb. Either the grain alone or the grain and the grass (that's the oatstraw) are **soothing** and nourishing. Regular use of either promotes a strong **nervous system** and a juicy **endocrine system.** Avena eases spasms and inflammation throughout your being, allowing engorged cells to relax, release fluid, and cool off. Oatstraw is ever ready to be your sweet sister, to give you heart, and to liven up your **love life**.

Use oats and oatstraw as a strength-giving food, a way to toughen up, a nerve tonic, a modern-day love potion, a rejuvenator, and a good friend in hot water.

- Dose of *fresh oatstraw tincture* is 20-125 drops a day, in water.
- Dose of *dried oatstraw infusion* is 1-4 cups/250-1000ml a day.

"Oatmeal made into a cake with water, baked and browned like coffee, then pulverized and made into a coffee, or infusion, forms a drink which will allay nausea and check vomiting in a majority of cases when all other means fail. . . ." Kings (1898)

*"**Rasayana karma** are rejuvenative tonics; oatstraw is one. Rasayana substances rebuild the body-mind, prevent decay, and postpone aging. . . . They do not simply add to the bulk or quantity of the body, but increase its quality. [They] are more subtle, more specific, and more lasting than simple nutritive substances."* V. Lad (1986)

Oats and Oatstraw are a Strength-Giving Food

(Numbers indicate milligrams per hundred grams oats and oatstraw)

Oatstraw herb includes the green stalk, leaves, and grain. The nutritive properties of oats and oatstraw are not very different, except that oatstraw is lower in calories and higher in vitamin A (carotenes) and vitamin C than the grain alone.

Since ancient times, the hardiest people have eaten oats and honored Avena.

Consistent use of oats and oatstraw in the diet usually brings about noticeable improvement in coordination, bone density, length of attention span, balance, memory, sensitivity to pleasant stimuli, clarity of thinking, ability to perceive connections and remedy misconnections, ease of achieving meditative and conscious dream states, and overall calmness and centeredness.

Avena combines well with slippery elm (Ulmus fulva), making a particularly valuable food for convalescents, feverish children, babes who fail to thrive, anorexics, anemics, and those with weak digestion or digestive distress including ulcers, dyspepsia, chronic constipation, bleeding colitis, and gastroenteritis.

Avena is high as well in calcium (1430), iron (4.6-57), phosphorus (240-425), the vitamin B complex, including thiamine (0.4-0.7), riboflavin (1.1-1.7), niacin (1.0-4.94), folic acid, and B_6 (.08), vitamins E (5), G, and K (.18), and fiber (17.3%).

Oatstraw and oats are also a source of potassium (352), carotenes expressed as vitamin A (5045 IU), vitamin C expressed as ascorbic acid (37), and protein (5-18%), including amino acids such as histidine, arginine, tryptophane (76), leucine (501), lysine (221), phenylalanine (275), isoleucine (275), valine (319), threonine (205), and methionine (86), the "limiting" amino acid (15% supplied). Oats is one of the most protein-rich grains generally available.

Avena is quite low in calories (less than 100 per cup of cooked grain, none in the infusion) and fat (2-7).

As a mild-tasting nutritional storehouse, oatstraw and oats are ideally suited for helping the wise woman healing/wholing herself or others with chronic illness such as AIDS/ARC, Crohn's disease, lupus, or multiple sclerosis.

Plain oatmeal, or "Wild'n'Oats Cereal" (see **Oatstraw Kitchen**), or oatstraw infusion—all mellow and very pleasant tasting—are effective forms of oats, used regularly. Oatstraw tincture has less nutritive value than the cereal or infusion, and is used only occasionally.

Oats and Oatstraw Make You Tough

Avena is a tough lady and she'll toughen you up too! Let oats and oatstraw help you build strong, pliable bones, firm and reliable teeth, a stable blood-sugar level, a powerful circulatory system, sturdy lungs, and rugged nerves.

Rich in bio-active minerals, Avena is an easily digested, inexpensive source of calcium used by wise women to mend bones, build flesh, and improve circulatory and nervous system functioning. Try Avena as your ally to nourish health/wholeness/holiness during pregnancy and lactation.

If you want a daily calcium supplement, try a cup of oatstraw infusion brewed with a pinch of shave grass (horsetail herb/Equisetum arvense). Within a month you'll notice the difference in your nails, teeth, and hair, and feel it in your bones. For those with severe gum disease, make your daily brew half oatstraw and half horsetail herb.

Oatstraw baths once or twice a week, in combination with oatstraw infusion taken by the quart/liter, is part of a wise woman's way of healing those with osteoporosis, rickets, bone cancer, and broken bones.

"A tincture made from Avena sativa (oats), fifteen to twenty drops four times daily, will stimulate the brain and spinal cord." H. Santillo (1984)

Oats and Oatstraw are a Nerve Tonic

Oatstraw and oats strengthen and nourish the nerves and the nervous system. Full of nerve-cell nutrients, oatstraw helps regulate nervous system and chakra energies. The emotional and subtle bodies benefit amazingly from regular use, and psychic abilities often improve. By nourishing and tonifying the nerves and helping to eliminate bio-electrical resistance, oatstraw opens the nervous system to a wide range of terrestrial and galactic energies. Pain reduction is virtually always a side effect.

When I'm edgy, under stress, stretching my limits, hysterical, exhausted, beyond help, grieving, or frazzled, I dring oatstraw infusion all day and take time for my Avena meditation (page 206).

When healing yourself or others dealing with chronic tension headaches, continuous eye strain, a high-stress lifestyle, and epileptic seizures, Avena is a reliable ally. For long-term health/wholeness/holiness, merely eat or drink oats daily; in the acute phase of these tumultuous situations, include an oatstraw bath or two.

Healing/wholing from nervous breakdown, emotional breakthrough, schizophrenic episodes, convulsions, and collapse is assured when you walk the Wise Woman way of spiraling transformation and use Avena baths and oatstraw infusions as your allies. Try weekly baths and copious amounts of the infusion for as long as needed.

Oatstraw tincture and oat cakes (see **Oatstraw Kitchen**) are calming and palatable for those withdrawing from drugs (including nicotine and caffeine). Ask Avena to come and bring you ease and freedom from your distress.

Symptoms of children's nervous distress such as bedwetting, colic, allergies, and hyperactivity are relieved with regular help from Avena and your Wise Woman ways.

Oat hull pillows and mattresses are recommended for nervous, high-strung individuals, and those recovering from war or natural disasters.

Those who are sleepless due to overwrought, highly-strung nerves or leg cramps are eased by Avena. Try a cup of infusion before or with breakfast and a cup, warm, before bed. Change will be obvious in about two weeks.

Oats and Oatstraw are a Modern-Day Love Potion

Love potions go right to the heart, and so does Avena. She helps clear your blood vessels of fatty deposits and eases the beat of your heart.

Avena's ability to clear cholesterol from blood vessels is much celebrated recently. In addition to lowering cholesterol levels, a cup or more of oatstraw infusion daily (or several oatcakes for breakfast) with your other Wise Woman ways, will support and rebuild the heart muscles and circulatory vessels, and ease those with heart spasms and palpitations.

Avena helps tighten and re-elasticize your veins, eliminating varicosities and hemorrhoids, when used as a bath and a food.

Love potions also make you want to hug and kiss and more, it is said. Avena's ability to help you improve your sexual appetite and performance has been touted, praised, and sung about for centuries.

Avena's effect is not specifically aphrodisiacal. Instead, oats and oatstraw nourish the nerves, so you receive more pleasure from touching; the glands, so your juices are on the move; your heart and blood vessels so blood can circulate freely to the pelvis; and your ability to be intimate with others, so your love-making is deeply satisfying.

Less well known, but of importance to lovers, is the ability of oats and oatstraw to stabilize blood sugar levels. Large swings in your blood-sugar level can make you sleepy when the action heats up and cranky when it's time for sweet talk. Let Avena help. Diabetics and hypoglycemics, as well as lovers, find Avena a powerful ally.

Oats and Oatstraw Rejuvenate

How does Avena rejuvenate? She increases your sensory sensitivity, restores your bone and muscle mass, strengthens your capillaries, clears your blood vessels, and nourishes your hormonal and circulatory systems to optimum performance. That's how!

Alliance with Avena will give you increased energy (especially sexual energy), a glowing vigor, and remarkable skin and hair. That's rejuvenation!

Avena infusion, and to some degree the tincture, nourishes, strengthens, regulates, and revitalizes the endocrine system. Avena especially nourishes the thyroid, ovaries, and uterus.

Try a cup of infusion weekly, or 10-20 drops of tincture daily, as a preventative of prostate problems.

Women weakened and tired by childbearing, repeated pregnancies, and extended lactations find themselves feeling spry again after becoming friends with oats and oatstraw.

Regular use of Avena can help you strengthen your adrenals as well, thus helping you heal yourself or others with allergies and some menopausal problems such as night sweats.

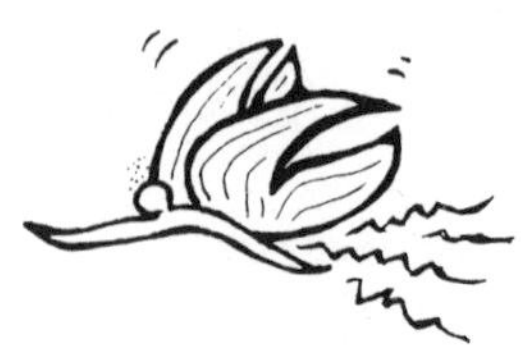

"The pericarp of Oats contains an amorphous alkaloid which acts as a stimulant of the motor ganglia, increasing the excitability of the muscles. . . ."
Maude Grieve (1931)

Oats and Oatstraw are Good Friends in Hot Water

An evening in a hot tub with Avena is a delicious experience.

Relax in a full oatstraw bath to soothe pain from any internal distress including cystitis, pelvic inflammatory disease, rheumatism, lumbago, digestive kinks, sore kidneys, nervous debility, gout, urinary gravel, kidney stones, neurasthenia, and neuralgias. Try repeated full oatstraw baths and your Wise Woman ways to heal those who are exhausted, paralyzed, and in emotional distress, or those dealing with liver ailments, scrofula, and bone diseases.

Use a sitz bath of oatstraw to ease bladder spasms and pain, uterine pain, and chronic intestinal distress.

Use an oatstraw footbath to soak away stink, sweat, cold, and pain from your tender tootsies.

Use oatstraw washes to nourish and heal those with skin diseases, flaky or dry skin, frostbite, chilblains, wounds, and eye irritations.

For chronic conditions, take your oatstraw bath twice a week or more, and drink the infusion freely, for as many weeks as needed. In acute situations, use hot oatstraw baths and poultices frequently until pain subsides, then once or twice a day, as needed.

Oatstraw Baths

Ingredients	Directions
2 qts/liters oatstraw infusion	Add reheated, strained oatstraw infusion to a tub of hot water. Immerse self and soak away tensions.
	or
2.2 pounds/1 kilo oatstraw 1 gallon/4 liters water	Boil water and pour over oatstraw in a large tub. When cooled sufficiently, bathe. (Yes, with the oats and all.)

". . . thousands of tons of oat husks . . . formerly . . . used as fuel or packing material, nowadays . . . [are the] raw material from which furfural is made. Furfural is [used] in making nylon, synthetic rubber, and antiseptics." *Oxford book of Food Plants*, Oxford U. Press, 1969

Avena Meditation

Put on some gentle, rippling music. Allow yourself fifteen minutes of uninterrupted time to read, remember, and follow the meditation on your own. Or, to listen to your own recording of these words:

I am Avena, your guide. Put yourself in my care. Rest now. Allow your muscles to relax. Allow your muscles to fall away from your bones. Allow yourself to feel the freedom of life without muscles. Sitting or lying quietly, let yourself become all bones. Let yourself be but a skeleton.

In your imagination, let yourself be made only of bones. And imagine that your skeleton, your bones, are at rest in a beautiful field of green grass with the sun warming them.

Raise the bones of your right arm and hand up in the air like an oatstraw. Gently lower those bones. Move the bones of your left arm and hand into the air, reaching for the sky. Gently lower those bones. Feel the double bone in your lower arm, the multiple small bones of your hands, and the easy gliding contact of bone on bone at your wrists, elbows, shoulders.

Pick up your knees, the bones of your knees, so the legs bend and the feet, the foot bones, come to rest near your buttocks, the lower edge of your pelvis. Relax your knee bones. Feel your thigh bone, how it rests in the hip socket. Feel the twin bones of your lower leg. Notice how the bones of the feet hold themselves.

Draw your knees up towards your chin and chest, your skull and ribs. Let the long bones of the legs relax and let your foot bones fall out to the sides. Imagine a breeze coming to shake these bones, gently, softly. Allow your foot bones to become oatstraw flowers, oatstraw seeds. Let the breeze make your flowers dance. Let the breeze ripple through you.

Notice your backbone. Begin to move your pelvis from side to side so the backbone sways right and left. Let the skull sway as it will, opposing the movement of the pelvis.

Feel the warm sun shining on you as you sway in the breeze. Hear the call of the birds and insects living in the grainfield. Smell the scents of wildflowers wafting on the breeze. Know yourself as part, an important part, of all this.

Stay here as long as you wish. When you are ready, return to the body you know (yourself with muscles on your bones) and gently open your eyes.

Notice the depth and brilliance of your vision, your hearing, your skin. Notice your ease. Thank Avena.

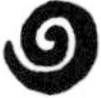

Oatstraw Pharmacy

Skin Soother

Tie a handful of oatmeal into a thin cloth and soak in warm water (in the tub with you is fine), squeezing now and then until the milky white oat cream appears. Use this, in a hot bath, as a cleansing rub, skin softener, complexion treatment, and itch reliever. Rub in spirals on joints. Rub on face. Leaves skin feeling marvelously nourished, cleansed, and softened.

Oatstraw Hair Rinse

Shampoo hair as usual, rinsing and applying creme rinse if wanted. Pour 1 cup/250ml strained oatstraw infusion over hair and massage in; don't rinse out. Towel dry hair for best results.

Oat Tonic

Nourishes and rehydrates

1 cup/250ml oats
1 cup/250ml water
1 teaspoon/5ml lemon juice
1 teaspoon/5ml raw honey
1 teaspoon/5ml water

Pour boiling water over oats and let stand overnight. In the morning add remaining ingredients. Mix well, then pour into cloth and wring juice out, saving it carefully. Take by the spoonful.

A little something extra for sick young ones, nauseated moms, those recovering from any gastro-intestinal problems, including surgery, and those healing from acid poisoning.

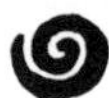

Oatstraw Kitchen

Wild Oatmeal Bread

serves 6-8

3 c/750ml whole wheat flour
1 cup/250ml rolled oats
5 tsp/25ml baking powder
2 Tbs/30ml dried greens*
1 egg
3 tablespoons/45ml honey
1 Tbs/15ml olive oil
1½ cup/375ml milk or water

*Try nettle, violet, or dandelion leaves

Mix dry ingredients together very well in a large bowl. Beat egg in a separate bowl; then beat in rest of wet ingredients. Pour wet stuff into dry and stir only until blended. Spoon into a greased 8 inch/23cm cake pan or cast iron frying pan. Bake at 350 F/80 C for one hour, or until center is dry. Top may be very brown and crusty.

Preparation time; About 1½ hours: 20 minutes plus one hour baking. Adjust flour/liquid ratio as needed so batter is neither too soupy nor too dry. Don't overstir, it toughens the bread.

Wild Oats 'n' Breakfast

serves 2

1 tsp/5ml slippery elm
1 tsp/5ml plantain seed/hulls
1 tsp/5ml sesame seed
½ cup/125ml steel-cut oats
2½ c/625ml boiling water*

*or use sassafras tea, sweet birch tea, or spicebush tea.

Mix dry ingredients together and add to boiling, salted water. Stir until boil resumes; lower heat and cook for 25-30 minutes. *Overnight method:* Put mixed dry ingredients in a thermos, and add boiling water. Cover and retire. Your cooked cereal awaits you next morning.

Preparation time: 30 minutes (overnight method—5 minutes). Watch out that it doesn't boil over. To use rolled oats instead: reduce water by ½ cup and cooking time to 5-10 minutes.

Oatcakes

makes 12-16 "cakes"

2 cups/500ml rolled oats
½ tsp/3ml baking powder
½ tsp/3ml salt
1 cup/250ml oats
2 tablespoons/30ml olive oil
6-8 Tbs/90-120ml hot water
½ cup/125ml rolled oats

Grind rolled oats to a fine meal in a blender or grinder. You'll get about 1½ cups/375ml meal. Mix this with baking powder, salt, 1 cup/250ml unground oats, and oil. Add just enough water to form a ball of dough. Make it two balls. Sprinkle just a little oats on your counter and roll out each ball (adding more oats as needed) to two hand-spans wide (9 inches/25cm). Cut each circle into 6-8 wedges. Cook on a cookie sheet at 350F/80C for fifteen minutes, or in a cast-iron skillet for eight minutes a side.

Preparation time: 30 minutes from conception to consumption. Serve hot with butter or cold with fruit conserves for a most elegant breakfast or tea.

"Instead of coffee, a drink made from equal parts Oat beards, roasted acorns, and chicory [root], in equal parts, is a welcome and beneficial change."
Alma Hutchens (1969)

Festival Oatcakes

makes 8 little "cakes"

¼ cup/60g butter
1 teaspoon/5ml honey
½ cup/125ml rolled oats
1 tablespoon/15ml wine*
more honey

*preferably elderberry or dandelion

Melt butter and honey carefully. Stir in oats, wine, and a pinch of salt. Add more honey slowly until taste and heft are to your liking. Form little cakes, put on an oiled baking sheet, and bake at 350 F/80 C for 15-20 minutes or until brown.

Preparation time: 30 minutes unless you taste the wine too frequently! These are a witchy sacramental bread and can be used for any ritual celebration.

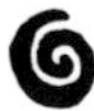

Oatstraw Fun and Facts

• Alma Hutchens is virtually the only writer of my ken who treats Avena as a medicinal, nutritional ally. *"An important restorative in nervous prostration and exhaustion after all febrile diseases, it [oats] seems to support the heart muscles and urinary organs."* Others cursorily mention her sexy ways and body-building abilities.

• Socrates says oats are choleric and fiery. Healers of later centuries were cautioned not to use oats "when the stomach is hot and overacid."

• There were at least twenty-five species of Avena cultivated in 1931; today only three. The USSR is the leading producer of oats, with USA second, and Canada third.

• Wild oat flower essence nourishes clarity in one's life direction.

• Thanks to *The Witches' Goddess,* by Janet and Stewart Farrar (Phoenix, 1987) for leads on Avena's story/myth, and the idea for festival oat cakes.

• Thanks to David and Nikki Goldbeck, *American Wholefoods Cuisine,* (NAL, 1983) for inspiration and that fabulous oatcakes recipe.

• Thanks to Robert Masters for the meditation that transformed itself into the "Avena meditation."

• The ancient ones knew oats as a weed. Avena's place of origin is unknown and virtually unguessable. Is it Sicily? A Chilean island? Atlantis?

• Organic oatmeal and steel cut oats are available from:
    Deaf Smith products
    North East Co-op (800-321-COOP)
    Walnut Acres, Penns Creek, PA 17862.

• Fresh oatstraw tincture is available from:
    Avena Botanicals, PO Box 365, West Rockport, ME 04865.

• Resources for nutritional breakdown of oats and oatstraw:
    Composition of Cereal Grains, Pub. 585, NRC, 1958
    Composition of Foods, Handbook 8, USDA, 1963
    Nutrition Almanac, Nutrition Search, McGraw Hill, 1975
    Nutritional Herbology, Pedersen, 1987

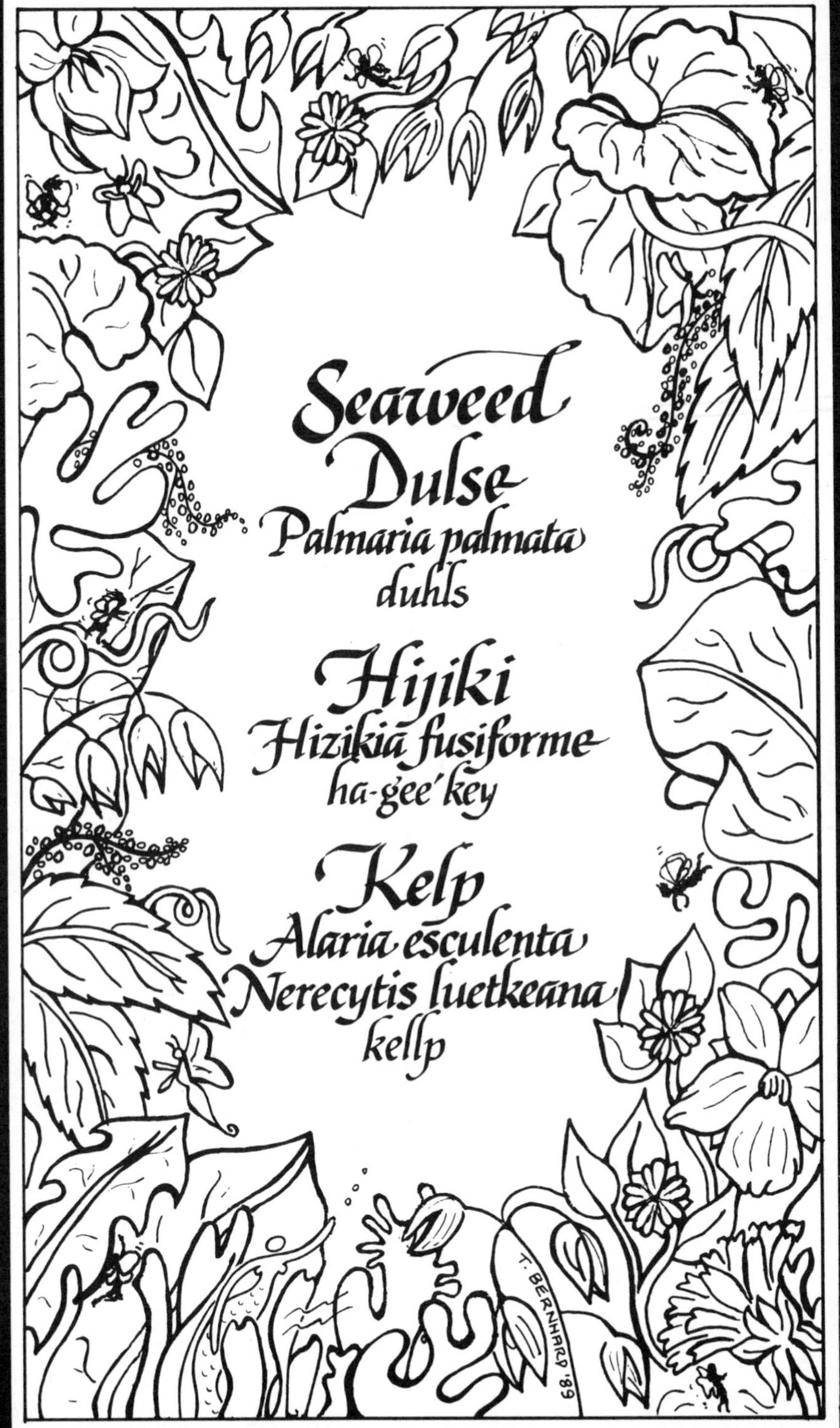
Seaweed
Dulse
Palmaria palmata
duhls
Hijiki
Hizikia fusiforme
ha-gee'key
Kelp
Alaria esculenta
Nerecytis luetkeana
kellp
T. BERNHARD '89

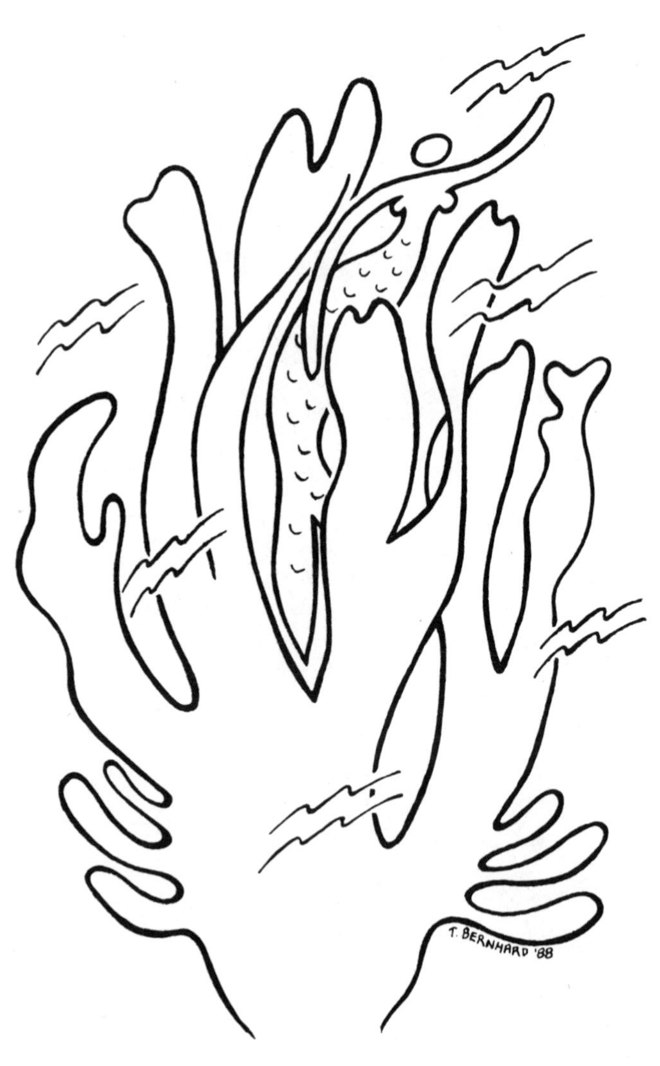
T. BERNHARD '88

Seaweed Speaks

Come dance with me.
Dance with me.
Flow with me.
Flow with me.
Move with me
Flexibly
In the sea's tides . . .

Warm wet moon womb tune I sing.
Deep full rich sun song I sing.
Sing with me now.
I am the sea's green hair.
I am the ocean's weed.
Be with me now . . .

Now flexibly
And flowingly
Be sensitive and
Dance with me.
Nerve net filigree be and
Dance with me
Here . . .

Warm wet moon womb tune I sing.
Deep full rich sun song I sing.
Sing with me now.
I am the sea's lush grass.
I am the ocean's dream.
Be with me now . . .

Come dance with me.
Feed on me.
Fill yourself
Full of me.
Eat now
In ecstasy,
Filled
With the flow . . .

Warm wet moon womb tune I sing.
Deep full rich sun song I sing.
Sing with me now.
I am the sea's salt feast.
I am the ocean's gift.
Come
Be with me now . . .

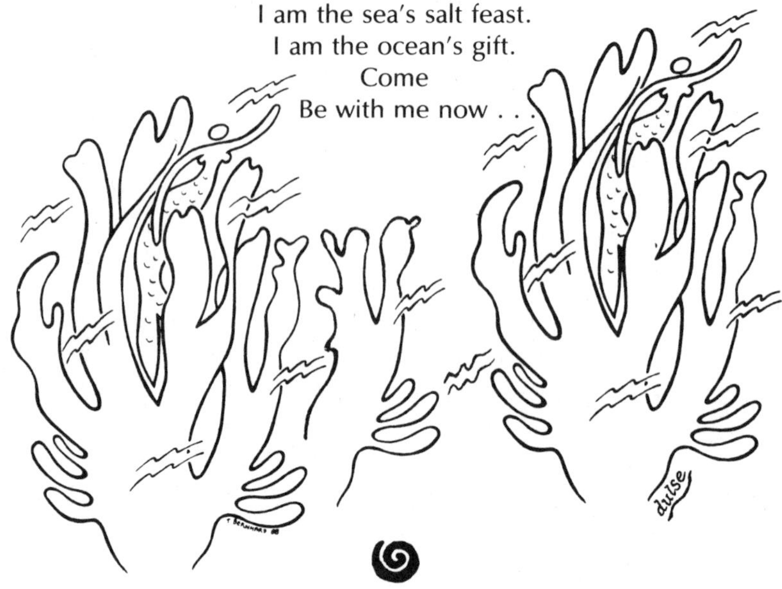

Hijiki Facts

Botanical name: *Hizikia fusiforme*. ***Other useful species:*** *Eisenia bicyclis*/Arame. ***Family:*** Phaeophyta/Brown algae. ***Chinese names:*** Hai tso, chiau tsai, hai ti tun, hai toe din, hai tsao, hoi tsou. ***Korean names:*** Nongmichae. ***Habitat:*** On rocks exposed at low tide. ***Range:*** Japan, China, Korea. ***Fun:*** Hijiki is the only plant in this book that I've never met alive and in person. So I can't say I love her, but I certainly have a mad crush on her! She's been my ally for introducing many to the delights of eating seaweed. Virtually everyone who dares taste hijiki (she does look like little black worms) wants more, then more, and more, and soon they're hooked on seaweed . . . heh, heh, heh.

Hijiki is a high protein seaweed. It also supplies excellent amounts of carotenes (vitamin A), the vitamin C complex, the vitamin B complex, and vitamins E and K.

The mineral content of hijiki is well balanced, with large amounts of iron, phosphorus, and calcium.

Hijiki is a very good source of algin. (See **Seaweed Facts: *Medical uses.***)

Dulse Facts

Botanical name: *Palmaria palmata*; palma (Latin) means palm of the hand and refers to the usual shape of dulse. ***Other useful species:*** *Rhodymenia palmata, Laurencia pinnatifida.* ***Family:*** Rhodophyceae/ Red algae. ***English names:*** Dulce, red kale, Neptune's girdle. ***French names:*** Gomon vache. ***Icelandic names:*** Saccha, sol. ***Irish names:*** Dillisk, dillesk, crannogh. ***Japanese names:*** Darusu. ***Norwegian names:*** Sou sol. ***Tlinket (Native American) names:*** Raa-ts. ***Habitat:*** On rocks, shells, other algae; from midtide mark to below low tide mark; in deep waters. ***Range:*** Northern and Southern hemispheres, all Atlantic and Pacific coastal waters. ***Fun:*** Dulse is fermented into an alcoholic beverage in Siberia, and baked into bread in Iceland.

Dulse is very high in protein (25.3%), and that protein is exceptionally digestible (75%). Dulse is also very high in iron (150), potassium (8060-8100), sodium (2085), and vitamin A. *(Figures are milligrams per hundred grams of herb.)*

As with all seaweeds, the vitamin composition varies quite dramatically from season to season, with highest carotene (vitamin A) concentration generally in the summer and highest vitamin C complex concentration usually in the fall.

Dulse is notably rich in iodine (8) and phosphorus (267-270).

Dulse is an excellent source of vitamins B_6, B_{12}, E, and C, as well as many other minerals and trace minerals including calcium (296-567), magnesium (220), bromine, sulphur, radium, boron, rubidium, and titanium. Folic acid and folinic acid are also present.

Dulse Cold Cure

Soak a handful of dulse for 10-15 minutes in enough hot water to cover. Then cook the dulse in that water, at very low heat, for 15-20 minutes. Strain. Save seaweed: add to soup or give it to the earth. Add honey and lemon juice, to taste, to the hot liquid. Old sea folk put in a glug of rum, too.

"The oldest book in Iceland makes reference to the rights and concessions involved before one might collect and/or eat fresh sol (Palmaria palmata) on a neighbor's land. The alga [seaweed] has been eaten there since the year 961 before the common era." Judith Madlener (1977)

Kelp Facts

Botanical name: *Alaria esculenta*; ala (Latin) means wing, esculenta (Latin) means edible. ***Other useful species:*** *Nereocystis luetkeana, Laminaria longicruris, L. longissima, L. angustata, L. japonica, L. ochotensis, Fucus versiculosis, Macrocystis pyrifera*, and *Pleurophycus gardneri*. ***Family:*** Phaeophyceae/Brown algae. ***Common names:*** *(Alaria)* Wakame, edible kelp, wing kelp, honeyware; *(Nereocystis)* Ribbon kelp, giant kelp, bull whip kelp, sea kelp, horsetail kelp, bladder kelp, sea otter's cabbage; *(Laminaria)* Kombu; *(Fucus)* Bladderwrack, rockweed. ***Scottish/Irish names:*** Bladderlochs, tangle. ***Icelandic names:*** Marinkjarni. ***Quileute (Native American) names:*** *(Nereocystis)* Xopiikis. ***Quinault (Native American) name:*** *(Nereocystis)* Kotka. ***Habitat:*** Rocky coasts, exposed locations; near and below the low tide mark. ***Range:*** *(Alaria)* North temperate to subfrigid zones of Atlantic coastal waters. *(Nereocystis)* South temperate to subfrigid zones of Pacific coastal waters. *(Fucus)* Atlantic and Pacific oceans, Arctic to temperate waters. ***Fun:*** *Macrocystis pyrifera* is the world's leading source of algin. *Fucus* species seaweeds are the most abundant and available for the casual gatherer.

Kelps *(figures indicate milligrams per hundred grams* Laminaria *and* Fucus *species)* are very high in calcium (800-3040), potassium (2110-5300), magnesium (760-867), sodium (3007-5610), and tin (2.4).

Kelps are also high in silicon (7.6), aluminum (63.1), bromine, and iodine (150-540).

Kelps are high in carotenes expressed as vitamin A (140-6600 IU), and also supply at least average amounts of virtually every other vitamin, including the B complex: thiamine (.08-.11), riboflavin, (.14-.32), niacin (5.70-10), B_6, B_{12}; the vitamin C complex expressed as ascorbic acid (25.8); K, and E.

Kelps are also mineral treasure chests and have been found to contain average or higher amounts of manganese (7.6), phosphorus (240-260), selenium (1.7), iron (8.9-100), silver, strontium, chloride, copper, barium, boron, radium, lithium, nickel, zinc (0.6), chromium (0.7), cobalt (1.6), vanadium, titanium, mercury (4.0), arsenic (6.8), lead (9.1), molybdenum, rubidium. (See **Seaweed Facts** for a discussion of toxicity of heavy metals found in seaweeds.)

Kelps are quite low in calories (249) and fat.

Kelps are superb sources of algin and alginic acids and contain average amounts of protein (6.5-12.7%).

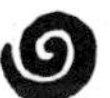

Seaweed Facts

Fiber uses: Dried stipes of *Nereocystis* can be used as fishing line. ***Food uses:*** Fresh and dried seaweed may be found for sale in many of the world's coastal markets, especially in the Philippines, Japan, Indonesia, Korea, China, and Hawaii. In North America, however, fresh seaweed is found only in ethnic oriental markets, and dried seaweed in specialty stores may be available only in pill form. Alginates from seaweed appear in many commercial foods, such as ice cream, to thicken and stabilize. ***Medicinal uses:*** Seaweed is the primary source of algin, which, as purified mucilage, is used in many pharmaceuticals and cosmetics, as surgical fibers, and in dentistry. ***Soil uses:*** Fertilizer beyond compare. ***Ocean uses:*** Water purifier. ***Animal uses:*** Sold as a dietary supplement recommended for virtually all animals, including birds. ***Toxicity:*** *Externally,* adverse reactions to seaweed are not reported. *Internally,* seaweeds are non-poisonous though there are two hazardous species. (See **Seaweed Fun and Facts**.) Heavy metals and natural radioactive elements are found in most seaweeds and there is serious controversy about the bio-availability of such toxins. Well-documented studies attest to the fact that the arsenic in kelp is not assimilated. Does this mean that the other heavy metals are not assimilated either? One author suggests that none of the minerals in kelps are bio-available! Australia has banned the sale of Japanese seaweeds due to the high toxic metal content. For my own peace of mind, I gather my own seaweeds from the least polluted ocean waters I can find; I support the efforts of other small-scale, conscientious seaweed gatherers; and I contribute to water conservation and quality improvement personally and through organizations.

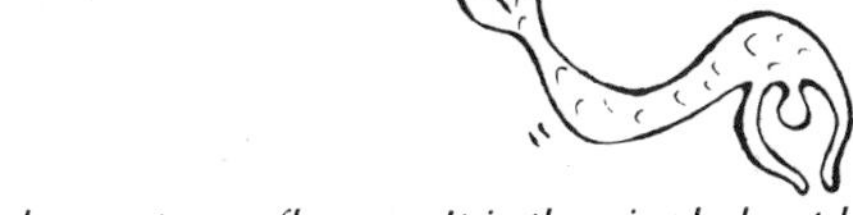

"Fucus has a strong flavour. It is the single best kelp to use (fresh, dried, cooked, ground, or steeped overnight) in restorative and healing situations." Ryan Drum (1988)

"A kelp's daily life is the deep flow-pulsation of the tides, changing direction approximately every six hours. If corn is ancient and wise on land, so is kelp in the sea." L. Hanson (1980)

Seaweed Weed Walk

Wake up. Put on some warm clothes and meet me downstairs.

Ready? OK. Grab a couple of those tofu buckets and follow me. We're off to gather some seaweed. The heart-healthy seasoning, the salty spice of life!

We'll walk to the beach, and talk about seaweed on the way. I left the pickup there yesterday and walked home, so we won't have to walk back later, when our buckets will be full of seaweed and heavy. The tide won't be out for several hours yet, so we can take our time and enjoy the walk and the early morning fog.

Seaweeds aren't, of course, really weeds. They're more like wild flowers, or more accurately, like underwater ferns. I think of them as ferns because they reproduce by spores; most of them are hardy perennials; and they're superbly graceful.

Unlike land plants, seaweeds don't have different tissues for root, stem, and leaves, but one sort of tissue that assumes somewhat analogous shapes: holdfasts are like roots, stalks like stems, and blades or fronds, like leaves. Floats give the seaweed buoyancy.

Holdfasts, as the name implies, hold the seaweed fast to the ocean bed, but do not gather nutrients as roots do. All of the seaweed's nourishment comes from the sun and the seawater, absorbed through the entire surface of the blade or frond. The stalk spans the distance (sometimes as much as a ten-story building) between the holdfast and the frond. Hear the surf over in the cove? We haven't much further now to walk.

Specialized tissues form at reproductive sites. There, particular cells thicken and swell, until a jelly surrounds the sexual bodies, which bear spores. This jelly protects thousands of spores until they ripen, float free of their parent, and drift off in search of a new spot to touch down. As soon as one lands on a site to its liking, it germinates immediately and starts to grow.

Here we are! We still have quite a bit of time before the tide has ebbed enough to reach the dulse. Let's go out in the rowboat and see the kelp beds. Somebody said kelp is the grandfather of the ocean, but I am reminded more of mermaids when I look into the dense expanse of rippling kelp fronds.

Get a life jacket, and bring that bucket. I can't resist coming home with a little fresh nereo, our favorite snack food. While you row, I'll tell you more about seaweed. The pull in your shoulders, the sun sparkling on the waves, will help you remember what you hear; row hard.

All varieties of kelp are safe to gather and eat, except one, called acid kelp, which burns a bit if you touch it. There is one other poisonous seaweed but it looks more like slime than weed. Between the sting and the slime no one is likely to try to eat either of them. So basically, we can say then that all seaweeds are edible.

All around the world, people eat them. By far the largest and most spectacular kelp, though not necessarily the best-tasting, is the one you're rowing us out to see: *Nereocystis*, giant kelp. Almost anyone who's been on a beach along the Atlantic or Pacific coast after a storm has seen the long tubular stalks, holdfasts, and thick ballon-like floats of nereo. Bull whips, the kids call 'em. Those floats make great bowls and toys of all sorts. But we're just going to harvest some of the fronds, which are quite delicious once dried.

If you have a hankering for something spicy, you can make a pretty good pickle out of stormwrecked nereo stalks and floats. It's one of the few seaweeds that not only can survive being tossed up on the beach after a heavy storm, but can still be appetizing despite the harsh treatment. Try substituting the stalk for cucumber or green tomato in your favorite relish or chutney recipe. But be careful to rinse it only in seawater to remove clinging sand. Freshwater washing before drying often makes the seaweed fishy tasting.

In the water, kelp is an enchanting dancer. Can you see her now? It's enough to make your mouth water! How are your arms? Need these sunglasses? Row just over there a bit more.

Great. Stop here. *Splash.* Now we're anchored and you can get a closer look. It's hard to see the size of this kelp bed from here, floating on the water. But take my word for it, it's big. Out from this edge grows a seemingly endless expanse of waving kelp blades where whales, sea lions and sea otters swim. The kelps form huge lush underwater fields, meadows, and forests which are home to myriad lives.

Rest now and let your hands dangle in the water. Let the kelp touch you. Close your eyes. Feel its story.

Feel the floats nudge you, each float the size of a newborn person's head, floating in the amniotic fluid of mother ocean. Each float is filled with half a gallon/two liters of air.

Feel the smooth, smooth, undivided blades undulate against your wrists and hands. Slide your hands along the blade. First this way, toward me, toward the float.

Feel these little attachments? The blades grow out of there; the further away from the float the frond part is, the older it is. You could feel it grow if you sat here for even a day. At this time of year it grows about a nose length in twenty-four hours.

Now slide your hands the other way; grab hold and slowly begin to pull. And pull and pull. Here, gather it into the buckets we brought. Keep pulling. Sure, you can open your eyes. It's a long pull. About fifty times your length, I'd say, on a big one.

Now, see how the blade gets thicker and tougher as we pull it in? This is the oldest part. See how the green fades and the brown color is more obvious? I use this older, tougher part for the garden and the younger, thinner part for eating. There! It's all in.

We'll each pull in a couple more and that'll fill the buckets and get us back in time to search out dulse. Remember to cut the blade an arm's length from that little attachment to the float, so the kelp will keep growing for its full year of life (yes, it is the rare annual seaweed)—nourishing and sheltering so many.

Silence except for sea sounds, bird cries, and boat creaks . . .

All right. Up anchor and on to dulse. I'll row for a bit. We want to get over there, into the turbulence.

Dulse, blood mystery of the sea. Dulse, daily, is a wonderful ally for strengthening women. With her dark purple-red color and her ever-changing shape, dulse is as red and changing as a woman's moon time. She is the image of uterine power and mystery. With her beneficial yeasts, proteins, and minerals, dulse is an optimum nourisher for uterus and nerves.

OK. Let's be careful of the boat in this water. Even at low tide, it's rough. There's the dulse. Right there in the crevice of the cliff. See how it hangs on? It loves to be dashed by the waves. There. Got it? It's such a fragile-looking seaweed, you wouldn't think she'd like to hang out in such a rough place!

Maybe I especially like dulse because I identify with her. She's tenacious, hardy, adaptable, and flourishes even in extreme situations. And she has a wise woman way of changing her form to adapt to specific micro-environments. Dulse is a wise woman, a shape-shifter, a bleeding woman, a changing women, a woman whose friend it is good to be.

That's the holdfast. That little disk. Hard to believe it could ever get a start, no matter how small, in this cliff face. There's hardly any stalk either. The whole thing is mostly blade. Look through it. What a color! Like stained glass. And she's so smooth and curves so gently, like a fragment of some tropical sunrise set adrift here in this cold water.

The little decorations all along the edge of the dulse, like little appendages, are secondary growths. See how the blade gets split and split again as it grows until it looks like a hand? Palmaria, like the palm of your hand. Most of them are hand-sized, too. Though some are baby hands and some are monster hands. Arrgh! Got ya!

Enough fun. Let's get busy before the tide changes. Check all along here on the other seaweeds, those wet rocks, even under ledges. Dulse likes to hunker down and go along for the ride. She plays hard to find and hard to get. Cut her properly, respectfully, with a knife, and it's likely she'll grow again. She's a long-lived crone of the sea. And one who gets around. You'll find dulse back home on the east coast, too.

We have a lot of work ahead of us still today. It takes longer to hang the seaweed to dry than it does to harvest it. Yup, we'll dry it all. Neither the dulse nor the kelp is great fresh . . . too rubbery.

No, no rinsing. Fresh water would burst the cell walls, and once dried, the seaweed, though not much different in looks, would smell fishy and taste unpleasant. Yeah, like the stuff you may have had in pills.

When we get home we'll spread the dulse on those screens you saw in the tall racks by the back door, where it's out of the direct sun. With a good breeze, it will be dry enough to put away this evening. It will still be pliable; dulse never really gets crisp and dry like other seaweeds and herbs. Sometimes I roast it or toast it before adding it to dishes, but mostly I like it as a chewy snack.

Then we'll hang the kelp: some outside on clothesline (secured with clothespins) and some inside from the nails I have hammered into all the rafters . . . but only after we carpet the house with newspaper to catch the drips! Then we'll light a fire in the woodstove so the nereo will dry as fast as possible. I'd dry it all inside, but I don't have room.

The kelp will get crunchy dry. In three or four days, I'll be able to take it down and store it in loose bundles to finish drying before final storage in paper or plastic bags. Enough of my talk. Let's harvest dulse and listen to her for a while!

Is that the laugh of my grandmother I hear?
Is that the song of the mermaid?

There, that ought to do us. The season's almost done on dulse. See how some of it is looking grey? I have enough harvested to last me to spring, though. OK. I'll row this time. Yup, back to dock. Breakfast is waiting! And I'm hungry.

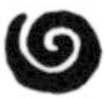

Seaweed Properties and Uses

- ***protective,*** anti-radiation, anti-cancer, anti-oxidant, anti-toxic, anti-rheumatic, antibiotic, antibacterial, alterative
- ***nutritive,*** trace mineral supplement, cardio-tonic, rejuvenative, aphrodisiac
- ***mucilaginous,*** emollient, demulcent, aperient, anti-constipative, diuretic
- ***anti-stress,*** analgesic, calmative, anti-pyretic

Seaweeds, especially the brown ones, are frequently a regular part of a wise woman's diet, to nourish and insure health/wholeness/holiness and to **prevent damage** to tissues from chemicals, heavy metals, and certain types of radioactivity. The potent **infection-halting** properties of the kelps combine with an **immune-stimulating** factor and **optimum nourishment** for repair of **glandular, cardiac, urinary,** and **nervous systems**. Kelps and other seaweeds help offset stress, boost stamina, lower blood pressure and cholesterol, restore sexual interest and enjoyment, and even ease sore joints.

Use seaweed as a body guard, an everyday miracle, an ally with lots of heart, a way to get your juices flowing, a gut greaser, an ally in women's mysteries, a great way to stay in shape, and a sleek finishing touch.

- Dose of *fresh or soaked seaweed* is ¼ oz–8 oz/5-220 grams a day.

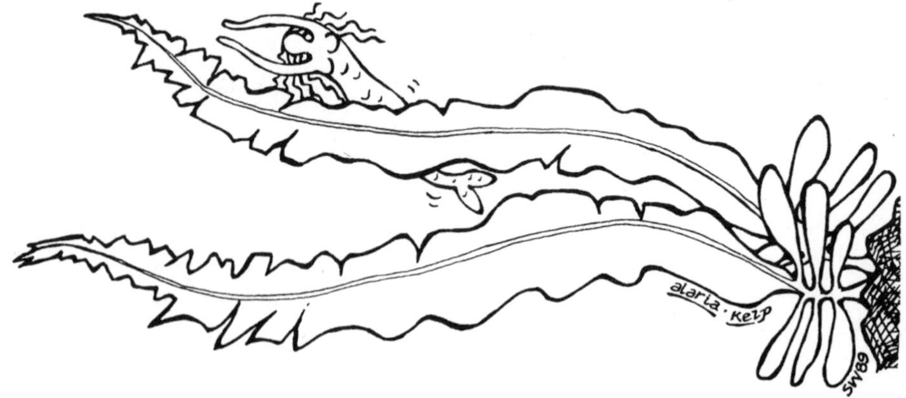

Seaweed is a Body Guard

Superb protection from modern pollutants, heavy metals, and accidental radioactive leaks is the gift of seaweed, the body guard. Regular use, especially of brown types, clears lead, arsenic, cadmium, mercury, chemical pollution, and radioactive strontium from the body, prevents absorption from new sources, and protects against damage caused by exposure to carcinogens and teratogens.

Workers at Swedish nuclear power plants eat seaweed to reduce and eliminate their absorption of strontium 90, a radioactive element. Research at McGill University finds that alginic acid, one of the main components of seaweed, binds with radioactive strontium to form strontium alginate, an insoluble compound, which is rapidly eliminated from the gastro-intestinal tract, reducing the absorption of strontium 90 by fifty to ninety percent.

Strontium 90, released in nuclear accidents as well as in the running of nuclear power plants, has a high affinity for calcium. When released into the air, it is easily concentrated in calcium-rich foods such as milk (including mother's milk) and leafy greens. Eat these contaminated foodstuffs and the radioactivity, now combined with calcium, enters the bone marrow where it can damage delicate immune and blood cells. Consistently eating seaweed helps eliminate any radioactive particles already absorbed, repairs damage to the bone marrow, and prevents further absorption of strontium 90.

Fucoidan and algin, components of brown seaweeds, diminish blood levels of lead in animal studies. Seaweeds have been shown to remove mercury, cadmium, lead, barium, tin, and other heavy metals from tissue, according to the Marine Technology Society.

In an environment increasingly contaminated with radioactive waste and chemical pollution, frequent use of seaweed is a Wise Woman way of maintaining health, providing anti-cancer insurance, and keeping your attention focused on mother ocean, her needs, and her abundance in maintaining the health/wholeness/holiness of us all.

Try using a sprinkle of seaweed on grains, even breakfast cereals, vegetables, and eggs. Serve seaweed as a vegetable in its own right once a week or more. Increase consumption as needed, such as when healing after radiation, chemotherapy, or extensive X-rays.

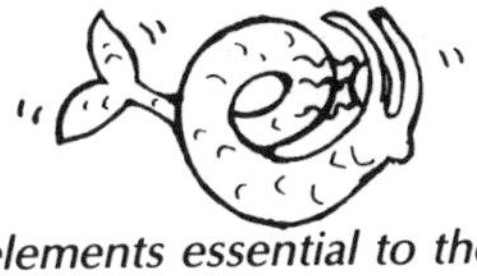

"Of the fourteen elements essential to the proper metabolic functions of the human body, thirteen are known to be in Kelp."

Dr. J.W. Turentine, USDA agricultural scientist (1974)

Seaweed is an Everyday Miracle

The benefits of including seaweed's optimum nourishment into your daily diet are extensive: increased longevity, enhanced immune functioning, revitalization of the cardiovascular, endocrine, digestive, and nervous systems, and relief from minor aches and pains. No wonder seaweed has been part of the traditional diet of all coastal cultures, including the people of Japan, Korea, China, Iceland, Denmark, Wales, Scotland, Hawaii, and South Pacific Isles, and all the peoples who had trading contacts with the coastal cultures.

In fact, remnants of Stone Age seaweed dinners have recently been discovered in South Africa. In my book that's as good a recommendation as four stars.

All seaweeds are high in fiber. Those in the brown family supply large amounts of algin as well. Each seaweed contains a wide range of essential nutrients, including enzymes, nucleic acids, amino acids, minerals, trace elements, and A, B, C, D, E, and K vitamin complexes. Seaweeds offer us zest for life and the perfect medium for electrical (nerve) flow.

Benefits from a Wise Woman alliance with seaweed—glossier hair, more luminous skin, less digestive distress, renewed energy and stamina, rekindled sexual desires, and reawakened delight in life—will be noticeable in about thirteen weeks.

Seaweed is an Ally with Lots of Heart

Seaweed is a full-hearted cardiovascular ally. Japanese research over the past several decades has found many cardiotonic and hypotensive (as well as nutritive) constituents in kelps like Laminaria.

Dancing, singing seaweed strengthens circulation, balances blood pressure, lowers cholesterol, builds healthy blood, increases the veins' and heart's contractile force, restores and increases cardiac efficiency, nourishes and prolongs the life of the heart muscle, and encourages rhythmical working of the heart in all its aspects: physical, emotional, and inspirational.

How can weeds with so much sodium (we all know salt raises blood pressure) be good for the heart and even hypotensive, that is, capable of lowering blood pressure?

Sodium is not to blame for high blood pressure. Sodium chloride may be. Table salt may be. But table salt contains sugar, aluminum salts, and several other agents as well as sodium chloride. This is an unnatural salt solution and one that creates cardiovascular stress.

The naturally-occurring sodium in seaweeds (and garden weeds) bathes the inner being with rich salty nourishment, like the amniotic fluid of our original home. This sodium relieves tension in blood vessels made brittle by immersion in the wrong saline solution, table salt. (Note that commercial sea salt is usually as full of free-flowing agents and other addenda as commercial table salt. Real evaporated sea water salt is pinkish in color. As usual, if it's white, you can't trust it.)

Seaweed is a wonderful green ally to use with other Wise Woman ways when healing those with problems of the heart and circulation including atherosclerosis, hypertension, chilly extremities, varicosities, heart infections, repressed feelings, and self-blame.

Seaweed is a Way to Get Your Juices Flowing

Juices in the hormonal system, juices in the glands, juices in the kidneys, juices in the gonads, juices in the digestive tract, juices in the brain: seaweed keeps your juices flowing smoothly by nourishing superbly.

Daily use of seaweed provides optimum nourishment for the hormonal, lymphatic, urinary, and nervous systems.

The hormonal system uses the minerals and trace elements so richly available from seaweed to repair tissue, build new cells, and create hormones responsible for regulating blood pressure, metabolism, fertility, sexuality, and reaction to allergens, to name but a few.

In addition to providing direct nourishment to the endocrine glands, seaweed functions as a communicator between the glands. Electrical activity flows smoothly in the medium seaweed provides. One herbalist describes the role of seaweed as "hormonal counselor or ambassador, maybe even a special messenger, to keep communication clear and balanced in the endocrine network."

As little as a teaspoonful/5grams of seaweed daily, combined with Wise Woman ways, helps heal those with goiter, impotence, infertility, delayed menarche (onset of menstruation after age 16), obesity, anorexia, prostate enlargement, lack of ovulation, thyroid malfunction (both hyper- and hypo-), menopausal distress, allergic reactions, and hives.

The lymphatic and immune systems are also avid partakers of seaweed's splendid feast of nutrients. Combined with this optimum nourishment, the communication-enhancing effects of seaweed further enhance response time and strength in the immune sytem. This reduces opportunistic bacterial and viral infections and helps prolong youth and vitality, not to mention joy and ease in life.

Seaweed also inhibits the growth of many viruses, as well as gram-positive and gram-negative bacteria. This directly assists the immune system, as does seaweed's anti-oxidant ability. Since some types of rheumatism and arthritis are the result of viral infections, seaweed's long-standing use as a joint easer and anti-rheumatic becomes clearer. The wise woman understands a holographic connection here: seaweed shows stiff joints how to flow.

The urinary system gets a special boost from seaweed's seeming excess of potassium and sodium. Those with cystitis, kidney weakness, gout, diabetic kidney ills, and bladder weakness find health/wholeness/holiness with seaweed and Wise Woman ways.

The nervous system relaxes in the presence of seaweed's mineral abundance. Seaweed creates an inner environment where nerve signals flow more smoothly and where brain chemicals are produced as needed: to maintain alertness, increase memory, reduce pain, and provide a sense of buoyant bliss. (Envision the head-sized floats of kelp bobbing on a gently undulating sea.)

Daily use of seaweed strengthens mental facility, increases sensory receptivity, and reduces the effects of mental stress. Ask seaweed to help restore neural sheaths and thus lessen the pain and debility of those with neuritis, multiple sclerosis, nervous tics, and so-called senility.

Seaweed is a Gut Greaser

Seaweed provides a multitude of gifts to the digestive system: soothing, disinfecting, and nourishing distressed surfaces, helping out with the metabolism of lipids, and maintaining a healthy balance of digestive yeasts and bacteria in the intestines.

Seaweed is an exceptional ally to the wise woman healing those with gastric ulcers, duodenal ulcers, ulcerated colon, colitis, constipation, watery stools, and other intestinal ills, thanks to its bio-available nourishment, high algin content, mucilaginous fiber, and rhythmical resonation.

The salt forms of alginic acids in seaweeds are known as alginates. These alginates are capable of absorbing and retaining large amounts of water, neutralizing over-acidic digestive secretions, and reducing internal bleeding. Enhanced by the mucilaginous fiber and the wave-like energy of seaweed, algin acts as a gentle regulator of intestinal action.

Lipid metabolism, or fat digestion, is one of the body's minor miracles, and it is no wonder that sometimes there are snags in the process. Seaweed not only helps smooth out glitches in fat digestion, it can dissolve fatty build-ups in the body and blood vessels, and help regulate levels of triglycerides, phospholipids, and cholesterols.

Yeast-sensitive people, or those diagnosed with candida overgrowth, find that the friendly digestive yeasts on dulse (dried without a fresh water rinse) rapidly restore digestive integrity.

Seaweed is an Ally in Women's Mysteries

Seaweed flows and shifts like the energy of a woman. Saline solutions of ocean and uterus rock in rhythm. Pulses of tide, menstruation, heart beat, and fertility join seaweeds and wombs. Nourishing breast milk merges with waves of green fronds . . . optimum nourishment and the salts of life . . . breasts, seaweeds.

Seaweed eaten daily is a powerful ally to a wise woman, for prevention and healing herself or others with osteoporosis, breast cancer, mastitis, uterine cancer, irregular menstrual cycles, ovarian cancer, fibroids, ovarian cysts, infertility, fibro-cystic breast distress, and premenstrual/menopausal problems such as water retention, emotional freak-outs, chills and hot flashes, fatigue, lack of lubrication, loss of calcium, and general irritability.

Seaweed is a Great Way to Stay in Shape

By providing optimum nourishment to the thyroid, helping to regulate metabolism, and increasing the effectiveness of the digestive system, seaweed helps you get in shape and stay that way.

Seaweed helps weight melt away, literally, by re-engineering fat metabolism. Wise Woman wisdom and recent studies strongly indicate that obese beings metabolize fat very differently than lean ones do. Seaweed, acting through the liver, intestines, glands, and nerves, readjusts lipid metabolism insuring long term weight reduction.

Any restricted diet is improved by the addition of even a little seaweed: your vitamin-mineral-wholeness supplement from mother ocean.

Digestive damage caused by repeated dieting, antibiotic overuse, or chemotherapy can be healed with Wise Woman ways and seaweed's soothing mucilage, absorbing algin, and beneficial bacteria and yeasts.

When weight gain is your intention, when anemia, emaciation, anorexia, or convalescence is the problem, seaweed is the Wise Woman ally to arouse the appetite, restore strong digestion, nourish calm nerve functioning, alter poor self-image, and regulate energy flow. Seaweed also heals digestive surfaces injured by repeated vomiting and purging.

Use sprinklings of seaweed at first, in well-liked foods, and increase up to several servings a day if desired.

And if you are satisfied with your weight, don't forget the extra energy, stamina, freedom from fatigue, and longevity that come from regular use of seaweed.

Seaweed is a Sleek Finishing Touch

Want thicker, bouncier, more lustrous hair? (Like a mermaid . . .) Eat seaweed.

Want even-textured, wonderful-feeling skin? (Like a dolphin . . .) Eat seaweed.

Want to have strong nails and healthy teeth? (Like a shark . . .) Eat seaweed.

Some folks claim it'll even regrow your hair! Eat seaweed.

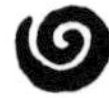

Seaweed Pharmacy

Plant Food Feast

especially for potatoes

Seaweed in the garden is a feast for sandy soils, a compost activator, and a particularly rich potash supplement for potato growing.

1 lb/500g fresh clover herb
1 lb/500g fresh comfrey leaf
1 lb/500g fresh seaweed *or*
4 oz/120g dried seaweed
1 lb/500g fresh d'lion herb
5 lbs/2 kilograms manure*
5 gallons/20 liters rain water

*horse, sheep, goat, or rabbit

Chop green herbs well and combine with seaweed, manure, and water. Do cover quite tightly before leaving it in a sunny spot to brew (and I do mean ferment) for several weeks. Sprinkle rock phosphate and granite dust on the potato patch while you wait. *To use,* dilute 1 part brew in 16 parts water and pour on potato plants. (Hold your nose!)

Preparation time: Several hours to gather the ingredients; another hour to chop and mix it; two weeks' wait; then you're set for the rest of the growing season.

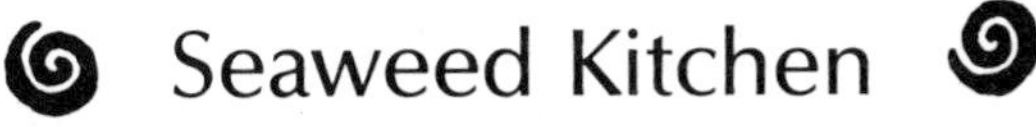

Seaweed Kitchen

Bladderwrack Tea

Gently simmer a handful of Fucus for 15 minutes in enough water to cover. Strain and enjoy. *Or*: fill a jar only a quarter full with dried bladderwrack; add boiling water to completely fill the jar; cap and let steep overnight. Next morning, strain (give the seaweed to the nearest patch of earth), warm, and enjoy, seasoned to your taste.

Old wives say a cup or two a day of Fucus tea, for no more than three months will melt excess pounds away. You may resume, if desired, after a break of six weeks.

Mother Earth/Mother Ocean Soup

serves 6-8

3 onions, chopped
3 tablespoons/45ml olive oil
6 potatoes, cubed
2 carrots, sliced
2 parsnips, sliced
½ c/125ml dried wild greens
½ c/125ml dried seaweed
12 cups/3 liters water

Sauté onion in oil until brown. Add all remaining ingredients. Cook until vegetables are done. Adjust seasoning, adding salt if desired, and let mellow overnight. Or serve immediately.

Preparation time: Under an hour. Seaweed doesn't need to be soaked first when cooked in soups.

Green and Purple Salad

serves 4

4 cups/1 liter watercress
1 cup/250ml dulse pieces
1 cup/225g goat cheese

Tear watercress and dulse into pieces. Arrange on four plates of brilliant hue. Sprinkle with crumbled goat cheese. Provide olive oil and lemon juice for at-table dressing.

Preparation time: With materials on hand, this salad is ready in 5-10 minutes. If you live near a stream, soak the dulse before you set out to gather the watercress. This salad is a tasty, nourishing, beautiful gift from the waters, both salt and fresh.

Sesame Seaweed Cornbread

serves 6-8

1 cup/250ml cornmeal
1 cup/250ml wholewheat flour
¼ teaspoon/1ml salt
4 tsp/12ml baking powder
1 Tbs/15ml dried seaweed
***
1 egg
1 cup/250ml milk or water
¼ cup/65ml sweetener
2 tablespoons/30ml oil
***
¼ cup/65ml sesame seeds

Sift dry ingredients together in a large bowl. Beat egg and add to other liquid ingredients. Grease a cast iron skillet or heavy cake pan & sprinkle sesame seeds evenly over bottom. Pour liquid mix into dry mix and stir only enough to blend; over-stirring toughens the bread. Spoon into pan. Bake in a very hot oven for 20-25 minutes or until dry in center. Call everyone to come eat just before bread is done so it can be served HOT from the oven.

Preparation time: 45 minutes the first time through; once you get the hang of it though, you can stir this up and have it ready for breakfast in 30 minutes. Blue corn meal and purple dulse are my special touches for this favorite fast bread.

"Seaweeds get their energy from the sun and their mystery from the moon." *Carol Petherbridge (1988*

Carrot/Onion/Hijiki

serves 4

½ cup/125ml dry hijiki
1 cup/250ml warm water
2 tablespoons/30ml olive oil
2 onions, crescent cut
2 carrots, diagonal cut
1 tablespoon/15ml tamari

Soak hijiki in water for 20-30 minutes. Cut onions in half from top to bottom; then cut top to bottom slices. Cook in oil until very brown. Put the carrots in an even layer over the onions. Top with a layer of hijiki. Add tamari and about half of the soaking water; cover tightly; cook until carrots are tender.

Preparation time: 20 minutes. This classic macrobiotic dish makes a seaweed lover out of the most skeptical adult or child. Arame can be used if hijiki is unavailable. The colorful contrast of orange carrot and black seaweed is spectacular at the table. This dish is an all-time favorite at the Wise Woman Center.

Not Fishy Chowder

serves 4

1 onion, chopped 1 stalk celery, thin sliced 1 tablespoon/15ml olive oil 2 potatoes, cubed 1 cup/250ml corn ½ carrot, diced ½ cup/125ml dry seaweed 8 cups/2 liters water	Sauté onion and celery in oil until tender. Add vegetables and water. If using tough seaweed like alaria, add that now, too. Bring to a boil, reduce heat and simmer until potato is soft. If using tender seaweed like dulse or nereocystis, add now. Serve when seaweed is cooked.

Preparation time: 10 minutes cutting and 30 minutes cooking. You can, of course, add fish of any sort, as well as other vegetables. Try it with two or more different types of seaweed.

Hijiki Caponata

serves 4

½ cup/125ml hijiki 1 cup/250ml warm water 2 tablespoons/30ml olive oil 10 lg cloves garlic, minced 1 onion, minced 1 Tbs/15ml chili powder 1 medium eggplant, diced 3 tablespoons/45ml olive oil 3 tablespoons/45ml tamari 1 Tbs/15ml dark sesame oil	Soak hijiki in warm water while you dice and cook onion and eggplant. Sauté onion in oil very slowly; when soft, add garlic and continue to cook until golden, not brown. Stir in the chili powder, then the eggplant, and another drizzle of oil. Cover well and cook slowly, stirring now and then and adding more oil as needed. When eggplant is dark and soft, drain hijiki and mix it (and tamari) into eggplant. Cover and cook over medium heat 2-5 minutes more. Add sesame oil, turn heat to high and, stirring constantly, bring to a boil and cook for one more minute. Serve with crackers, olives, goat cheese, and a wild green salad.

Preparation time: 25 minutes if you have help peeling the garlic. This recipe was created by an Italian who claimed to despise seaweed until he tasted hijiki. It is equally good served chilled.

Rare and Common Soup

serves 4

8 shitake
1 cup/125ml dried Fucus
hot water
6 cups/1.5 liters water
1 teaspoon/5ml garlic oil
6 oz/175g soba noodles
1 Tbs/15ml tamari or miso

Soak shitake and seaweed separately in hot water for at least 30 minutes. Reserve liquid when draining. Slice shitake caps, saving stalks for later use. Bring water to a boil and add seaweed, mushrooms, garlic oil (made by soaking sliced garlic in oil to cover for several days), reserved soaking liquid (minus grit) and noodles. Cook uncovered at high heat until noodles are done; then cover and cook at low heat until bladderwrack is soft. Add tamari or miso after removing soup from heat.

Preparation time: 45-50 minutes including soaking the dried mushrooms and seaweed. This filling one-dish meal requires very little of the cook. If shitake are unavailable, any other mushrooms will do.

Vietnamese Healing Soup

serves 6-8

1 cup/250ml uncooked rice
10 cups/2.5 liters water
2 ounces/60g dry seaweed
1 onion, chopped
3 stalks celery
3 carrots
3 green onions
2-3 Tbs/30-45ml tamari
2 Tbs/30ml dark sesame oil
1 Tbs/15ml hot sesame oil

Begin cooking the rice in 8 cups/2 liters water. (Traditionally, white rice is used, but brown rice may be substituted.) Snip the seaweed into bite-sized pieces and add to cooking rice. Chop the onions, celery, and carrots and add them to the pot. Simmer for 45-60 minutes, adding more water as needed. Add sliced green onions and other seasonings after the soup is off the heat, just before serving.

Preparation time: Ready to eat in an hour, but it can keep cooking if need be. The essence of the healing is in the seaweed and the hot oil, but I'm too sensitive to peppery stimulants, so I serve the hot oil separately and let each diner add their own.

Anne's Marinated Hijiki

serves 13

1 cup/250ml dry hijiki
3 cups/750ml hot water
4 cups/1 liter sliced celery
2 cups/500ml bean sprouts
4 cups/1 liter bok choy
dressing:
4 oz/125ml dark sesame oil
4 tablespoons/60ml tamari
2 Tbs/30ml rice vinegar
fresh ginger to taste

Soak hijiki in hot water while making dressing and cutting celery and bok choy. When hijiki is tender to the tooth, drain it well and combine with everything else (dressing too). Stir well and refrigerate overnight.

Any crisp vegetables may be used in this marinade: sunchokes, water chestnuts, burdock stalk pith, cattail roots, and so on.

Preparation time: About 30 minutes in the kitchen the night or morning before you plan to serve. Do try this easy dish at a party and prepare to be surprised by the empty bowl. (Thanks to Anne Georges.)

Alaria Minestrone

serves 20

4 tablespoons/60ml olive oil
2 c/500ml chopped onion
2 whole heads garlic
12 cups/3 liters vegetables
1 Tbs/15ml dried basil
2 Tbs/30ml dried wild greens
1 cup/250ml dried alaria, cut
2 teaspoons/10ml salt
10 cups/2.5 liters water
10 cups/2.5 l chopped tomato
2 cups/250ml leftover beans
2-4 cups leftover pasta

Sauté onion in olive oil while peeling and mincing garlic; sauté garlic. Add basil, greens, alaria, chopped vegetables, and water and bring to a boil. Lower heat and simmer until vegetables are done. Add tomatoes, beans, pasta, and adjust seasoning. Cook for at least another half hour.

If leftover beans and pasta are not available, use canned beans, and cook pasta in soup, allowing sufficient time for it to soften and merge with other ingredients.

Preparation time: At least 90 minutes. This soup is a great excuse to clean out your refrigerator. Spend a pleasant half-hour outside peeling garlic and listening to the birds. Then figure on an hour in the kitchen and you'll have a pot of soup and all the leftovers jars washed, too. The longer this soup simmers, the better. Minestrone gets tastier and tastier as it ages.

Seaweed Facts and Fun

• The seaweed weed walk was inspired by an exquisite afternoon of kelp harvesting with Ryan Drum. Any nautical mistakes are my own invention.

• The one poisonous type of seaweed is *Lyngbya* (mermaids' hair). It is a bright green, slimy-looking mass of hair-thin strands matted together in loose or irregular layers. *Desmarestia* (acid kelp) is not poisonous, but can cause stomach ache if eaten.

• Bradford Angier's *Field Guide to the Wild Plants,* a long-cherished companion, has full-page spreads on kelp, dulse, and laver, with lovely color drawings.

• My seaweed bible is *The Sea Vegetable Book*, by Judith C. Madlener, Potter Pub., 1977. Great identification guide and cookbook, with nearly two hundred seaweed recipes. Out of print, but worth looking for.

• Thanks to the *Sea Vegetable Gourmet Cookbook,* by the Lewallens (address below) for the Vietnamese Healing Soup.

• Buy seaweed by mail from:

Ryan Drum, Waldron Island, WA 98297
Nereo kelp, fucus, alaria. Catering to the seaweed addict.

Eleanor and John Lewallen, PO Box 372, Navarro, CA 95463
Mendocino nori, wakame, dulse, and sea palm fronds, with loving care.

Mt. Ark Traders, 120 SE Ave., Fayetteville, AR 72701
Wild wakame and nori as well as excellent quality cultivated hijiki, kombu, kelp, alaria, arame, nori, dulse, and sea palm.

• Before contact with whites, the Hawaiians ate more than six dozen different varieties of seaweed. They kept special seaweed gardens as well. Today, only a few Hawaiians know this art of cultivating ocean weeds.

• The kelp referred to in books written in England on health, diet, and gardening is always Fucus, unless otherwise noted.

• For further information on heart-healthy seaweeds read "Isolation and identification of cardiac principles from laminaria," by T. Kosuge, H. Nukaya, T. Yamamoto, & K. Tsuji in *Yakugaku Zasshi,* 103(6), 683-685, 1983.

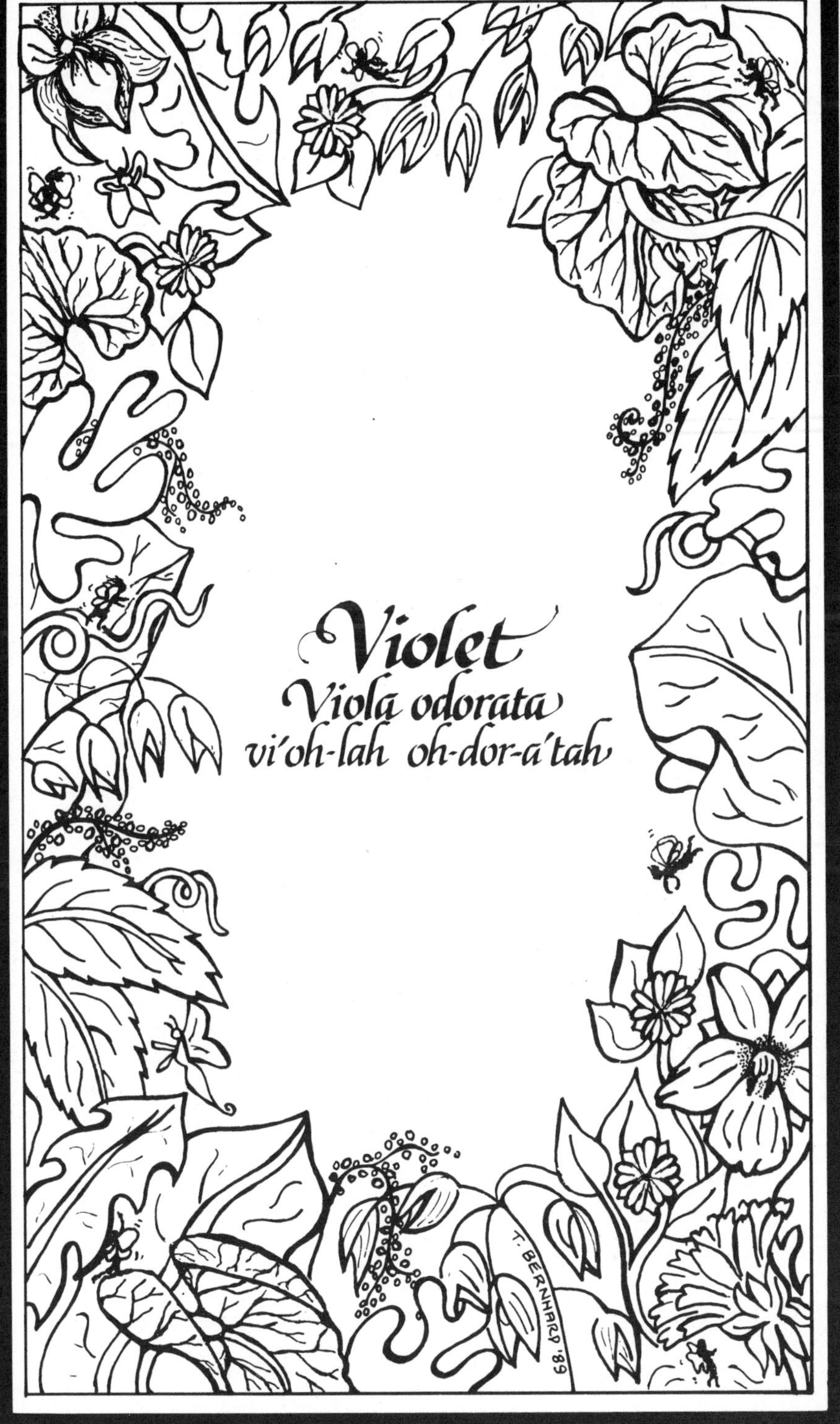
Violet
Viola odorata
vi'oh-lah oh-dor-a'tah
T. BERNHARD '89

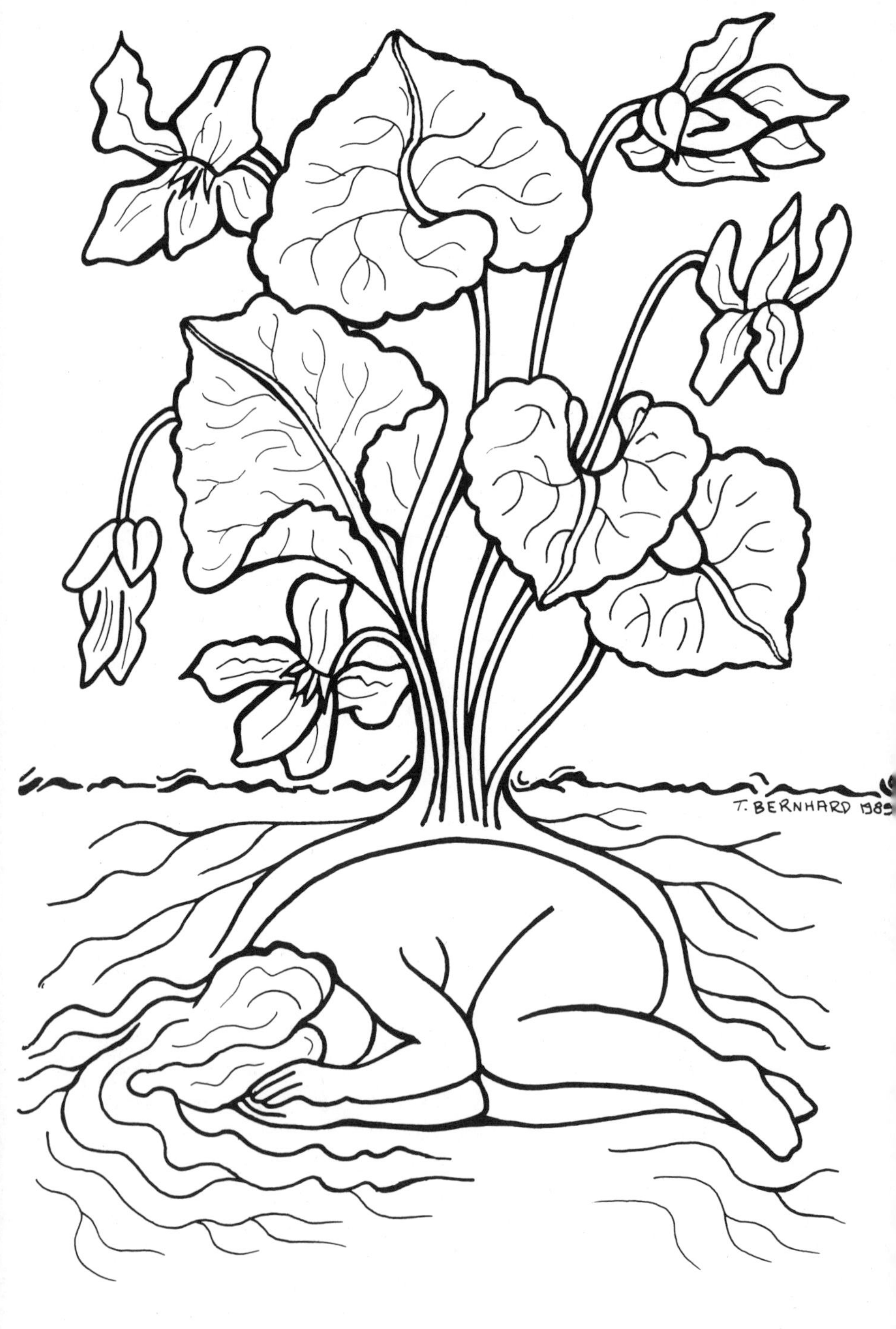
T. BERNHARD 1989

Violet Speaks

"And then my grandfather stopped, and told me to ask permission of the forest spirits before we entered," I heard her say. By the brightness of her own white hair, I knew her grandfather was himself one of the forest spirits by now.

"I waited until I knew we could enter; I was about ten, powerful, certain, aware, alive; it was easy then to know the right way immediately and seize it. We walked on along the path silently, aware of the breathing and beating of life within and without us. I would say I felt joyous and glorious, yet without any introspection; I was, I existed, in wholeness," she continued.

I'm so glad she decided to sit here with her friends and tell her story. How attractive and sweet smelling she is. I wonder what her name is; perhaps I'll never know. I would like to know more about her.

"We walked, without hurry, stopping to refresh ourselves and amuse ourselves with the gurgling, chilly stream, who was relaxing now from her early spring rushes, and chuckling a bit at her earlier haste. We splashed each other gently. I felt fully blessed by the universe and the water spirits."

She has closed her eyes, as if to enjoy anew the tremulous feeling of tiny cold water drops on her so-receptive skin. How alike we are! The early morning mist suits me and the stream bank, too. Though I do try to grow high up on the banks, at least high enough to miss those springtime rushes she mentioned. Yes, I like to live where I'm moist and shaded, like here along this streamside path. So good for the complexion. I wonder where she lives? I wonder what her name is? She is so fine to look at, to listen to, to smell.

"We walked until we reached the high meadow, and stopped at the edge of the clearing. I heard my grandfather whisper in my ear, 'A sacred place; a holy place. A place of great medicine. A place of power.' The meadow was filled with translucent, numinous light . . . light shining from within the throats of hundreds of bright small

wildflowers . . . light singing from the feathers of birds and the wings of butterflies . . . light welling up out of the earth and out of my own body as well."

I do enjoy her voice. It is so refined and crisp, yet so juicy, soothing, and easy. If I could talk, I think my voice might be very like that. Full of heartfelt emotion, bold, resourceful, yet gentle and caring. Yes, my voice would be very like hers. I wonder what her name is?

"My eyes seemed to open more and more to the light. My skin extended for yards all about me, it seemed; I could feel the breezes of the flights of the insects. Then, resonating in my head, came grandfather's voice, 'You are here today to find your first green ally.' Green filled my entire vision; a mysteriously moving, glimmering, constantly changing pattern of green. I was to find a green ally? A green ally. My first green ally."

Green ally? I wonder what that is? I wonder where she lives? I've never seen her here before. I wonder if she'll come back again? I wonder what her name is? What a delicate fragrance emanates from her. A scent that opens my nose, opens my eyes, opens my head, wakes me up, but so very discreetly. A noticeable scent, a scent of power, yet a humble scent. I wonder what makes her smell that way? I am almost intoxicated by the headiness of her smell.

"In the midst of this green pattern, purple lights glowed softly. I found myself drawn to those gentle, lambent lights. I felt that I myself had existence in those purple lights. No, it was some far older part of myself that existed there and called to me. Some part of myself that reached through the generations right back to the ancient mother of all, calling to me. And some part of me from the future called as well. Some part of myself that I would be when I was old (perhaps even myself of today), calling to me. Calling to me."

Could I call to her? Would she hear me? Would she stop her story and look around if I called to her? How can I call her if I don't know her name?

"Calling to me. I answered with my presence. I heard her calling. I went to her. She was calling now with voice and with searingly sweet scent. I settled to the ground beside her, on top of her, within her. She called me further and further into her. I gazed into purple passages lined with shimmering golden floors. I entered her world. I answered her call. I felt her roots as my own and I knew of my poisonous protection, rarely needed, and so hidden in my roots. I felt her leaves as my own and I knew my abundant green power to nourish, accessible

and available. I felt her flowers as my own and I knew my mind was majestically purple and open to resplendent glory."

Purple! Why, we are a lot alike. My favorite color is purple: purple with a little yellow, purple with a little white, or several shades of purple all together. If I must, I'll wear white or yellow, but I do try to keep a touch of purple present. Subdued purple. And startling purple. If it's purple, I love it! She has on a nice purple scarf, and a purple hat as well. I wonder what her name is? Would she respond if I called to her? How can I call her if I don't know her name?

"Purple. And in honor of my first green ally, my first and still favorite friend, my favorite sweet aunt of a plant, I always wear some purple. And, as you know, I took her name as well."

Name? Took her name?

"Violet."

Violet! Violet?

"Like these right here. . . ."

Violet! That's me!

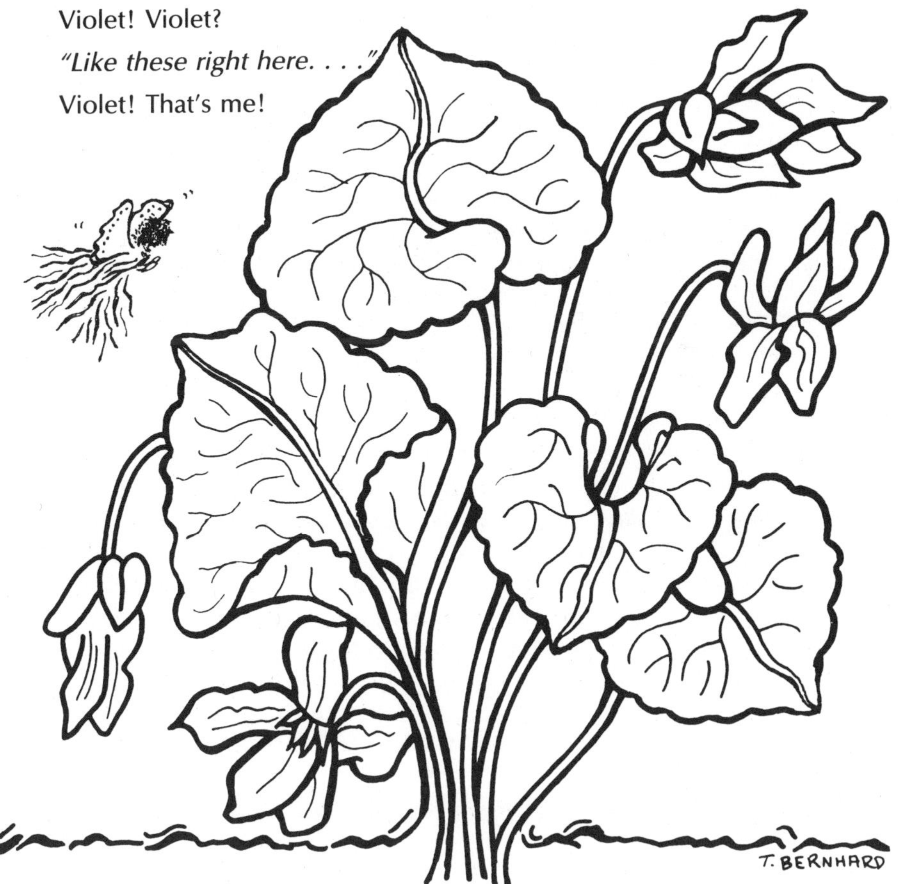

Violet Facts

Botanical name: *Viola odorata; V. tricolor* (Note: names for *V. tricolor* follow names for *V. odorata* in this list; separated by a semi-colon.) Ion (Greek) means violet and becomes viola/violet and violaceus/purple in Latin; odorata (Latin) means sweet smelling; tricolor (Latin) means three colors. ***Other useful species:*** *V. hederacea, V. arvensis, V. papilionacea, V. calcarata, V. canadensis, V. diffusa, V. japonica, V. kauaiensis, V. clandistina, V. palmata, V. pedata, V. rotundifolia, V. pubescens, V. heterophylla*, virtually all of the hundred or more species of *Viola*. ***Natural order:*** Violaceae/Violet family. ***English names:*** Purple violet, garden violet, sweet violet; Pansy, heart's ease, jump-up, three color violet, trinity violet, wild pansy, hens and roosters; butterfly violet. ***Chinese names:*** Hu-chin-ts'ao, huang-hua ts'ao, kuan-t'ou chien, ti-ts'iu ts'ao. ***French names:*** Violette odorante; pense sauvage. ***German names:*** Veilchen, Wohlriechendes Veilchen; Ackerveilchen, Steifmütterchenkraut, Freisamkraut. ***Ancient Greek names:*** Ione. ***Indian names:*** Banaf shah. ***Russian names:*** Fialka polevaya; anutini glazki, Ivan da Maria. ***Spanish names:*** Violeta. ***Perfume uses:*** Though little oil exists in the violet to be extracted, it is an exquisite scent and a perpetual favorite in toiletries, perfumes, and flavorings. ***Food uses:*** Candied violets are commercially available, especially in England; violet syrups are sold in the Mideast, where they flavor sherbets. ***Medicinal uses:*** Commercial cough syrups in Europe contain violet root. ***Soil uses:*** Biodynamic fertilizer for leaf crops; the Cherokee soaked corn seed in tea made from violet roots to help prevent insect damage during germination. ***Habitat:*** Shady woods' edges, moist gardens, meadows, grassy verges, sandy soils. ***Natural range:*** Europe. ***Current range:*** North America, Europe, Russia, India, Pakistan, Australia, New Zealand. ***Toxicity:*** *Externally,* the leaves can cause itching, stinging, burning, and minor eruptions on sensitive skins. *Internally,* the leaves are without toxicity; large doses of violet root (or seeds) can cause severe stomach upset, nervousness, and trouble with breathing and blood pressure regulation. ***Best identified by:*** shiny green heart-shaped leaves with edges rolled in, especially on young leaves; five-petaled irregular flower (like a little orchid) of purple, yellow, white, or a combination of these colors; sweet, bland-tasting leaves.

"Viola is cold and wet in the first degree . . . cools sweetly the body and gives sleep."

Icelandic ms (1475)

Violet Weed Walk

We won't have to go far to find violet, so we can complete our walk in a second. See, there's our first violet right here, at the edge of the lawn. This is the familiar purple-flowered sweet violet, harbinger of spring and sturdy perennial provider of soup and salad greens. We eat Aunt Violet all spring and summer.

And here's the little heart's-ease, also known as johnny jump-up or wild pansy. She's a welcome garden annual here ever since I brought a few plants home from a weed walk I did in an old-fashioned herb garden.

If you don't mind walking for a bit, though, we can find more varieties along the path in the woods. Bring a basket; we'll certainly want to bring back lots of leaves. They'll keep for up to a week in a cloth bag, well cooled. And we'll harvest lots of flowers, too. They won't last past the evening, but we'll have eaten them all by then.

My favorite spring breakfast is simply wild violet blossoms, eaten one by one, so I can savor the delicate differences in pollen taste, coloration, and smell of each little violet blossom miracle.

Keep on the lookout for heart-shaped leaves. On the small side. Not tiny, but not so big, either. Some cultivated garden violet leaves will grow as big as your outspread hand, but the whole plant of most of these woodland wildlings would fit in your hand.

Here we are. Notice how moist the ground is here. And how this spot stays cool and damp all summer, but receives lots of sunlight both spring and fall.

Don't be afraid to pick all the violet blossoms. Really. They are fake flowers! I mean, they don't set any seed. The familiar purple, white, or yellow violet flowers are "just for fun" and "out of sheer exuberance," botanists say. The real flowers, the ones that make seeds, come later, in autumn. They are green and well hidden in the mass of foliage. So enjoy all the violet blossoms you want every spring. Seems to me that the more of them I pick, the more the plant produces.

Come close. Sit on this rock and look into this violet plant. See how all her leaves come up from one place and spread out in a circle? Can you see or feel the slightly downy texture of each leaf? Look at the youngest leaves here in the middle of violet's circle. They are tightly curled into the center, rolled up from each side into the middle of the leaf. As the leaves grow larger and older, the coils relax and open into a heart shape.

It is said that plants with heart-shaped leaves comfort and strengthen the heart. But the heart isn't heart-shaped, is it? Not like this, I mean. What does have this shape? Right: the pelvis. In fact, female genitalia are heart shaped if you gently draw back the outer lips.

Yes, violet is a powerful ally for reproductive problems, dissolving and gently removing tumors, cysts, and even some cancers.

These small forest violets don't have purple flowers or heart-shaped leaves, but they are violets nonetheless. The color of the flower and the shape of the leaf is quite variable in the violet family. What remains the same is the healing slimy stickiness of the leaves. Chew this one. Now spit it into your hand and rub your hands together. Do you feel it? The more slippery the violet is when I chew it, the better medicine I find it to be.

It is a chore to harvest the little leaves of the wild violets here in the woods, so I usually eat my fill of them, but gather the larger leaves of the garden violets for my pharmacy.

Let's sit here now and listen to the soft murmur of the spring seeping from the cliff. Let's sit here for a while and breathe in the lush scent of the violets and the clean air. Someone told me that violets won't grow where the air isn't clean. Let's sit here for as long as we like, open to messages from the violets. And then we'll go home and make a beautiful salad with Aunt Violet's gifts.

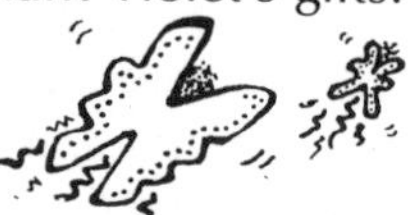

"The salicylic acid found in [all parts of fresh] Violets is an active disinfectant and tissue solvent. . . . It is applied externally in ointments to soften hard skin, corns, and warts; it is also fungicidal."

Charlotte Erichsen-Brown (1979)

Violet Leaf Properties and Uses

- ***nutritive,*** alterative
- ***dissolvent,*** anti-neoplastic, depurative, suppurative
- ***mucilaginous,*** expectorant, demulcent, laxative, diuretic
- ***anodyne,*** vulnerary, antiseptic, emollient

Violet leaves contribute plentiful greens to the salad bowl for months, **nourishing** and gently **altering** the functioning of **nerves, lungs, immune system,** and **reproductive system.** Violet has a special affinity for the **breasts** and is my favorite ally for **fibrocystic** breasts, breast cancer, and mastitis. Aunt Violet probably already grows by your door; seek her out and you'll be rewarded delightfully.

Use Violet leaves as superb nourishment, a cancer care ally, a bosom buddy, a head easer, a respiratory ally, and a wound healer.

- Dose of *fresh or dried violet leaf infusion* is 2-4 cups/500-1000ml a day.

Violet Leaves Are Superb Nourishment

Aunt Violet sees to it that you are nourished. She nourishes so superbly that thousands of years ago every wise woman from Atlantis to ancient Greece knew of her. Why, Aunt Violet was so well known in those days that even men knew of her: Homer and Virgil sang of her and even Pliny spoke of her wise, nourishing, healing ways.

Violet's perennial roots gather minerals and pass them to the leaves, where they are safely available to us. (The roots themselves are toxic in large amounts.) Count on violet leaves to provide you with a goodly amount of vitamins as well. One hundred grams of fresh spring leaves contain 264mg of ascorbic acid (a component of vitamin C) and 20,000 IU of vitamin A.

Violet's optimum nourishment supports the liver, gall bladder, and digestive and urinary systems every day, even when aggressive cancer treatments are administered. Because she supports and nourishes digestion, violet's nutritive value is increased: stronger digestion makes more nutrients available to the cells.

The taste of the fresh leaves or infusion of dried leaves is bland and slightly sweet, with a pleasant slipperiness.

Why not go outside right now and munch a violet leaf?

Violet Leaves Are a Cancer Care Ally

Some of the earliest herbal literature, especially from India and Egypt, notes Aunt Violet's ability to dissolve skin and reproductive system cancers (and tumors)—most notably breast cancers. The medical literature of the early 1900s included at least five scientific studies demonstrating violet's dissolvent and anti-cancer abilities. In some cases, the cancer resolved within a fortnight.

Fresh violet leaves, with their high salicylic acid content, are preferred for cancer treatment, and a must when dealing with external cancers. Steep a quart/liter jar full of fresh chopped leaves and boiling water overnight, and drink at least two cups of the resulting strained liquid each day. Use the remaining softened plant material to poultice the growth.

Try Aunt Vi, along with your Wise Woman ways, when healing yourself or others with swollen glands, growths, tumors, and cancers of the stomach, lungs, breasts, tongue, mouth, skin, bladder, kidneys, colon, larynx, throat, or tonsils.

Continuous compresses, baths, or poultices with Aunt Violet, especially her fresh leaves, ease and may eliminate the ever-present pain of those with terminal cancers.

Violet Leaves Are a Bosom Buddy

Violet has a special sympathy for breast tissue. She likes to smooth things out when there are fibrous cysts, lumps, infections, or growths, including cancers, in the breasts.

Two or more cups/500ml of violet leaf infusion daily at the first sign of soreness ease those with monthly breast swelling and tenderness, fibrocystic distress, and mastitis. Use violet poultices in addition if there is pain or inflammation.

A woman whose fibrocystic breasts bothered her for a full week premenstrually drank violet infusion for that week of distress and asked the Wise Woman questions: "How is this my ally? What gifts does it bring me of my greater wholeness?" Within two months, the premenstrual soreness was reduced to no more than two days.

Personal experiences of other close friends attest to violet's willingness and power to help when there's a lump in a breast. I have seen numerous (undiagnosed) breast lumps steadily decrease in size and tenderness with Wise Woman ways and Aunt Violet's assistance.

Violet Leaves Are a Head Easer

Violet has a very soothing, cooling effect on the head, mind, brain, nervous system, and crown chakra.

Try sipping a cup or more of violet leaf infusion throughout the day when you are bothered by nervous headache, hangover, epileptic memory loss, insomnia, deranged nerves, weak memory, restlessness, fevered fantasies, and inability to stop thinking.

Poultices or compresses of fresh violet leaves on the back of the neck are as easing as Aunt Violet's cool hand on your brow. Try them alone or in combination with violet leaf infusion to soothe and heal those with head pain from sun exposure, too much studying, eye strain, chemical exposure, sinus infections, fevers, or ear infections.

Violet Leaves Are a Respiratory Ally

Aunt Violet is a cool drink in the midst of overheated congestion, blocked grief, traumatic rememberings, and feverish fears. When mucus discharge is thick, yellow, sticky, and rattling, think of Aunt Violet's cool ways.

Try several cups of the infusion daily and experience Aunt Violet's soothing, healing effect on those with inflamed throat and bronchial surfaces. Use in conjunction with other Wise Woman ways for helping yourself or others with coughs, especially whooping cough, pulmonary ails, congestion, colds, shortness of breath, difficulty in breathing, flu, pleurisy, quinsy, tonsilitis, sore throat, and hoarseness.

Violet Leaves Are a Wound Healer

Antiseptic and dissolvent, cooling and healing, violet leaves (especially the smaller, wild ones) are decidedly helpful for a wide variety of skin woes, from traumatic to chronic.

I use poultices of the fresh leaves, then frequent applications of violet or hypericum oil for healing myself and others with wounds, pimples, abscesses, sores, swellings, old festering wounds, chronic and persistent skin diseases, herpes, sore breasts, red sore eyes, and mastitis. Soothing relief is felt at Aunt Violet's first touch. Inflammation often recedes overnight. And complete healing proceeds smoothly and painlessly when we walk the Wise Woman way hand-in-hand with violet.

For those with boils and burns, blend or crush fresh violet leaves with honey and apply. Replace with a fresh poultice when signaled by pain.

Use the leaf infusion as a gargle/mouthwash for those with inflammation, swelling, ulceration of the mouth, pain from mouth cancers or herpes sores. Try frequent hot fomentations, along with your other Wise Woman ways, to ease and heal those with mumps, laryngitis, malignant tumors, swellings from injuries (such as sprains and broken bones), and acute conjunctivitis.

"It is recorded that during the nine weeks that a nurseryman supplied a patient suffering with cancer in the colon—which was cured at the end of this period—a violet bed covering six rods of ground was almost entirely stripped of its foliage." Maude Grieve (1931)

Violet Flower Properties and Uses

• ***antiscorbutic,*** aperient

Violet flowers eaten are a treat to the senses and a **vitamin C** boost to the entire body. Preserved as an oil or syrup, they treat the **sensory organs.**

Use violet flowers to delight your senses.

• Dose of *violet syrup* is 1-5 teaspoons/5-25ml a day.
• Dose of *V. tricolor tincture* is 2-5 drops a day, in water, for children;
15-100 drops a day, in water, for adults.

Violet Flowers Are a Delight to the Senses

Violet flowers nourish your senses when prepared in the kitchen and help heal those with ear, throat, head, and skin maladies when prepared in the pharmacy.

Violet flowers, wild or cultivated (including pansies), are all edible. Their bright colors, subtle flavors, and evocative aromas are a constant joy to all the senses. Use them to garnish other dishes or strew them liberally in green salads. Crystallize some violets and you'll have fairy-like decorations to lift spirits in winter.

Violet flower oil in the ears can relieve tinnitus. Repeat as needed.

Violet flower syrup soothes those with sore throats, coughs, even whooping cough, and children's digestive complaints such as stomach ache and constipation. A spoonful before bed, along with Wise Woman ways, helps those troubled with nightmares, insomnia, and distressed sleep.

Tincture of *V. tricolor,* whole herb in flower, is specific for cradle cap, impetigo, and scabies. (If only it killed lice, too.) Use it daily, internally, for up to a week, for prompt relief from the first two problems. Use it longer, and with stronger allies (such as baths in green soap and sulphur ointment) to deal with scabies.

Pansy (*V. tricolor*) tincture is also tonic and pain-relieving to the heart.

"Violets have long symbolized young love and springtime, recalling street vendors in Paris and many other nostalgic memories." Connie Krochmal

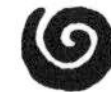

Violet Root Properties and Uses

- ***anti-pyretic,*** tonic, diuretic, expectorant, emollient
- ***emetic,*** cathartic

Violet root, fresh or tinctured, is a potent ally for reducing **coughs,** cooling **fevers,** and soothing sore **feet**. See caution on internal use under **Violet Facts: *Toxicity***.

Use violet root as a fierce blast of cool relief.

- Dose of *V. odorata root tincture* is 5-15 drops a day, in water.
- Dose of *V. tricolor root tincture* is 5-25 drops a day, in water.
- Dose of *violet root decoction* is 1-3 tablespoons/15-45ml a day.

Violet Roots Are a Fierce Blast of Cool Relief

If your garden sprouts more violets than you can keep up with, harvest some of the roots in early spring or late fall for your pharmacy.

The fresh or dried roots, crushed and soaked several hours in vinegar, are used to poultice hot, sore, even infected feet injured from overuse, or from chronic problems such as diabetes.

The tincture or decoction of *V. tricolor* root, taken in frequent small doses until the desired effect is achieved, breaks up and removes respiratory congestion, cools fevers, and moves urine.

The tincture or decoction of *V. odorata* root also dissolves respiratory mucus, reduces inflammation in the lungs and mouth, calms nervous coughs, clears lingering effects of whooping cough, and reduces hysteria.

"[Violets] are good for all inflammations, especially of the sides and lungs; they . . . allay the extream heate of the liver, kidneys, and bladder; mitigate the fierie heate of burning agues; temper the sharpness of choler, and take away thirst." Gerarde-Johnson (1633)

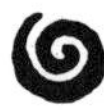

Violet Pharmacy

Violet Vinegar

for sumptuous salad dressings

Apple cider vinegar takes on not only a brillant tint, but a sweet odor from having violet flowers steeped in it for several weeks. See **Herbal Pharmacy** (tincture section), for specific instructions on making herbal vinegars.

Rosemary's Violet Moon Dreams Brew

a ritual drink

Place an amethyst in a crystal goblet. Fill the goblet to the top with violet blossoms and pure water. Sit the violet-amethyst goblet in the full moonlight. Drink half on arising and half before going to sleep.

Violet Complexion Lotion

especially for oily skin

1 cup/250ml violets
1 cup/250ml milk*
(*raw, goat preferably)

Steep violets in warm fresh milk overnight. Soak wash cloth in very hot water; wring out. Soak in violet milk and apply to face and neck.

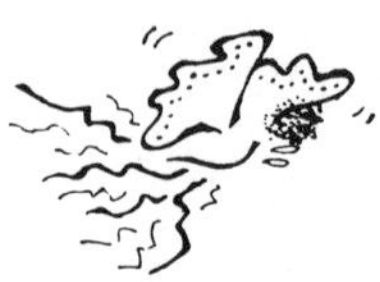

"Violet leaves proved to have an almost unbelievably high ascorbic acid content, but they were tested, retested, then tested again with a fresh supply of leaves, and we could only come to the conclusion that this rich vitamin C value is really there." Euell Gibbons (1966)

Violet Syrup

yields 3 cups/750ml

½ lb/225g fresh violets
2 cups/500ml water
2 cups/500ml honey

Enlist all the help you can to pick violet blossoms. Boil water; pour over blossoms; cover. Let steep overnight in non-metallic container. Strain out flowers. Reserve purple liquid.

Alternate method for loners: pour 2 cups/500ml boiling water over as many flowers as you can get. Strain liquid. Reheat and pour over the next day's harvest. Do this daily until your liquid is pleasingly violaceous (purple).

Combine mauve-colored liquid and honey. Simmer gently, stirring, for ten or fifteen minutes, until it seems like syrup. Fill clean jars. Cool. Keep well chilled to preserve.

Preparation time: Hours and hours of picking await you, and all in pursuit of some purple-colored sugar water. Or is there more to it than that? Perhaps Aunt Violet will open a gateway to ecstasy for you. Uncle Euell Gibbons pours his on hot broiled grapefruit and proclaims, "Utterly delicious!"

Sweet Aunt Vi

1 cup/250ml packed violets
¾ cup/190ml water
juice of 1 lemon
2½ c/625ml sugar or honey

Make a thick paste of violet blossoms, lemon juice, and water in blender or with mortar and pestle. Blend sweetener in very, very well. Store very cold; freezer is fine.

Use ¼ teaspoon/1ml at a time, every hour or so, as needed, to ease those with coughs, constipation, headaches, and grief.

"The influence of the dissolving properties [of violet] seem to have intricate inward skill, reaching places only the blood and lymphatic fluids penetrate."

Alma Hutchens (1969)

Biodynamic Fertilizer

for lettuce, cabbage, chard

2 qts/2 liters dry manure*
1 lb/500g fresh violet leaves
1 lb/500g cabbage leaves
1 lb/500g nettle leaves
3 gallons/12 liters water
*cow/horse

Chop leaves finely. Mix with dry manure in a large container. Add water, cover tightly and steep for at least two weeks. Use about a cup of this concentrate to a gallon of water as a foliar fertilizer.

Biodynamic Fertilizer

for beets, broccoli, kale

2 qts/2 liters dry manure*
1 lb/500g violet leaves
1 lb/500g amaranth leaves
8 oz/250g shepherd's purse
8 oz/250g fresh seaweed *or*
2 oz/60g dried seaweed
3 gallons/12 liters rainwater
*fowl/horse

Chop leaves and stalks of fresh plants and mix with dry manure in a large plastic container such as a tofu bucket. Add water, cover well; steep for 2 or more weeks. 1 part of this concentrate diluted with 16 parts water is used to feed seedlings, transplants, and larger plants.

Homemade Litmus Test

yields just enough

2 jarsful of violet blossoms
boiling water
lemon juice
baking soda

Fill any size jars with violet blossoms; fill with boiling water to top, seal and steep overnight. Divide contents of one jar into three containers. Add lemon juice to one. It will turn purple/red; this is your acid indicator. Add baking soda to the other. It will turn green/yellow; this is your base indicator. Pour contents of second jar into as many small containers as you have soil samples to test. Match colors to indicators.

Violet Kitchen

Violet Vision Salad

serves 6

6 large violet leaves
3 tangerines
3 oranges
1 cup/250ml yogurt
1 handful violet blossoms
maple syrup (optional)

Line serving vessel with violet leaves. Arrange tangerine and orange sections artfully on leaves in waves, spirals, or circles. Pour yogurt just into center, so lots of oranges show. Add a puddle of maple syrup in the very center if you have a sweet tooth. Toss violet blossoms gaily over all.

Preparation time: 10 minutes when everybody helps; more like 25 when you're on your own. This will hold well chilled, but that's ruinous to the vitamin C content of the citrus. Throw on the violets just before serving.

Creamy Violet Green Soup

serves 6

2 Tbs/30ml olive oil
1 cup/250ml sliced wild leeks
4 cups/1 liter violet leaves
4 cups/1 liter water
salt to taste
4 cups/1 liter fresh milk

Sauté leeks in oil for three minutes. Add chopped violet leaves, stir for a minute. Add water and salt and bring to a simmer. Cook about fifteen minutes, then purée in blender or through a sieve. Reheat, adding milk. Garnish with a few violet blossoms and a dust of nutmeg before serving. Also nice cold.

Preparation time: 30-40 minutes in the kitchen; another hour to walk out to the leek patch, get my hands muddy digging leeks, rinse us all off in the stream, and walk back; 5 minutes collecting violets unless I get distracted.

Aunt Violet's "Chicken" Soup

serves 8

2 tablespoons/30ml olive oil
1 large onion minced
1 entire head garlic
10 mushrooms, sliced
2 stalks lovage or celery
2 carrots, thick slices
2 large potatoes, diced
4 c/1 liter fresh violet leaves
1 c/250ml strawberry leaves
8 c/2 liters water or broth
1 teaspoon/5ml salt
1 tsp/5ml dried marjoram
1 Tbs/15ml dried dill
½ tsp/3ml dried thyme
2 tablespoons/30ml miso

Sauté onion in olive oil until soft. Add sliced garlic and stir; add the mushrooms and sauté another few minutes, while chopping vegetables. Add all the vegetables, including chopped greens. Add water and salt; bring almost to a boil. Simmer 30-45 minutes. Add dried herbs. Reduce or eliminate heat. Just before serving, heat soup until very hot. Dissolve miso in a couple of spoonfuls of broth, add that to the soup, and take the whole pot to the table.

Preparation time: Say an hour. Who can say exactly how long to cook a soup? The longer the better, I say, as with love.

First Blush Greens

serves 4

2 c/500ml young brassicas*
2 c/500ml violet leaves
2 cups/500ml young nettles
splash tamari & lemon juice
*kale, collards, cabbage, shepherd's purse greens, watercress

Wash greens and chop without drying. Cook over medium heat, adding water if necessary, until suitably limp and warm. Season, garnish with dandelion blossoms, and serve.

Preparation time: No more than fifteen minutes in the kitchen; up to an hour gathering greens and blossoms; longer, much longer, on exquisite spring days.

"When Catherine Booth, wife of the founder of the Salvation Army, was dying from cancer, an appeal was made for violet leaves, since they alone could ease the agonizing pain." Richard Lucas (1977)

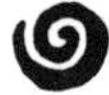

Violet Fun and Facts

• Billy Joe Tatum has violet recipes, lots of violet recipes, in her *Forager's Field Guide.* Don't miss Aunt Vi appearing as "Violet Cloud"!

• Connie and Arnold Krochmal give four pages of their booklet *Cooking with Wild Plants* to Aunt Violet: three recipes for flowers, four for leaves.

• Euell Gibbons has listened closely to Aunt Violet and tells us what he heard in *Stalking the Healthful Herbs.* I'm tickled that he calls her "Nature's Vitamin Pill," but never dreamed that anyone could find so many violet recipes calling for two cups/half a kilo of white sugar.

• Maude Grieve's *Modern Herbal* opens an inviting doorway to the world of Aunt Violet, quoting from many sources and including recipes for many medicinal applications. The horticultural directions are incredibly extensive.

• Violets are mentioned by Shakespeare in *Hamlet* and in *Pericles.*

• Milton calls upon violet in *Lycidas,* as do Homer and Virgil in their songs.

• Violets were the emblem of the Imperial Napoleonic party.

• Wear a wreath of violet blossoms and leaves as a way to ward off drunkenness; and if that doesn't work, it will prevent a hangover.

• Violet is the flower of Aphrodite and the symbol of Athens.

• Violets were created by Jupiter as a special food for his lover Io after he changed her into a white calf. He changed her thus to prevent his wife Juno from catching him cheating on her.

• Violets grown by your doorstep offer you powerful psychic protection and ease for your heart.

• Crystallized violets are sold by mail at $17 for 3½ ounces/100 grams. Order from S.E. Rykoff, PO Box 21467, Los Angeles, CA 90021.

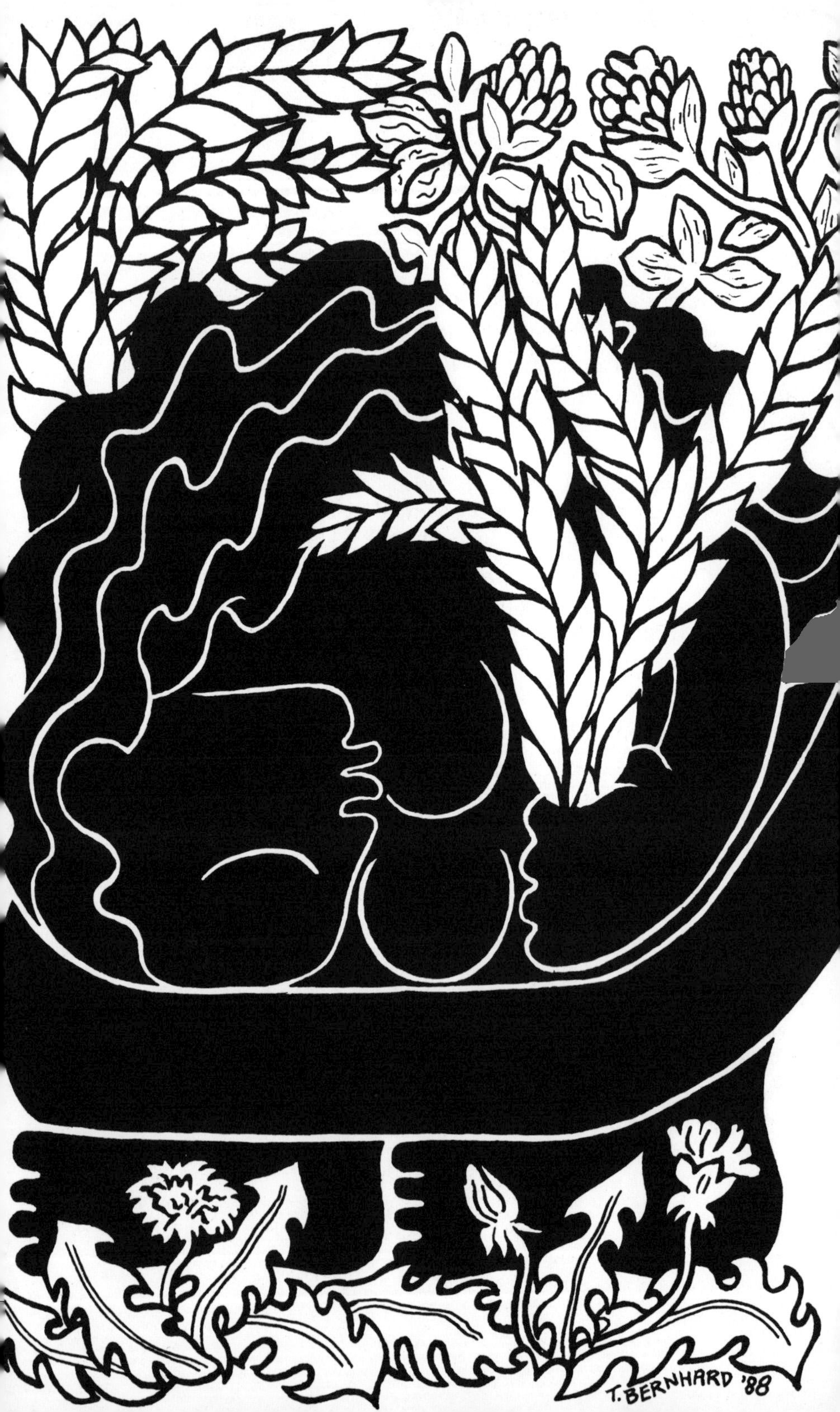
T. BERNHARD '88

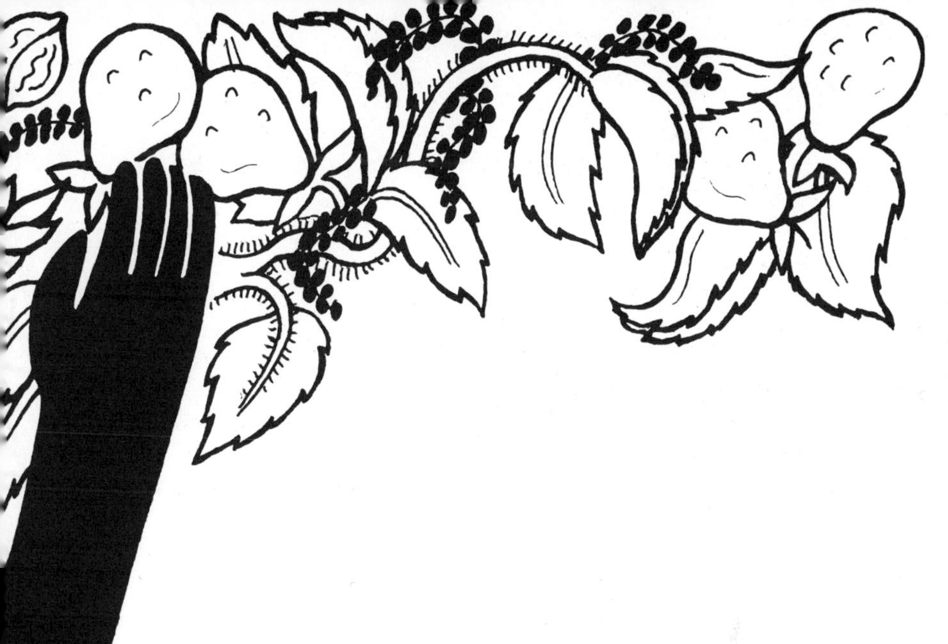

Herbal Pharmacy

In your herbal pharmacy you transform fresh and dried plants into herbal medicines. Learning to identify and use the common plants around you is easy and exciting, beneficial and safe. Making your own medicines saves you money if you follow the Wise Woman tradition of using local herbs, free for the taking. Even one day's work in field, forest, and kitchen can provide you with many years' worth of medicines. When you make your own, you know for sure what's in it, where it came from, when and how it was harvested, and how fresh and potent it is.

Dried herbs are best for the infusions recommended in this book. Stock your herbal pharmacy with your own foraged or cultivated dried herbs; expand your resources and experiment with new herbs by buying dried herbs from reputable sources.

Fresh herbs are best for the tinctures and oils recommended in this book. If you can't make your own, buy from sources who wildcraft or grow their own herbs to use fresh in preparations.

Whether you buy or make your medicines, remember, **herbal remedies may not work or may work incorrectly if they aren't prepared correctly**. Read this chapter carefully; it contains easy-to-follow instructions for every remedy and preparation mentioned in this book.

Meeting the Plants

Start by noticing the plants that live with you, along your driveway or sidewalk. Don't assume that medicinal plants are hard to find. Burdock, chickweed, and dandelion (to name only a few) are as common in cities and suburbs as in the country.

Learn more about the weeds around you directly from the plants, from a personal guide, and from field guides and herbals.

When we open all our senses, including the psychic ones, to the green world, we learn to hear and understand plant language. Through shape, color, location, scent, texture, taste, and energy, plants tell us how they will affect our bodies, which plant parts we can use, and how we can prepare them. Some wise women converse with the plant fairies and the devas. Some hear the song that each plant sings. Some feel the dances of the leaves, breezes, and insects. All are means of learning the ways of herbs. Though the Scientific tradition scoffs at such knowledge, the Wise Woman tradition honors the plant as the ultimate authority on its uses.

A personal guide into the plant world will show you plant features which ensure positive identification. A personal guide will introduce you to the foods, medicines, dyes, fibers, decorations, and delights hidden in common plants, and instruct you in wise harvesting and preparation. Check local garden clubs, botanical gardens, and nature centers for contacts with personal guides.

Field guides are indispensable references once your taste for herbal identification is whetted. I find the line drawings in the Peterson guides more helpful than color photographs when I have to distinguish between similar looking plants.

Herbals concentrate on the specifics of using plants as medicines and are rarely illustrated well enough to serve as a guide to identification. Field guides hardly ever include information on medicinal value. The link between your field guide and your herbal is the botanical binomial, or Latin name, of each plant. The binomial is (usually) consistent in all references, unlike common names which overlap and vary from region to region. Once you have identified a new plant, you can look it up by finding the binomial in herbals and other references. This can increase your confidence and ability to find and use safe herbal medicines.

My years of leading Weed Walks and helping people identify wild plants have shown me that learning to recognize herbs in the field is far easier, and much less fraught with danger, than most people realize. As Euell Gibbons is quoted as saying: "You don't learn all the plants at once; you learn them one at a time."

Even if you never pick your own herbs, knowing how the live plants look will be a great asset when you go to buy them.

Picking Herbs

When you have positively identified the plant you wish to use, center yourself by sitting next to the herb in silence. Take several deep breaths. Feel the earth under you, connecting you to all the plants. Listen to the sounds and songs all around you. Can you hear the song of your herb?

If you are picking only one plant, ask that plant to share its power with you. Tell it how you intend to use it. If you are harvesting many plants, look for a grandmother plant. Talk with her about using her grandchildren. Visualize clearly how you intend to use the plants. Sing. Thank the earth and begin your gathering.

Take care to preserve and contribute to the well-being of the plant community. Take no more than half of the annuals or biennials, no more than a third of the perennials. Walk gently and with balance.

Harvest plants when the energy you want is most concentrated. Roots store energy in the form of sugar, starch, and medicinal alkaloids throughout the cold or dormant season; pick them when above-ground growth of the plant has died back. Leaves process energy to nourish roots and flowers; pick them at their most lush, before flowers have formed, after all dew has dried, and before the day's heat wilts them. Flowers are fragile, pollen-filled, joyous; harvest them in full bloom, before seeds form, and before bees visit them. Seeds are durable, but likely to shatter and disperse if left on the plant too long; harvest seeds when still green and before insects invade. Barks (inner barks and root barks) may be harvested at any time but are thought to be most potent in spring and fall. Look carefully at the plant you wish to pick and you will see where the energy is highest; let this guide your harvesting.

Deal with your harvest immediately. Allowing the cut plants to lie about dissipates their vital energies, encourages mold and fermentation, and results in poor quality preparations. If you intend to eat your harvest, refrigerate the plants, or wash and cook them and sit down and eat. If you intend to make a tincture or oil, cover the herbs with alcohol or oil as soon as possible; don't refrigerate them. If you intend to dry the herbs, it is vital to lay them out to dry or tie them up to dry as soon after harvest as possible.

Drying Herbs

To dry herbs and maintain their color, fragrance, taste, energy, and medicinal potency, you need only:

• Pick when there is no moisture on the plant and do not wash the plant (roots are the exception).

• Dry the herbs immediately after picking, in small bunches or spread out so parts don't touch.

• Dry them in a dark and well-ventilated area.

• Take down the herbs and store in paper bags as soon as they are crisply dried. If insect invasions force you to store dried herbs in glass or plastic, air-dry them for two weeks, then dry in paper bags for another two weeks before sealing in tight containers.

• Keep the herbs as whole, cool, and dark as possible during storage. Under optimum storage conditions, well-dried volatile, delicate herbs last about six months; roots and barks maintain potency for six or more years.

Problems with Foraging

Are you concerned about contamination of wild plants with lead, chemicals, and dog doo?

Avoid harvesting herbs from roadsides where lead concentration is high; plants growing by busy roads will accumulate more lead. The nearer the plant is to the road, the higher the level of lead concentration. If you can't find a particular herb anywhere except by a road, pick at least eight feet from the road edge; lead levels drop sharply in the first few feet. In cities, pick from parks and other out-of-the-way places. Be wary of vacant lots which may be contaminated with lead paint.

Avoid picking under power lines and along roads where the weeds are controlled by spraying instead of cutting. Suburban lawns that have been doused with weed killers rarely grow medicinal weeds, but if you suspect chemical warfare (distorted, mutated, sparse weeds are good clues), avoid that area.

Avoid gathering herbs where canines gather. Dogs can pass parasites to humans.

Allow yourself to be guided by your intuition, as well as your senses and your intelligence, and you will know which areas to avoid when picking wild plants. Given the amount of chemical contamination on commercial herbs (and fruits and vegetables, for that matter), I honestly feel safer taking risks in the wild.

Open your eyes and observe the green abundance. Open your heart and feel the green joy. Come with respect for green power. The devas of the green nation welcome you.

Buying Herbs

Knowing how to buy herbs is as necessary a skill as learning to identify them. It is my personal goal to find or grow all the herbs I use. But even with access to a garden and hundreds of acres of Catskill country, I haven't yet achieved my goal. I, too, buy herbs collected, grown, and prepared by others.

Many practices in the commercial herb trade are appalling. Grossly substandard wages are paid to harvesters in Third World countries. Pesticide and herbicide chemicals banned in the United States are used on herbs grown overseas (and 80% of commercial herbs are imported). Dried herbs may be legally irradiated with the equivalent of hundreds of chest X-rays, yet there is no labeling visible to the consumer as to which herbs have been so treated. All commercial herbal warehouses, even those storing organic herbs, must legally be fumigated several times a year with chemical sprays.

I protect myself by purchasing herbs from individuals I know and trust. Their names and addresses are included in the References and Resources following this chapter.

Whatever the source, dried herbs should be brightly colored, fresh smelling, and as whole as possible. Powdered herbs, and herbs in capsules, lose medicinal value rapidly.

When you look at a dried herb, envision it as it was when alive. The only thing that should be missing is the water content. Dried seaweeds are vibrant purple, green, or black, not brown. Nettle leaves are a rich blue-green, *not* light green or yellowed. Burdock root smells fresh and tastes sweet, not rank or moldy. Smell dried herbs carefully and reject those which lack scent and those which smell of chemicals or molds.

The energy, or life force, of an herb can be sensed even when the plant has been dried. Absence of energy means that the herb is old, or has been handled incorrectly. If you can, hold the dried herb in your hands: feel for tingle, look for sparkle. A pendulum will react to the life force present in dried herbs; dowsing can confirm your sensory impressions.

If you are buying by mail, return herbs that do not look, smell, and feel alive. If you buy from a store, bring poor quality to the attention of the owner and demand unpowdered and unencapsulated herbs. Say what you want and what pleases you. Consumer desires do have power in the herb market. Interest in organically grown herbs has resulted in increased availability of organic medicinals.

Making Herbal Medicines

The art of making herbal preparations is fascinating and complex. Each herb has one or more optimum methods of preparation; each method extracts different properties from the herb. Each type of preparation affects the body in different ways. The quality of an herbal preparation is dependent on the quality of the herb used. The quality of the herb is affected by the weather during the growing season, the thoughts of the gatherer or grower, the time of harvest, and the conditions surrounding handling and storage. The moon sheds her subtle influence on all of this, adding to the variables. It's no wonder that every herbalist creates unique herbal preparations, and that non-herbalists feel confused.

After years of experimenting and teaching, I offer these easy, foolproof instructions for home preparation of herbal medicines. All the equipment you need is probably already at hand: canning jars with lids, small jars with lids or corks, a sharp knife, a grater, several pots and pans, water, oil, vodka, labels, and a ball-point pen.

I prepare herbal medicines in three bases: water, spirit, and oil. Water-based products are teas, infusions, decoctions, syrups, baths, enemas, fomentations, eyewashes, and douches. Spirit-based products are tinctures, liniments, vinegars, and essences. Oil-based products include essential oils, infused oils, ointments, and salves.

In all bases I use no direct heat. No herbs are ever boiled or baked. This virtually eliminates burned, fried, and ruined medicines. And the finer vibrations of the plants appreciate the care.

In a water base, dried herbs produce the best potency. Spirit bases produce superior medicinals when fresh herbs are used, although dried roots and barks are often acceptable. Oil bases absolutely require fresh plant material. Don't assume that you have no access to fresh medicinal herbs. Weed walks in city neighborhoods and along suburban sidewalks have never failed to provide an abundance of fresh medicinal plants.

Water Bases

Our bodies are based on water and so are plants. We digest in a water base. In most instances, I prefer herbal medicines in a water base. Nourishing herbs such as nettles, oatstraw, and seaweeds are at their best when prepared in water bases, for water is best able to extract and make accessible their full range of vitamins, minerals, and nutrients.

Water-based herbal medicines spoil rapidly and must be prepared at or near the actual time of use. However, you can store dried herbs for long periods, ready to use in a water base.

Water-based preparations are called teas, tisanes, infusions, decoctions, and syrups. They may be used as soaks, baths, douches, enemas, eyewashes, poultices, compresses, and fomentations. They are all made by soaking fresh or dried plant material in water (usually boiling).

Tea is the standard water-based herbal preparation; even restaurants know how to make it. At fancy ones they call it tisane.

Use one teaspoon dried herb per cup of boiling water. Add an extra spoonful for the pot. Let it steep in your cup or the pot for up to twenty minutes. Honey, lemon, and milk are medicinal additions. (Don't give infants honey.)

Volatile herbs are easily extracted into water and therefore prepared as teas. Chamomile, and aromatic seeds, are best prepared as teas.

Infusion is the most medicinally potent water-based herbal preparation. There are a great many definitions and recipes for preparing infusions; some herbalists use the term interchangeably with "tea."

My medicinal infusions contain a great deal of herbal matter and are steeped for a long time. The result is a liquid much thicker and darker than an herbal tea, leaving no doubt that you are dealing with a medicine, not a breakfast drink.

Prepare infusions in pint and quart canning jars. A teapot or cup is impractical for the long brewing an infusion requires and their openings allow volatile essences and vitamins to escape. Canning jars rarely break when filled with boiling water. They make it easy to measure the amount of water used in the brew. An infusion brewed in a jar is convenient to carry along to work, school or wherever, and this increases the probability that the infusion will be consumed.

Herbal infusions are the starting point for all the other water-based preparations mentioned in this book: decoctions, syrups, soaks, compresses.

Making Herbal Infusions

Roots: Use **one ounce/30 grams** (a big handful of cut-up root, or half a dozen six-inch pieces of whole root) of **dried root** in a **pint/500 ml jar**. Fill the jar to the top with **boiling water**. Put the lid on the jar and let it sit at room temperature for **eight hours**.

Roots are the most dense and usually the most potent part of perennial and biennial plants. The medicinal virtues of roots are often found in their alkaloids and minerals, which dissolve quite slowly into water. This is why many herbals suggest boiling roots; the rapid movement of the water molecules bouncing against the alkaloids and minerals frees them from the cells and extracts them into the water. I have found, however, that a very long period of infusion extracts all the useful medicinal substances from the roots, without the careful watching necessary when they are boiled.

Barks: Prepare the same as roots.

"Bark" is a misleading word, as the usual part of the tree or shrub actually used for herbal medicines is the **inner bark**, or cambium layer, which lies between the true bark and the wood. All the nourishment and life force of the tree, passing between roots and leaves, moves through this layer, making it a rich source of valuable resins, sugars, and astringents. The wood and the bark are dead cells and thus contain little that is medicinally useful. Cambium cell walls are tough, requiring long brewing for full extraction of medicinal virtues.

Leaves: Use **one ounce/30 grams** of **dried leaves** (two handfuls of cut-up leaves or three handfuls of whole leaves) in a **quart/liter jar**. Fill the jar to the top with **boiling water**, put the lid on and let it steep for **four hours** at room temperature.

Leaves contain the potent healer chlorophyll. Long steeping extracts all the chlorophyll, as well as the vitamins, minerals, and other medicinal components of the leaves. Steeping in a closed jar keeps the water-soluble vitamins from escaping in the steam.

Flowers: Place **one ounce/30 grams** of **dried flowers** (two big handfuls of crumbled-up flowers) in a **quart/liter jar**. Fill the jar to the top with **boiling water**, put on the lid and infuse for **two hours**.

Flowers are the sexual expression of the plant. They are generally delicate and volatile. Chamomile is exceptionally volatile and should be infused for no more than thirty minutes. When the stalk and leaves of the plant are used along with the flowers, as with yarrow, infuse for four hours, as though using leaves alone.

Seeds: Use **one ounce/30 grams** of **dried seeds, berries, hips**, or **haws** (one to three tablespoons/15-45 ml) in a **pint/500 ml jar** and fill it to the top with **boiling water**. Screw on a lid and infuse for **no more than thirty minutes**.

Seeds are the embryo of the plant. Though they are hard and dense, like roots, they are engineered to open and release their properties immediately upon contact with water, so they do not need to be infused for a long time. In fact, if seeds are brewed for too long, bitter oils and esters are leached out into the water and a foul-tasting brew results. Rosehips and hawthorn berries are exceptions; they may be steeped for up to four hours.

Combination Infusions: When preparing infusions containing several herbs, it is generally best to brew the components separately so that each herb infuses for the proper length of time. (This is unnecessary if the combination is all roots or all leaves.)

If you buy herbs which are already mixed and wish to infuse them, brew for the shortest time needed by any ingredient; for instance, a mix containing chamomile should be steeped for no more than thirty minutes. Some medicinal potency will be lost this way, but you will avoid extracting bitter esters, oils, and resins which may cause unwanted side effects.

The Wise Woman tradition focuses on the use of **simples**. A simple is a medicine made from a single herb. When combinations are used, they rarely exceed three herbs. This allows for maximum feedback on the effect of each herb.

Dosage: Two cups (sixteen fluid ounces)/500 milliliters of an infusion per day is the standard dose for a person weighing 125-150 pounds/60-70 kilograms. Use one cup/250 ml if you weigh 65-75 pounds/10-20 kilograms. Half a cup/125 ml for 30-40 pounds/10-20 kilograms. A quarter cup/4 tablespoons/60 ml for 15-20 pounds/under 10 kilograms.

Summary of Infusion Data

Plant Part	*Amount*	*Jar/Water*	*Length of Infusion*
Roots/barks	1 oz/30 g.	**pint/500 ml**	8 hours minimum
Leaves	1 oz/30 g.	**quart/liter**	4 hours minimum
Flowers	1 oz/30 g.	**quart/liter**	2 hours maximum
Seeds/berries	1 oz/30 g.	**pint/500 ml**	30 minutes maximum

Herbal Decoctions and Syrups

Decoction, or simple decoction, is my term for an infusion which has been reduced to one-half of its volume by slow evaporation. A double decoction is an infusion reduced to one-fourth of its original volume. Some herbalists use "decoction" to refer to what I call an infusion; others use it to mean something closer to tea.

Decoctions keep longer than infusions if carefully stored under refrigeration. Decoctions are more potent than infusions; this makes them invaluable when dealing with children and animals—a smaller dose is more easily administered.

Decocting is an excellent way to prepare an herb with a strong or bitter taste, such as dandelion, so it can be consumed without gagging. Adding a bit of some nice-tasting brandy or liqueur to decoctions enhances the taste and the keeping qualities.

Decoctions of roots and barks are often prepared; decoctions of leaves, flowers, or seeds are rarely prepared. Since decoctions are made by evaporation, the volatile essences and water-soluble vitamins in the leaves, flowers, and seeds are lost in the process.

I always make decoctions when I have to be in the same room as the stove for the entire evaporating time. With such a low heat, decoctions rarely burn, but if you become involved in something else, there is the danger of reducing the liquid to a scorched nothing. For a pint of infusion/500 ml, about an hour is needed to reduce it by half.

Making a Decoction

• Begin by straining the plant material out of the infusion and discarding it.

• Measure the liquid.

• Heat the liquid until it begins to steam; this is before it simmers and long before it boils. Stand right there and watch for the steam to start rising. When it does, turn the heat down very low.

• Steam until the liquid is reduced to half or one-quarter of what it was in the beginning. A little stainless steel pan with measuring marks on the side is of invaluable assistance in this process, but you can also judge by the mark left on the side of the pan as the liquid level falls. Or you can measure it.

• Pour the decoction into a clean or sterile bottle.

• Label with the contents, strength, and date. Example: Simple decoction of dandelion root, fall, 1988.

• Optional: Add one tablespoon of brandy or spirit per four ounces/125 ml of decoction.

• Cap well.

• Cool at room temperature, then store in the refrigerator. Some decoctions may keep for as long as a year, others ferment and sour within a few months.

Dosage: A simple decoction is four times as potent as an infusion. One cup (8 ounces/250 ml) of infusion is equal to one-quarter cup (2 ounces/60 ml) of a simple decoction. Use up to one tablespoonful/15 ml for an infant.

• Double decocting increases the strength of the infusion by a factor of sixteen (four times four). So the dose equivalent of one cup/250 ml is only one tablespoon (½ ounce/15 ml). The usual infant dose is half a teaspoon/3 ml of double decoction.

Making a Syrup

Add sugar or honey to any type of decoction, and you have a syrup. The extra sweetness makes some herbs more palatable, soothes the throat, and can improve keeping qualities. Sugar, however, increases calcium loss, nourishes yeast infections, and reduces your resistance to all infection.

How much sugar or honey should you add? The exact amount is determined by weight. A standard for syrups is an equal amount, by weight, of sugar and decoction.

One cup (8 fluid ounces/250 ml) of water or decoction weighs 8 ounces/250 grams. So one cup/250 ml of decoction requires half a pound/250 grams of sugar.

Honey is about twice as sweet as sugar. Use a quarter of a pound (4 ounces/125 grams) of honey to every cup of decoction. One level tablespoon/15 ml of honey weighs about one ounce/30 grams.

• Add the sweetener to the hot liquid.

• Increase the fire until the brew just comes to a boil.

• Pour the boiling hot syrup into a bottle and cap it. Sterilized bottles reduce the risk of producing unexpected herbal fermentations. But boiling liquid kills many yeasts in an unsterilized bottle.

• Optional: Add a tablespoon/15 ml of brandy, vodka, etc., to further stabilize the syrup.

• Store the syrup in the refrigerator once it cools. Syrups keep for 3-6 months.

Dosage: Generally, one teaspoon/5 ml of syrup is a dose for a 125-150 pound/60-70 kilogram person. The dose is repeated as needed, up to 8 times daily. Use a half teaspoonful/3 ml for 60-75 pound/20-40 kilogram children and a quarter teaspoonful/1 ml for children under 30 pounds/10 kilograms.

☆

Summary of Syrup Proportions

• Begin with one pint (16 oz/500 ml) of infusion.

• Reduce the liquid to half its original amount (8 oz/250ml).

• Add an equal amount, by weight, of sugar (8 oz/250 grams), or half the amount, by weight, of honey (4 oz/125 grams or 4 soupspoonfuls).

External Uses of Infusions

A **soak** consists of an infusion that has been rewarmed after the plant material has been strained out. The affected body part is then soaked in the warm infusion.

If you soak your feet in an herbal infusion, it's a **foot bath**, an excellent way to soothe and heal the entire body, and absorb herbal benefits.

A **sitz bath** is a big soak! Two or more quarts/liters of infusion are usually needed to fill a shallow bowl or pan big enough for you to "sitz" in.

A **bath** is an enormous soak, like steeping your body in an infusion. You can prepare an herbal bath by putting the herbs directly in the tub, but my plumber made it clear to me that herbs and drains are incompatible. Some herbals say to put the herbs in a cloth and allow the bath water to run over them but I find the resulting bath too weak. If you want a strong herbal bath, try it this way: infuse two quarts/liters of your favorite bath herb, strain, and add the liquid to your hot bath. Ahhhhh!

Enemas, douches, and **eyewashes** are herbal infusions carefully strained and inserted into the proper body cavity.

Plant material strained out of an infusion still contains healing qualities and can be used to **poultice**. Simply place the damp plant material, warmed if desired, or fresh plant material grated, chewed, or crushed, directly on the body. Poultices are preferred for first aid and infections.

Make a **compress** by putting macerated fresh or infused dried plant material into a cloth. Compressing is recommended when using hairy herbs which may irritate sensitive skin. They are less messy than poultices, and are often the choice when dealing with internal organs and growths.

For a **fomentation**, take a clean washcloth or small cotton towel, soak it in a heated infusion, ring it out, and apply. Fomentations treat breast congestion, sprains, muscle aches, and the like.

Spirit Bases

Herbs prepared in vodka, brandy, or other liquors, or vinegar, are called **tinctures**. Tinctures can be used internally or externally. Herbs prepared in rubbing alcohol are called **liniments**. Liniments are for external use only.

Tinctures

Tinctures are a popular way of using medicinal herbs. They have the following advantages over water-based preparations:

- Tinctures remain potent for many years.
- Small quantities of tinctures are effective, sometimes as little as one drop, making them more portable and potable.
- Tinctures act very rapidly, especially when administered under the tongue.
- Certain herbal alkaloids and resins are extractable only into alcohol, not water.
- A small amount of plant material produces a tincture consisting of many medicinal doses.

Nourishing factors found in herbs, such as vitamins and minerals, are poorly extracted into tinctures, and, since only small amounts of tinctures are taken, only small amounts of these nutrients are ingested. The Wise Woman tradition focuses on the excellent nourishment available in wild foods and herbs to support the body's ability to repair and heal itself. Thus, water-based preparations are usually my first choice as herbal medicines. I use tinctures when I travel, when I need immediate medicinal effect, or when I am dealing with rare, horrible tasting, or expensive plants.

People who refrain from using all alcohol can still take tinctures. Since alcohol-based tincture doses are small (20 drops is an average dose) and diluted in water, the taste and effect of the alcohol is virtually non-existent. Many ex-alcoholics indicate that herbal tinctures react like medicines in their bodies, not like alcohol. To further mitigate the effect of the alcohol, let it evaporate somewhat by adding the tincture to some water and letting it sit exposed to the air for several hours.
Dosage: Tincture dosage is widely variable. Experiment with caution and consult references.

Making a Tincture From Fresh Plant Material

The best tinctures are made from fresh plants. These tinctures are so far superior to commercial tinctures made from dried plants that they almost appear to be different medicines! Homeopaths call these "mother tinctures."

Tincturing is amazingly simple:

- Identify and pick the plant parts you desire to tincture.
- Look through the plant material and discard any damaged parts.
- Do not wash any part of the plant except roots, and those only when necessary.
- Chop the plant material coarsely, except flowers and delicate plants.
- Fill a jar to the top with the chopped plant material.
- Then fill the jar to the top with 100 proof vodka, vinegar, or the spirit of your choice. (Yes, you can fill a jar to the top twice!)
- Cap the jar tightly.
- Label the jar with the name of the plant, the part of the plant used, the type of spirit used, and the date. Example: Chickweed, whole plant in flower, 100 proof vodka, 12 May 1988.
- Top up the liquid level the next day. (The plant fairies come by and take a little taste of each new tincture.)
- Allow plant and alcohol to mingle together for six weeks or more.
- Decant the tincture and it is ready to use.

Making a Tincture From Dried Plant Material

Most dried plants are unsuitable for tincturing, with the exception of dried roots, resins, barks, and leathery leaves (such as rosemary, uva ursi, and wintergreen). Powdered herbs are never suitable for tincturing. The procedure is similar to making a tincture from fresh plants:

- Put two ounces/60 grams dried root or bark in a pint/500ml jar.
- Add ten fluid ounces/300 ml of 100 proof vodka or other spirit.
- Cap well and label (plant, part, type of spirit, date).
- Watch the alcohol level closely for the first week and top it up as necessary. (Those fairies get very thirsty.)
- Decant the tincture after six or more weeks.

Making a Vinegar Tincture

Vinegar tinctures are not very potent, don't last for as long as alcohol tinctures, and have an aggravating tendency to rust the lid onto the tincture bottle. A few medicinal herbs, such as lobelia and wintergreen, are commonly tinctured in vinegar. Many flowers, such as dandelion blossoms and violets, are put up in vinegar. Make full strength tinctures with a variety of edible flowers and seasoning herbs, and you'll be thrilled with the marinades and salad dressings you'll be able to create.

Follow the above tincture instructions for fresh and dried plants, with these changes:

- Fill your jar to the top with room temperature, not boiling,vinegar.
- Use apple cider vinegar, wine vinegar (or wine), rice vinegar, but not white vinegar.
- Use cork or plastic to cap all your vinegar tinctures. A piece of waxed paper or plastic wrap between the jar and a metal lid is acceptable.
- The usual dose of a medicinal vinegar tincture is one teaspoon/ 15 ml per hundred pounds/50 kilograms of body weight.
- In cooking, use your vinegar tincture just as you would regular vinegar. Heavenly!

Tips for Making All Tinctures

- Choose a jar that will be filled to the top by the plant material and the alcohol; if an empty "head space" is left, some of the plant material oxidizes. This is unsightly but not spoiled.
- For extra potency, put up tinctures when the moon is dark or new; decant them when the moon is full. This helps oils, too.

• Keep your tincture in a place where you can watch the interesting changes of color, and occasionally poke your finger in to get a taste. There is no need to shake it daily or keep it in isolation or the dark. Avoid strong direct sunlight though. Occasionally tinctures will ooze; protect your furniture.

• Although the tincture is ready to use in six weeks (that's one reason why you labeled it with the date—so you know when it is ready), there is no need to decant it then. I have kept some herbs sitting in their vodka for years with no problems or decrease of potency.

• To decant the tincture, just pour off the alcohol, put it into a brown glass bottle, and cap tightly. You will notice that the plant material remaining is still wet. Put small handfuls of it in a cotton cloth and wring, hard! (This also builds good muscles in the hands.) Add this extra tincture to your bottle.

• If your tincture is made from dried roots, much of it remains in the roots after decanting, because dried plant material absorbs alcohol. There are various ways to retrieve that extra tincture. The easiest way is to put the plant material through a centrifugal juicer (minus the cutting blade) such as an Acme or Braun. If you don't have access to a juicer, you can use a salad spinner. Wringing is also possible.

• Label the bottle of decanted tincture with the same information you put on the original tincture.

• When you're ready to use the tincture, put some of the decanted tincture in a small brown glass bottle with a dropper top. Please use only glass droppers, as residues from plastic droppers will interfere with the medicinal actions of the herbs (and your continued good health). Label the dropper bottle clearly and keep it in a safe place. Buy dropper bottles at your local pharmacy or by mail. (See References and Resources.)

• It is advisable to respect the potency of herbal tinctures; although it is unlikely that ingestion of even an entire ounce/30 ml bottleful could kill someone, the likelihood of unsettling effects from such a large dose is great.

Choosing Your Spirit

I prepare nearly all of my tinctures in 100 proof vodka. Other herbalist friends wouldn't think of making a tincture in anything but brandy. Pharmacists and homeopaths make their tinctures in pure grain alcohol (198 proof).

I suggest 100 proof vodka because it is readily available and fairly inexpensive, clear, and exactly half water and half alcohol. Most books which give recommendations on dosages of tinctures assume that the tincture you are using is a 50% tincture, that is, half water and half alcohol. Preparing a tincture in 100 proof vodka eliminates the need to do fancy math to determine the correct dose.

Summary of Tincture Proportions

• Tincture **one ounce/30 grams fresh** plant material in approximately **one ounce/30 ml** spirit for 6 weeks.

• Tincture **one ounce/30 grams dried** plant material in **five ounces/ 150 ml** spirit for 6 weeks.

Oil Bases

There are two very different types of oil-based herbal medicines. They are known as essential oils and infused oils.

Essential oils cannot be made easily at home. They are the pure plant oil, usually extracted by chemicals or hot steam. Hundreds of pounds/kilograms of fresh plant material may produce only a few ounces/cl of essential oil. Essential oils are readily available commercially but their quality differs greatly. They are used in aroma therapy, as insect repellents, and to increase local circulation. Distrust inexpensive essential oils.

Essential oils are intended for external use, but only after being diluted. They can be fatally poisonous if taken in quantity internally. They are also highly irritating to the mucus surfaces of the body (genitals, mouth, eyes, etc.) and may cause allergic skin reactions in some people. Be certain to keep all essential oils well out of the reach of children.

Infused oils can be made at home. They are usually reserved for external uses, but could be taken internally without disastrous results. Infused oils are much less potent than essential oils and have none of the associated side effects. Infused oils are made only from fresh plants, with the exception of some dried roots which can be coaxed into an oil base if baked in the oven for many hours.

Infuse herbs in any type of oil: olive, safflower, coconut, almond. The lighter, clearer oils are expensive; they produce delicate and beautiful infused oils. Olive oil is my personal choice; it rarely turns rancid, is absorbed easily into the skin, adds its own healing benefits to the preparation, and is available inexpensively.

Making Infused Oils

• Pick the plant on a dry, sunny day.

• Discard any diseased or soiled parts. **Do not wash any part of the plant**. If there is dirt on the plant, scrub it off with a stiff, dry brush.

• Chop the plant coarsely.

• Completely fill a clean, very dry jar with the chopped herb.

• Slowly pour oil into the jar, poking with a chopstick or knife to release air and make sure oil penetrates into all layers of the herb.

• Add enough oil to thoroughly cover all the plant material and fill the jar to the very rim. (As with preparing a tincture, it is really possible to fill that jar twice: once with herb and then again with the vehicle.)

• Cork the jar or screw on a lid.

• Label the jar with the name of the plant, the plant part used, the kind of oil used, and the date. Example: Burdock seeds, olive oil, October 1988.

• Keep the jar of infusing oil at normal room temperature and on a surface that will not be ruined by seeping oil.

• Decant the infused oil in six weeks. The plants can be left in the oil longer, but have a tendency to mold and spoil if not kept very cool.

• Oil held in the plant material after the decanting can be extracted. Put small handfuls into a clean kitchen towel or cotton cloth; squeeze and wring out the oil.

• Allow the decanted oil to sit for several days while the water in it (from the fresh plant material) settles to the bottom of the jar. Then carefully siphon or pour off the oil, leaving the water behind.

• Store at cool room temperature or refrigerate.

Troubleshooting Infused Oils

Mold grows readily in infused oils. The presence of any moisture on the herb or in the jar encourages mold growth.

• If the jar is not filled to the top, mold will grow in the air space left. To save your preparation, completely remove the mold, and fill the jar to the top with fresh oil.

• If the jar was not totally dry when you filled it, mold will grow along the inside of the jar. Save your preparation by carefully pouring the oil and plant material into a dry jar. Jars dried in the oven for five minutes immediately prior to use prevent this problem.

• If the jar is put in the sun or left near a heat source, the warmth will cause condensation inside the jar, providing the moisture necessary for colonies of mold. Remove the mold and pour oil and plant material into a fresh jar.

• If the plant material was wet when combined with the oil, mold will grow throughout the oil. Saving it is impossible. Start again.

Some herbs release **gas** as they infuse. You may notice bubbles moving in the oil; this is not a problem and does not indicate spoilage. Chickweed is notable in its gas production when infused in oil. The gas will force some of the oil out of the jar (yes, even if tightly capped). Corked jars go pop!

Rancidity occurs when there is plenty of heat and oxygen. Infused oils in an olive oil base resist rancidity at cool room temperature for several years. In very warm climates, adding the contents of a capsule or two of vitamin E to the decanted oil helps prevent rancidity. Tincture of myrrh or benzoin added to ointments also checks rancidity; use about ten drops of either per ounce/30 ml of oil.

Making Ointments

Ointments and salves are easily made from infused oils.

• Pour one ounce/30 ml of infused oil into a very small pan.

• Grate a tablespoon/15 ml of beeswax and add it to the oil. (Buy beeswax from a local beekeeper, craft supply shop, or marine supply store.)

• Place the pan on low heat; a candle flame will suffice.

• Stir constantly until the beeswax is totally melted. This rarely takes more than a minute or two.

• Pour the liquid into your ointment jar and allow it to cool and solidify.

• If the consistency is too hard, remelt and add more infused oil.

• If the consistency is too soft, remelt and add more beeswax.

References & Resources:

Green Allies and Deep Roots

*★indicates book quoted from
(and page number in this book where quote appears)*

★ *American Indian Herbology of North America* (pages 97, 209, 249)
Alma Hutchens; 1969, Arco

★ *American Medicinal Plants* (page 101)
C.F. Millspaugh; 1892 and 1974, Dover Publications Inc.

★ *Australian Weeds* (page 143)
Gai Stern; 1986, Harper & Row

★ *A City Herbal* (page 102)
Maida Silverman; 1977, Knopf

★ *Common Herbs for Natural Health* (pages 115, 145, 173)
Juliette Levy; 1974, Schocken Books

• *Compassionate Herbs*
Hilda Leyel; 1946, Farber & Farber

• *Composition of Foods*
USDA #8, 1963

• *Eating Garden Weeds*
Nancy Bubel; Country Journal, July 1977

• *Field Guide to Edible Wild Plants*
B. Angier; 1974, Stackpole

• *A Field Guide to Weeds in Australia*
C. Lamp & F. Collet; 1976 (revised '79), Inkata

• *A Field Guide to Wildflowers of Northeastern North America*
R.T. Peterson & Margaret McKenny; 1968, Houghton Mifflin

• *Grandmother's Secrets–Her Green Guide to Health from Plants*
J. Palaiseul; 1974, G.P. Putnam's Sons

★ *Guide to Medicinal Plants of the U.S.* (page 246)
Connie & A. Krochmal; 1973, New York Times

• *Guide to Medicinal Plants*
Schauenberg & Paris; 1977, Keats

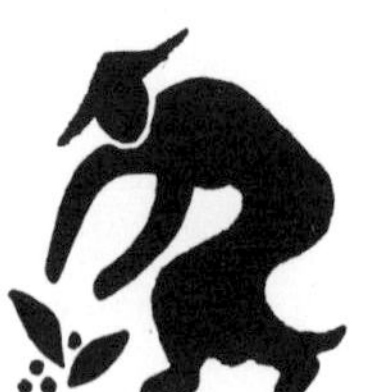

• *Handbook of Proximate Analysis–Tables of Higher Plants*
J.A. Duke & A.A. Atchley; 1986, CRC

★ *Healing with Herbs* (pages 99, 140)
Henrietta Rau; 1980, Arco

★ *Health, Happiness and the Pursuit of Herbs* (page 180)
Adele G. Dawson; 1980, S. Greene Press

★ *Health through God's Pharmacy* (page 179)
Maria Treben; 1982, Ennsthaler

• *Herb Walk*
Mary Ann Chai; 1978, Gluten

• *Herbal Bounty*
S. Foster; 1984, G.M. Smith

• *Herbal Medications*
D.G. Spoerke; 1980, Woodbridge

★ *Kings American Dispensatory* (page 122)
H.W. Felter, MD, & J.U. Lloyd, PhD; 1983, Electic Medical Publications

• *Medical Botany*
Memory & W.H. Elvin-Lewis; 1977, Wiley

• *Medical Doctor's Guide to Herbs*
J. Heinerman; 1977, Bi-World

★ *Medicinal Plants of the Mountain West* (pages 95, 144, 176)
M. Moore; 1979, Museum of New Mexico Press

★ *Modern Herbal* (pages 142, 204, 245)
Maude Grieve; 1931, Dover Publications Inc.

★ *Natural Healing with Herbs* (page 202)
H. Santillo; 1984, Hohm Press

• *New Generation Guide to Wild Flowers of Britain & Northern Europe*
A. Fitter, D. Attenborough (ed.); 1987, University of Texas Press

• *New Zealand Medicinal Plants*
S.G. Brooker, R.C. Cambie, & R.C. Cooper; 1987, Heinemann

• *Nutritional Herbology*
Mark Pedersen; 1987, Pedersen

• *Nutrition Almanac*
1975; McGraw Hill

• *Nutritive Value of Foods*
USDA #72, 1971

★ *Roots* (page 107)
Doug Elliot; 1976, Chatham

★ *The Sea Vegetable Book* (page 215)
Judith Cooper Madlener; 1977, Clarkson N. Potter Publishing

• *Scientific Validation of Herbal Medicine*
D.B. Mowrey; 1986, Cormorant

★ *Secrets of the Chinese Herbalists* (page 252)
R. Lucas; 1977 and 1987, Parker Publishing

★ *Stalking the Healthful Herbs* (page 127, 248)
Euell Gibbons; 1966, Van Rees

★ *Use of Plants for the Past 500 Years* (page 242)
Charlotte Erichsen-Brown; 1979, Breezy Creeks Press
Box 104, Aurora, Ont. Canada I4G3H1.

• *Way of Herbs*
M. Tierra; 1980, Unity

★ *Weeds and What They Tell* (page 121)
E.E. Pfeiffer; (no date), Bio-Dynamic Literature

• *The Weed Cookbook* (p. 148)
Adrienne Crowhurst; 1972, Lancer Books

• *Weeds: Guardians of the Soil*
J.A. Cocannouer; 1950, Devon Adair

★ *Weed Herbal* (pages 128, 157, 184)
Audrey Wynne Hatfield; 1969 & 1983, Sterling; Rupert Crew Limited

• *Wild Food in Australia*
A.B. & J.W. Cribb; 1987, Fontana/Collins

★ *Yoga of Herbs* (page 200)
V. Lad, D. Frawley; 1986, Lotus Press

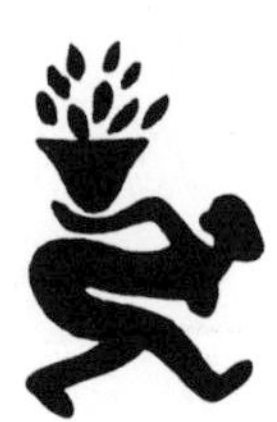
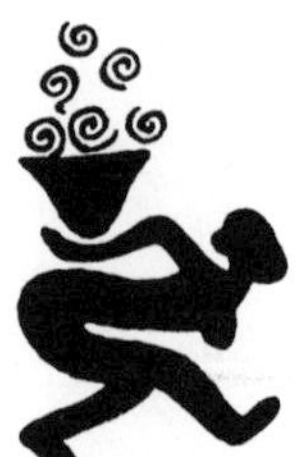
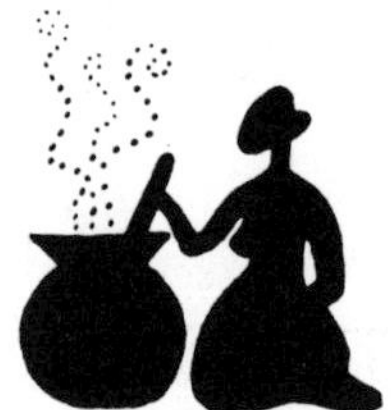

Wildfood Cookbooks

Billy Joe Tatum's Wild Foods Cookbook
Billy Joe Tatum; 1976, Workman Pub.
1 West 39 Street, NYC, NY 10018

Cooking with Wild Plants
Connie & A. Krochmal; no date, Pamphlet Productions

Edible Garden Weeds
Nancy Turner & A. Szczawinski; 1978, U. of Chicago Press
5801 S. Ellis Ave., Chicago, IL 60637

Edible Sea Vegetables of the New England Coast
L. Hanson; Box 15, Steuben, ME 04680

Exploring Nature's Uncultivated Garden
Deborah Hoog; 1987, Rainbow Montage

Field Guide to Edible Wild Plants
Lee Peterson; 1978, Houghton Mifflin

Foraging for Dinner
Helen Ross Russell; 1975, Thomas Nelson

Lawn Food Cookbook
Linda Runyon; 1985, Runyon Publishing Co.
PO Box 450, Warrensburg, NY 12885

Sea Vegetable Gourmet Cookbook
Eleanor and J. Lewallen; 1983, Mendocino Sea Veg. Co
PO Box 372, Navarro, CA 95463

Shoots and Greens of Early Spring
Wildman Brill; 1987, Brill
143-25 84th Dr., #6C, Jamaica, NY 11435

The Wild Gourmet
Babette Brackett & Maryann Lash; 1975, Godine

Mail Order Sources for Herbs

Unless otherwise noted, all herbs are wildcrafted and organically-grown.

Amrita Herbals
Rt. 1, Box 737
Floyd, VA 24380
"From the fairies to you."

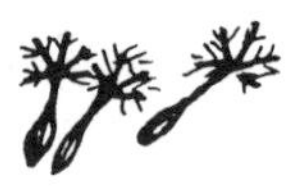

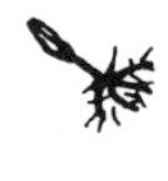

Avena Botanicals
PO Box 365
West Rockport, ME 04865
"Carefully wildcrafted and organically-grown herbal products."

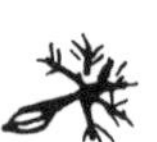

Blessed Herbs
Rt. 5, Box 1042
Ava, MO 65608
"A family business in service to the highest spirit in us all."

Equinox Botanicals
Rt. 1, Box 71
Rutland, OH 45775
"The combined experience of a physician, an herbalist, and a midwife."

Frontier Cooperative Herbs
Box 299
Norway, IA 52318
Commercial supplier with some organic herbs, including oatstraw.

Green Terrestrial
Box 41, Rt 9W
Milton, NY 12547
"In co-creation with the devas, I offer these green blessings."

Herb Pharm
Box 116
Williams, OR 97544
"The highest quality, chemical-free, herb products available."

Ryan Drum
Waldron Island, WA 98297
Incredible kelp! "Better herbs for better medicines."

Wish Garden Herbs
PO Box 1304
Boulder, CO 80306
"Attention to detail and love for women in every bottle."

Glossary

Abortive: induces expulsion of a conception, usually only during the first two months of pregnancy.

Absorbent: aids in the absorption of fluids.

AIDS/ARC: acquired immune deficiency syndrome / AIDS-related complex.

Alterative: promotes a gradual and benefical change in a being.

Analgesic: relieves pain without slowing healing; not *narcotic*.

Anodyne: allays or soothes pain, usually externally.

Anthelmintic: injures or kills intestinal parasites/worms.

Anti-anaemic: corrects or prevents a shortage of red blood cells.

Anti-asthmatic: corrects or prevents asthma.

Antibacterial: kills and prevents the growth of all bacteria.

Antibiotic: kills or prevents the growth of living organisms, especially viral and bacterial infections.

Anti-cancer: prevents the formation and growth of cancer cells.

Anti-catarrhal: diminishes inflammation and congestion of all mucus membranes.

Anti-constipative: prevents and relieves hard, slow-moving feces.

Anti-depressant: prevents or relieves depression.

Anti-diabetic: helps prevent or moderate diabetic tendencies and symptoms.

Anti-diarrheal: relieves and prevents diarrhea.

Anti-hemorrhagic: stops and helps prevent loss of a large amount of blood in a short period of time, either outside or inside the body.

Anti-neoplastic: controls, damages, or kills cancer cells.

Anti-onchotic: reduces swelling.

Anti-oxidant: prevents oxidation. In metal, oxidation produces rust. In humans, oxidation is in part responsible for signs of aging.

Anti-pyretic: reduces inner fires; cools fevers.

Anti-purine: prevents and allievates gout, usually through reduction of uric acid.

Anti-radiation: removes and prevents further absorption of radioactive elements.

Anti-rheumatic: relieves and prevents rheumatic conditions and gout.

Antiscorbutic: counteracts deficiencies of the vitamin C complex (usually refered to as ascorbic acid).

Antiseptic: kills or damages septic (infective) bacteria.

Anti-spasmodic: eases or prevents spasms, convulsions, and rigidity, especially in the muscles.

Anti-stress: reduces or eliminates the effects of stress on a person.

Anti-toxic: removes and prevents absorption of poisonous substances.

Anti-tumor: reduces and checks continuing, uncontrolled growth of new cells.

Aperient: gentle opener of the bowels; promotes easy, regular bowel movements.

Aphrodisiac: increases sexual desire and ability, usually by providing optimum nourishment to the endocrine system.

Appetizer: sharpens the appetite, especially for food.

Astringent: contracts organic tissue; can reduce secretions and diminish swelling.

Bactericide: kills and destroys bacteria.

Bacteriostatic: restrains the development of bacteria.

Bitter: contains bitter principles which nourish and often stimulate the mucus membrane of the digestive system.

Calmative: nourishes the nervous system and calms the whole person.

Cardio-tonic: nourishes and strengthens the functioning of the heart; may increase the force of contractions and slow the beat.

Carminative: expels gas (carmen = to sing); relieves, prevents flatulence.

Cathartic: a harsh laxative producing a copious, unformed stool; irritates and excites the large intestine.

Chi: Chinese term for vital force; the same as *ki*/Japanese, *prana*/Hindu, *mana*/Kahuna, *bioplasmic energy*/Russian, and *bioenergy*.

Cholagogue: stimulates flow of bile from gallbladder and through the bile ducts.

Cooling: reduces overheating; thins mucus, increases urine, moderates inflammation.

Demulcent: sooths and reduces irritation internally and externally; protects against further irritation.

Deobstruent: slowly loosens and removes obstructions to health/wholeness/holiness, that is, the flow of life, whether material, psychic, energetic, or emotional.

Depurative: removes impurities.

Diaphoretic: promotes diaphoresis (copious, profuse sweating), usually by acting on the nervous system.

Discutient: dissolves and absorbs diseased tissue, tumors, and abnormal growths.

Digestive: promotes and strengthens, but does not stimulate, digestion; often increases enzymatic action in the digestive system.

Dissolvent: disintegrates and disrupts growths and swellings.

Diuretic: promotes, sometimes stimulates, the formation and release of urine.

EBV: Epstein-Barr virus, a herpes virus.

Emetic: causes intense vomiting.

Emmenagogue: promotes normal flow of menstrual blood.

Emollient: softens and soothes, usually externally.

Epispastic: stops and helps prevent nosebleeds (epistaxis).

Erysipelas: a skin infection caused by a species of streptococci bacteria; characterized by redness, swelling, blisters, fever, pain, and swollen lymph nodes.

Estrogenic: supplies hormonal precursors, usually in the form of complex sugars, which allow the person to produce needed estrogens.

Exthanematous: heals eruptions and diseases of the skin such as roseola, rubella, chicken pox.

Expectorant: encourages, sometimes stimulates, expulsion of mucus or fluid from the bronchial tubes, lungs, and respiratory system.

Febrifuge: reduces and dispels fevers; literally, makes fevers flee.

Female tonic: nourishes and strengthens the functioning of the uterus and ovaries.

Fungicide: kills fungal infections.

Fungistatic: stops the spread and growth of fungal infections.

Galactagogue: increases the quality and quantity of breast milk.

Hepatic: strengthens and nourishes the liver and its functioning.

Hemostatic: stops or controls bleeding (*hemo*), internally or externally.

Hypnotic: induces or encourages sleep and sleepiness.

Hypoglycemic: decreases the amount of sugar in the blood; usually tonifies the pancreas and the liver.

Keratolytic: softens the skin, may cause shedding of the outer layer.

Laxative: mildly promotes bowel evacuation by increasing the bulk of the feces, softening the stool, or lubricating the intestinal surfaces.

Lithotriptic: dissolves kidney and bladder stones.

Male tonic: nourishes and strengthens the functioning of the testes; may help prevent prostate enlargement.

Mucilaginous: glue-like, gelatinous, sticky, viscid, moist; mucilaginous herbs coat, soothe, and heal the skin and internal mucus surfaces.

Nervine: nourishes, soothes, and restores the nervous system; alleviates nervous irritability.

Nutritive: provides biologically-active optimum nourishment in the form of vitamin complexes, minerals and trace minerals, amino acids, sugars, starches, and the resonance of health/wholeness/holiness.

Parturient: initiates and encourages the birthing process.

Pectoral: nourishes and strengthens the chest; relieves lung diseases.

Pityriasis: a common skin disease marked by round or oval finely-scaling, itchy patches. P. alba is without pigment and occurs mostly on the cheeks of children. P. rosea is pink, preceded by a large herald patch, and spreads over unexposed parts of the body, with many small sores following the normal creases of the body. Usually lasts four to eight weeks.

Protective: minimizes damage from environmental pollution.

Pulmonary: aids lung functioning, assists breathing.

Purgative: promotes rapid and extreme bowel evacuation; drastic.

Refrigerant: cooling.

Rejuvenative: restores youthful qualities, increases stamina, encourages *joie de vivre.*

Relaxant: eases tension and pain without sedating.

Restorative: brings back usual functioning; not as strong as a *rejuvenative.*

Rubifacient: promotes or causes reddening (*rubi*) of the skin, usually by dilating capillaries and increasing surface circulation.

Sedative: decreases or slows excessive activity; may repress healing functions.

Sexual tonic: strengthens and improves the functioning of the internal and external sexual organs; not an *aphrodisiac.*

Stimulant: increases or speeds up functional activity; often pushes one past normal limits.

Stomachic: a tonic to the action of stomach; nourishes and strengthens.

Styptic: slows or stops bleeding by contracting tissue and blood vessels; usually used externally.

Suppurative: promotes the formation of pus; draws infected matter to a head.

Tonic: nourishes the functioning (*tonus*) of a muscle, organ, or system; invigorates and strengthens all activity.

Urinary tonic: nourishes and strengthens the activity of the urinary organs.

Vermifuge: causes the expulsion of parasitic intestinal worms without necessarily killing them.

Vulnerary: promotes and quickens the scar-free healing of wounds (vulnerabilities).

Wen: a cyst of the sebaceous gland; a protuding abnormal growth. Derived from OE *wund*, a wound. Also a *rune* corresponding to "w".

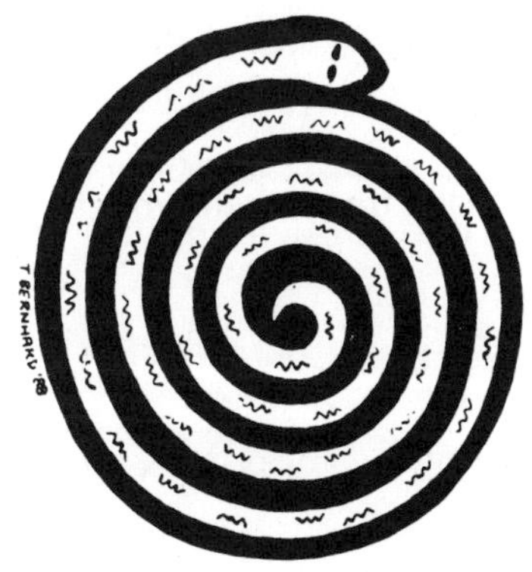

Nutritional Values

• The levels of nutrients below and in **Green Allies' Properties and Uses** sections are milligrams per 100 gram sample of the plant.
• The range in parentheses following each nutrient in the text (not here) relates both to the range found within the plant at different seasons and to the differences between actual methods of presenting the information. Many of the references I consulted converted information to a zero moisture basis (ZMB); some did not.
• Statements of very high (vhi), high (hi), and average (av) levels refer to the following ranges. RDA is the recommended daily allowance; where none is listed, the RDA has not been set.

- Aluminum: vhi (206-66), hi (66-30), av (30-7)
- Calcium: vhi (4300-1900), hi (1900-975), av (975-500), RDA (1000+)
- Chromium: vhi (3.9-1.9), hi (1.9-1.3), av (1.3-0.7)
- Cobalt: vhi (15.3-14.5), hi (14.5-10), av (10-3.5)
- Iron: vhi (253-100), hi (100-45), av (45-7.3), RDA (10-18)
- Magnesium: vhi (1960-500), hi (500-250), av (250-140), RDA (350)
- Manganese: vhi (146-14), hi (14-6.3), av (6.3-4)
- Niacin: vhi (43.5-12.5), hi (12.5-6.7), av (6.7-3.0), RDA (6.6)
- Phosphorus: vhi (2030-600), hi (600-320), av (320-150), RDA (800+)
- Potassium: vhi (8060-2500), hi (2500-1350), av (1350-1000), RDA (2.5)
- Protein: vhi (71-28%), hi (28-15%), av (15-10%)
- Riboflavin: vhi (4.6-1.5), hi (1.5-0.4), av (0.4-0.16), RDA (1.2+)
- Selenium: vhi (14.3-3), hi (3-1.5), av (1.5-0.9), RDA (0.2)
- Silicon: vhi (38.6-15), hi (15-6.5), av (6.5-2)
- Sodium: vhi (9917-300), hi (300-60), av (60-20)
- Thiamine: vhi (5.1-1.0), hi (1.0-0.4), av (0.4-0.2), RDA (1+)
- Tin: vhi (6.7-2.4), hi (2.4-2.0), av (2.0-0.9)
- Vitamin A (in International Units): vhi (80,000-24,800), hi (24,800-6200), av (6200-1000), RDA (5000)
- Vitamin C: vhi (15,000-450), hi (450-65), av (65-20), RDA (60+)
- Zinc: vhi (8.6-3.5), hi (3.5-1.5), av (1.5-0.5), RDA (15)

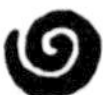

Index

Abortifacients, 101, 279
abscesses, 96, 122, 176, 245
absorbents, 119, 279
acetylcholine, 181
acid poisoning, 207
Achillea millefolium, 263
acne, 96, 101, 148, 176
acupuncturists, 71
adrenals, 173
age spots, 149
AIDS, 174
AIDS/ARC, 173, 180, 201, 279
alcohol, in tinctures, 268
alcoholic beverages, 215
algae, *see* seaweed
algin, 216, 223, 224, 226
alkalanizer, 146
Alaria esculenta, 211-234
allergies, 121, 172, 173, 181, 189, 197, 225
  children's, 203
alteratives, 95, 100, 119, 171, 222, 242, 279
alternative health care, *see* Heroic tradition
aluminum, 96, 120, 143, 216, 284
AMA health care, *see* Scientific tradition
amino acids, 201
analgesics, 222, 279
anemia, 120, 147, 175, 201, 227
animal feeds, 115, 135, 167, 197, 217
anodynes, 95, 146, 149, 150, 242, 279
anorexia, 144, 147, 201, 225, 227
anthelmintics, 177, 279
anti-anaemics, 171, 279
anti-asthmatics, 171, 279
antibacterials, 222, 279
antibiotics, 32, 95, 222, 279
  overuse, 227
anti-cancers, 222, 279
anti-catarrhals, 279
anti-constipatives, 222, 279
antidepressants, 200, 279
anti-diabetics, 171, 279
antidiarrheals, 179, 279
anti-hemorrhagics, 171, 279
anti-neoplastics, 242, 279
anti-onchotics, 95, 279
anti-oxidants, 222, 279
anti-purines, 171, 280
anti-pyretics, 95, 119, 222, 247, 280
anti-radiation, 222, 280
anti-rheumatics, 95, 171, 222, 280
antiscorbutics, 95, 119, 171, 246, 280
antiseptics, 171, 177, 181, 242, 280
anti-spasmodics, 200, 280
anti-stress, 222, 280
anti-toxics, 222, 280
anti-tumor, 95, 280
aperients, 95, 141, 146, 222, 246, 280
apéritifs, 151
aphrodisiacs, 95, 222, 280
appendicitis, 143
appetizers, 280
Arctium lappa, 86-110
Arctium minus, 90
Arctium tomentosum, 90
Arctostaphylos uva-ursi, 269
arsenic, 216, 217, 223
arteries, hardened, 173
arteriosclerosis, 144
arthritis, 96, 121, 124, 144, 150, 181, 225
ascorbic acid, *see* vitamin C
asthma, 121, 174-175
astringents, 95, 141, 171, 179, 280
atherosclerosis, 225
Avena Meditation, 206
Avena sativa, 191-210
  see also: A. barbara, fatua, nuda, orientalis, stringose, 197

Back pains, 96, 99, 102, 121, 124, 150
bacteria, 122, 225-226
bactericides, 141, 280
bacteriostatics, 95, 150, 280
barium, 216, 223
bark, preparation, 262
baths, 96, 122, 205, 266
bed sores, 102
bedwetting, 203
bee stings, *see* insect bites
beer, 151, 152, 189
bile ducts, 142
birthing energy, 99, 204
birthing tinctures, 38
bitters, 280
black cohosh *(Cimicifuga racemosa)*, 38
blackheads, *see* pimples
bladder, 99, 100, 225
    see also urinary system
blisters, 96, 122, 150
blood cleansing, 98
blood loss, 175
blood mysteries, 5, 15-17
blood poisoning, 122
blood pressure, 144, 173, 224-225, 240
blood sugar levels, 99, 144, 172, 204
blood volume, 14
blue cohosh *(Caulophyllum thalictroides)*, 38
body
    Heroic tradition, 49
    Scientific tradition, 61, 65-66
boils, 96, 102, 122, 176, 245
bone cancer, 202
bone density, 201
bones, broken, 96, 102, 148, 202, 245
boron, 215, 216
botulism, 143
bread, 215
breasts, 145
    cancer, 96, 227, 244
    milk, 146-147, 175-176
bromine, 215, 216
bronchitis, 121, 144, 174-175, 178
bruises, 102, 122, 148
burdock *(Arctium lappa)*, 86-110
    common names, 90
    dosages, 95, 97, 100-102
    facts, 90
    habitat, 90
    identification, 90
    leaf, 102-103
    life cycle, 91-94
    pharmacy, 103
    preparation, 104-105
    properties, 95-103
    range, 90
    recipes, 104-108
    root, 91-93, 95-99
    seed, 100-101, 109
    taste, 91, 93
    toxicity, 90
    uses, 95-103
    weed walk, 91-94
burdock speaks, 87-89
burns, 96, 101-102, 176, 245
bursitis, 96, 124
butterflies, 190
buying herbs, 259-260

Cadmium, 223
calcium, 96, 120, 143, 147, 172, 201-202, 215-216
    loss, 265
    RDA, 284
calmatives, 149, 222, 280
calories, 96, 147, 201, 216
Capsicum frutescens, 57
cancers, 99, 121, 144, 180, 243-244
    see also individual organ entries
candida, 98, 227
cardio-tonic, 149, 222, 280
cardiovascular system, 144, 148, 173, 224, 246
carminatives, 95, 119, 200, 280
carotenes, *see* vitamin A
cathartics, 247, 280
Catholic church, 40
Caulophyllum thalictroides, 38
cayenne *(Capsicum frutescens)*, 57
chemotherapy, 179, 227
chakra, 15, 202, 244
chamomile *(Matricaria* species), 261, 263
change, 20-22, 27
chapped skin, 149
chi, 171, 173, 280
chicken pox, 101, 122, 176, 197
chickweed *(Stellaria media)*, 111-128, 273
    common names, 115
    dosages, 119, 120, 121, 122, 124
    facts, 115
    habitat, 115
    identification, 115
    pharmacy, 124-125
    properties, 119-124
    range, 115

recipes, 125-127
taste, 117
toxicity, 115
uses, 119-124
weed walk, 116-118
chickweed speaks, 113-115
chicory *(Cichorium intybus)*, 137-138
chilblains, 205
childbirth, 38, 99, 145, 204
hemorrhage, 177
trauma, 173
chills, 227
chiropractors, 71
chloride, 216
chlorophyll, 120, 172
cholagogues, 95, 102, 141, 146, 281
cholesterol levels, 144, 147, 203, 224, 227
choline, 147
chromium, 96, 120, 143, 172, 216, 284
Cichorium intybus, 137-138
Cimicifuga racemosa, 38
circle, Heroic tradition, 49-50
cirrhosis, 143
cobalt, 96, 120, 143, 172, 216, 284
coffee substitutes, 135
cold sores, 96-97, 122
colds, 173-174, 245
chest, 121
cures, 215
colic, 203
colitis, 98, 121, 201, 226
collapse, 203
colon, 53, 226
cancer, 98, 244
see also intestinal system
comfrey *(Symphytum* species), 70
compost activators, 184
compresses, 267
congestion, 142
Conium maculatum, 178
conjunctivitis, 102, 123, 245
constipation, 121, 142, 144, 174, 201, 226
in children, 246
contraceptives, 145
convulsions, 203
cookbooks, 277
cooling, 97, 103, 119, 121-122, 200, 247, 281
copper, 120, 172, 216
corns, 150
cough syrups, 240
coughs, 101, 103, 121, 174, 180, 245-246
bloody, 177
nervous, 247
cradle cap, 246
Crataegus oxyacantha, 263
Crohn's disease, 201
croup, 121
curing, *see* healing
cystitis, 100, 121, 173, 179, 205, 226
cysts, 96, 102, 120

Dandelion *(Taraxacum officinale)*, 129-162
and burdock, 99
common names, 135
dosages, 141, 144, 146, 149
facts, 134-135
flower, 149-150, 269
habitat, 135
identification, 135
leaf, 146-148
pharmacy, 151-152
properties, 141-151
range, 135
recipes, 153-160
root, 138-139, 141-145
sap, 150-151
taste, 264
uses, 141-151
vinegar, 269
weed walk, 136-140
dandelion speaks, 131-134
dandruff, 97, 179
daydreaming, 37
death, 12-13, 21-22, 62-63
decoctions, 264-265
demulcents, 95, 100, 119, 200, 242, 281
deobstruents, 141, 281
depression, 150
depuratives, 95, 102, 146, 171, 242, 281
dermatitis, 197
from burdock, 90
Desmarestia species, 234
detergents, 146
diabetes, 99, 121, 144, 160, 204, 225, 247
water retention, 173
dialysis, 65-66, 173
diaper rash, 122
diaphoretics, 95, 200, 281
diarrhea, 174, 178, 180, 226
dieting, 123-124
digestion, 174, 243
digestive stimulants, 141

digestive system, 142, 201, 205, 240
  see also intestinal system
    and specific organs
digestives, 281
discutients, 102, 150, 281
disease, 29
disinfectants, 167
dissolvents, 242, 281
diuretics, 95, 100, 102, 120, 200, 222, 281
  dandelion, 141, 146
  nettle, 171, 179
  violet, 242, 247
Doctor D's appendix, 162
dog bites, 178
dosages
  decoctions, 265
  infusions, 263
  tinctures, 268
  see also individual herbs
dropsy, 99, 100, 145, 179
drying herbs, 258
dulse *(Laurencia pinnatifida, Palmaria palmata, Rhodymenia palmata)*, 211-234
  common names, 215
  facts, 215
  habitat, 215
  range, 215
  see also seaweed
dyes, 135, 167
dysentery, 180
dyspepsia, 142, 201

E. coli *(Escherichia coli)*, 174
ear infections, 244
Echinacea tincture, 99
eczema, 96, 101, 148, 176, 189
edema, 99, 145
Eisenia bicyclis, 214
emetics, 247, 281
emmenagogues, 281
emollients, 119, 149, 222, 242, 247, 281
emphysema, 121
endocrine system, 204, 225
  see also individual glands
epilepsy, 203, 244
epispastics, 171, 281
Epstein-Barr virus, 144, 173, 180, 281
Equisetum arvense, 202
erysipelas, 122, 281
essential oils, 271
estrogenics, 95, 281
ethylene gas, 161
expectorants, 171, 242, 247, 281
exthanematous, 95, 281
eye lotions, 124-125
eye strain, 203, 244
eyes, sore, 102, 123, 149, 205, 245

Fatigue, 172-173, 175, 204, 227
fats, 96, 120, 201, 216
  metabolism of, 226-227
febrifuges, 95, 200, 281
feelings, repressed, 225
feet, 181, 247
female tonics, 281
fertilizers, 103, 167, 184, 217, 228, 240
fever blisters, 96, 122
fevers, 99, 121, 148, 178, 244, 247
  intermittent, 180
fiber content, 96, 120, 201, 224
fibers, 167, 197, 217
fibrin, 190
fibrocystic distress, 244
fibroids, 227
fishing line, 217
flowers, preparation, 263
flus, 99, 121, 173-174, 178, 245
folic acid, 201, 215
folinic acid, 215
fomentations, 267
foraging, 257-258
  problems, 258-259
formic acid, 181
freckles, 149
French glossary, 162
frostbite, 205
fucoidan, 223
Fucus versiculosis, 216
fungicides, 141, 282
fungistatics, 95, 150, 282
fungus infections, 97, 176

Galactagogues, 141, 146, 171, 282
gall bladder, 122
gall stones, 99, 142
gas, 273
gastroenteritis, 201
Gaultheria procumbens, 269
ginger *(Zingiber officinale)*, 38
glands, swollen, 120, 244
goiter, 178, 225
goldenseal *(Hydrastis canadensis)*, 57
gout, 101, 124, 145, 181, 225

green thumb, 31
green witches, 40, 85
    references, 44-45
gum disease, 202

Hair, 101, 176, 179, 182-183, 207
hallucinations, 180
hangovers, 244
harvesting, 257-258
hawthorn berries *(Crataegus oxyacantha)*, 263
hay, 197
hay fever, 115, 121, 173
headaches, 99, 103, 150, 203, 244
    nettle, 172-173, 181, 189
healers, 33-34, 56, 66-67, 71
healing, 20, 32-33, 53-54, 61
health, 5, 12, 20, 47, 55
    Scientific tradition, 61, 63, 66, 67-69
health care options, 1
heart pain, 246
    see also cardiovascular system
heat rash, 102
heat stroke, 244
heavy metals, 217, 223
hemlock *(Conium maculatum)*, 178
hemorrhages, 175, 177
hemorrhoids, 97, 121, 174
    bleeding, 177
hemostatics, 171, 177, 282
henbane *(Hyoscyamus niger)*, 178
hepatics, 141, 149, 282
hepatitis, 142
herbs
    buying, 259-260
    harvesting, 257-258
    preparation, 258, 260-273
    sources, mail-order, 278
herbalism, 56-57, 69-70
Heroic tradition, 1-3, 47-59
    healing, 21, 32
    references, 59
    spiral of transformation, 75, 78-79
    symbol, 49-50
herpes, 96, 99, 122, 245,
hijiki *(Eisenia bicyclis, Hizikia fusiforme)*, 211-234
    common names, 214
    facts, 214
    habitat, 214
    range, 214
    see also seaweed
histamines, 181
hives, 122, 176, 181, 225
Hizikia fusiforme, 211-234
hoarseness, *see* coughs
holdfasts, 218
holograms, 18
horsetail herb *(Equisetum arvense)*, 202
hot flashes, 227
Hydrastis canadensis, 57
hydrochloric acid, 147
Hyoscyamus niger, 178
hyperactivity, 203
hypertension, 99, 225
hypnotics, 141, 177, 282
hypoglycemia, 99, 144, 204
hypoglycemics, 95, 282
hysteria, 247

Immune system, 176, 178, 180, 224-226
impetigo, 97, 246
impotence, 178, 225
indigestion, *see* digestive system
infertility, 173, 225, 227
infused oils, 271-273
infusions, 261-264
    combination, 263
    external uses, 266-267
insect bites, 122, 149, 150, 176, 178, 181
insecticides, 184, 240
insomnia, 144, 203, 244, 246
insulin, 32, 173
intentions, 85
intestinal system, 98, 121, 144, 174, 205
    see also colon
inulin, 96, 140
iodine, 215, 216
iron, 120, 143, 147, 172, 175, 189, 201, 215, 216
    RDA, 284
itches, 122

Jaundice, 142
joints, stiff, 102, 193
    see also arthritis, bursitis, gout, rheumatism

Kelp
    see also Alaria esculenta, Fucus versiculosis, Laminaria species, *Macrocystis pyrifera, Nereocystis luetkeana, Pleurophycus gardneri*
kelp, 211-234
    common names, 216

facts, 216
habitat, 216
range, 216
see also seaweed
keratolytics, 102, 150, 282
ketosis, 98
kidney stones, 145, 179
kidneys, 14, 99-100, 171, 173, 225
see also urinary system

Lactation, 146-147, 175-176
lappin, 96
Laminaria species, 216, 224
Laportea canadensis, 167
laryngitis, 245
Laurencia pinnatifida, 215
laxatives, 135, 141, 171, 177, 242, 282
lead, 216, 223
leaves, preparation, 262
leg cramps, 203
Leontodon taraxacum, 134
leukemia, 189
liniments, 267
lipids, *see* fats
lithium, 216
lithotriptics, 141, 171, 282
litmus test, 250
liver, 14, 99, 121, 142-143, 147, 160
lobelia *(Lobelia inflata)*, 57, 269
Lobelia inflata, 57, 269
longevity, 139-140, 224
love, 24-27, 37
love potions, 203-204
lubrication, lack of, 227
lumbago, 173, 205
lungs
cancer, 244
hemorrhage, 177
see also respiratory system
lupus, 201
lymphatic system, 144, 148, 173, 225-226
Lyngbya species, 234

M*acrocystis pyrifera*, 216
magnesium, 96, 120, 143, 147, 172, 215, 216
RDA, 284
malaria, 180
male tonics, 119, 282
manganese, 96, 120, 143, 147, 172, 216, 284
mastitis, 102, 148, 227, 244, 245
Matricaria species, 261, 263
measles, 101, 122, 176
measurement, 64-65
medicines
patent, 55, 57
preparation, 260-273
meditation, 206
men, 40-41, 52-53
menarche, delayed, 225
menopausal problems, 172, 225, 227
menstrual
cramps, 30-31, 145, 150, 175
cycles, 227
flow, 103, 175, 177
powers, 5
mercury, 216, 223
metabolic disturbances, 160
midwives, 71
mind, Heroic tradition, 48-49
mold, 272-273
Mollugo verticillata, 115
molybdenum, 120, 216
mononucleosis, 144
mouth cancer, 244, 245
mucilage, 96, 217
mucilaginous, 222, 242, 282
mucus surfaces, 97
multiple sclerosis, 201, 226
mumps, 245
muscle tightness, 181
mushroom mistakes, 143

Narcotics, slight, 146
nephritis, 99
Nereocystis luetkeana, 211-234
nervines, 200, 282
nerve inflammation, 173
nervous breakdown, 203
nervous system, 201, 202-203, 226, 244
nervousness, 226, 240, 244, 247
nettle *(Urtica dioica)*, 163-190
common names, 167
dosages, 171, 173, 175, 176, 177, 178, 179
facts, 167
habitat, 167
identification, 167
leaf, 171-177
pharmacy, 182-184
properties, 171-181
range, 167
recipes, 185-189
root, 179-180
seed, 177-178
stalk, 171-177
sting, 169, 181
toxicity, 167, 180

uses, 171-181
weed walk, 168-170
nettle speaks, 165-166
neural sheaths, 226
neuralgia, 205
neurasthenia, 205
neuritis, 181, 226
niacin, 120, 143,147, 172, 201, 216
RDA, 284
nickel, 216
night sweats, 175, 204
nightshade *(Solanum* species), 178
nose bleeds, 177
nourishment, 8, 13-14, 18-19, 35-38
nutritives, 95, 119, 141, 146, 171, 200, 222, 242, 282

Oatstraw *(Avena sativa)*, 191-210
common names, 197
dosages, 200
facts, 197
habitat, 197
identification, 197
pharmacy, 207
properties, 200-206
range, 197
recipes, 208-209
uses, 200-206
weed walk, 198-199
Oatstraw speaks, 193-196
obesity, 178, 225
see also dieting, weight
oil bases, 271-273
oil glands, 103
ointments, preparation, 273
ophthalmia, 123
options, 23, 24
oral tradition, 9
orchards, 161
osteoporosis, 202, 227
ovarian cancer, 120, 227
ovarian cysts, 227
ovulation, lack of, 225

***P**almaria palmata*, 211-234
palsy, 181
pancreas, 144
paper pulp, 167
paralysis, 115, 181
parturients, 282
patent medicines, 55, 57
pectorals, 119, 171, 282
pelvic inflammatory disease, 205
perfumes, 240
pertussis, *see* whooping cough
pharmacies, 255-273
burdock, 103
chickweed, 124-125
nettle, 182-184
oatstraw, 207
references, 274-276
seaweed, 228
violet, 248-250
see also **Recipe Index**
phospholipid levels, 227
phosphorus, 96, 120, 143, 147, 172, 201, 215, 216
RDA, 284
pimples, 96, 97, 101, 122, 150, 245
pinkeye, 123
pityriasis, 176, 282
placenta, expulsion, 145
Pleurophycus gardneri, 216
pleurisy, 121, 174, 245
pneumonia, 121, 144, 174-175, 178
poison ivy, 102
poison oak, 102
poisons, *see* toxins
pollen, 115, 161, 197
pollution protection, 223
postpartum hemorrhage, 175
potash, 147
potassium, 96, 120, 143, 145, 147, 172, 201, 215, 216
RDA, 284
potassium chloride, 190
potassium phosphate, 190
poultices, 103, 124, 267
pre-eclampsia, 100
pregnancy, 38, 99-101, 142, 147, 175
premenstrual problems, 99, 145, 227
prevention, 10
prickly heat, 102
prostate gland, 179, 204, 225
protectives, 222, 282
protein, 96, 120, 143, 147, 172, 201, 215, 216, 284
Pseudomonas, 174
psoriasis, 97
puke weed, *see* lobelia
pulmonaries, 95, 282
punishment, 50-51
purgatives, 282

Quinsy, 245

Racism, 52-53, 68
radioactive elements, 217, 223
radium, 215, 216
rancidity, 272, 273
rashes, 96, 97, 122, 176
  itchy, 181
  weepy, 148, 150
RDA (Recommended Daily Allowance), 284
recipes
  burdock, 104-108
  chickweed, 125-127
  dandelion, 153-160
  nettle, 185-189
  oatstraw, 208-209
  references, 277
  seaweed, 229-233
  violet, 251-252
  see also **Recipe Index**
Recommended Daily Allowance (RDA), 284
refrigerants, 119, 282
rejuvenatives, 95, 177, 222, 282
relaxants, 100, 283
relaxation, 150
  see also Avena Meditation
renosis, 145
respiratory system, 101, 121, 144, 174-175, 240, 245, 247
  see also lungs
restlessness, 244
restoratives, 119, 283
rheumatism, 96, 99, 124, 144, 172, 173, 181, 205, 225
Rhodymenia palmata, 215
riboflavin (vitamin B_2), 120, 143, 147, 172, 201, 216
  RDA, 284
rickets, 120, 202
ringworm, 102
roots, preparation, 262
Rosa species, 263
rosehips *(Rosa* species), 263
rosemary *(Rosmarinus officinalis)*, 269
Rosmarinus officinalis, 269
roundworms, 174
rubidium, 215, 216
rubifacients, 181, 283
rules, 33, 47, 51
Rumex crispus, 108

Salt, and blood pressure, 224-225
saponins, 119
Sassafras albidum, 70
sassafras root *(Sassafras albidum)*, 70
scabies, 102, 246
scabs, 122
scalds, *see* burns
scalp, 97
  infections, 176, 179
  tonic, 178
scarletina, 101
schizophrenic episodes, 203
sciatica, 96, 173, 181
Scientific tradition, 1, 2-3, 61-73
  healing, 21, 32
  pharmacy, 256
  references, 73
  spiral of transformation, 75, 76-77
scurvy, 120
seaweed, 211-234
  common names, 214-216
  dosages, 222, 225
  facts, 217
  pharmacy, 228
  preparation, 219, 221
  properties, 222-228
  recipes, 229-233
  toxicity, 217, 219, 234
  uses, 222-228
  weed walk, 218-221
  see also dulse, hijiki, and kelp
seaweed speaks, 213-214
sedatives, 141, 283
seeds, preparation, 263
selenium, 96, 172, 216
  RDA, 284
self-blame, 225
senility, 68, 226
sensory receptivity, 226, 246
sexism, 52-53, 67-69
sexual appetite, 203-204
sexual tonics, 283
Shigella, 174
silica, 147
silicon, 96, 120, 143, 172, 216, 284
silver, 216
simples, 38-39, 263
sinus infections, 244
skin, 101, 148, 149, 160, 176, 183
  cancer, 244
  disease, 205
  eruptions, 173
  flaky, 205
  helpers, 96-97, 178, 207, 248
slippery elm *(Ulmus fulva)*, 143, 201
snake bites, 178

sodium, 96, 120, 143, 145, 147, 215, 216, 224-225, 284
Solanum species, 178
sore throat, *see* coughs
spider bites, 178
spiral, Wise Woman tradition, 11, 22
spirals of transformation, 74-81
spirit bases, 267-271
spirit/soul, Heroic tradition, 48
spleen, 160, 180
  cancer, 189
splinters, 122, 176
sprains, 96, 102, 148, 245
Staphylococcus aureus, 174
Stelllaria media, 111-128, 273
Stellaria pubera, 115
sties, 102, 123
stiff neck, 124, 150
stimulants, 181, 283
stinging nettle, *see* nettle
stings, *see* insect bites
stomach, 103, 160
  aches, 150, 246
  cancer, 121, 189, 244
  see also digestive system
stomachics, 95, 141, 146, 283
stools
  bloody, 177
  watery, 226
stress, 173, 181
  mental, 226
strontium, 216, 223
styptics, 171, 283
substance abuse, 142
sulphur, 147, 172, 215
sunburn, 149
suppuratives, 242, 283
surgery, 32
sweat glands, 103
swellings, 96
Symphytum species, 70
syrups, 264-266

Taraxacerin, 147
taraxacin, 147
Taraxacum magellanicum, 134
Taraxacum mongolicum, 134
Taraxacum officinale, 129-162
teas, 160, 261
testicular problems, 120, 178
  cancer, 122
thiamine (B_1), 96, 120, 147, 172, 201, 216
  RDA, 284
thistle, 145
thread, 167
thread worms, 174
throat cancer, 244
thyroid, 120, 178, 225, 227
tics, nervous, 226
tin, 143, 172, 216, 223, 284
tincture preparation, 267-271
tinnitus, 246
tisane, 261
titanium, 215, 216
tongue cancer, 244
tonics, 95, 100, 102, 171, 179, 200, 247, 283
  dandelion, 141, 143, 146
tonsilitis, 99, 245
toothaches, 176
toxicity
  burdock, 90
  chickweed, 115
  dandelion, 135
  essential oils, 271
  nettle, 167, 180
  oatstraw, 197
  seaweeds, 217, 219, 234
  violet, 240, 243
toxin neutralizers, 98, 119, 143, 178
trace minerals, 172, 222
triglyceride levels, 227
truth, 27, 28, 61, 63
tuberculosis, 121, 144, 174
tumors, 96
typhoid, 101

Ulcers, 121, 174, 201, 226
ulcers, external, 96, 97, 102, 122, 176
Ulmus fulva, 143, 201
uniqueness, 9, 27-28
uric acid output, 101
urinary system, 100, 121, 145, 173, 179, 205, 226
  cancer, 244
  see also bladder, kidneys
urinary tonics, 95, 283
urine flow, 247
Urtica dioica, 163-190
  see also U. canadensis, gracilis, pilulifera, procera, urens, 167
urtication, 181
uterine pain, 205
uterine prolapse, 99

uterine cancer, 227
uva ursi *(Arctostaphylos uva-ursi)*, 269

Vanadium, 216
varicose veins, 96. 102
varicosities, 225
veneral infections, 99
vermifuges, 174, 177, 283
vinegar tinctures, 248, 269
Viola odorata, 235-253
  See also V. arvensis, calcarata, canadensis, clandestina, diffusa, hederacea, heterophylla, japonica, kauaiensis, palmata, papilionacea, pedata, pubescens, rotundifolia
Viola tricolor, 240, 246, 247
violet *(Viola odorata)*, 235-253
  common names, 240
  dosages, 243, 246, 247
  facts, 240
  flower, 246
  habitat, 240
  identification, 240
  pharmacy, 248-250
  properties, 242-247
  range, 240
  recipes, 251-252
  root, 247
  toxicity, 240, 243
  uses, 242, 247
  vinegar, 269
  weed walk, 241-242
violet speaks, 237-239
viruses, 225-226
vitamin A, 96, 120, 122, 143, 147, 172, 201, 215, 216, 243
  RDA, 284
vitamin B complex, 147, 172, 201, 216
  B_6, 201, 215, 216
  B_{12}, 215, 216
  see also riboflavin, niacin, and thiamine
vitamin C complex, 64, 65, 96, 120, 122, 143, 147, 172, 201, 215, 216, 243, 246
  RDA, 284
vitamin D, 172
vitamin E, 201, 215, 216
  and rancidity, 273
vitamin G, 201
vitamin K, 172, 175, 201, 216
vulneraries, 100, 102, 119, 146, 149, 242, 283

Warts, 119, 150
water bases, 261-267
water retention, 100, 173, 179, 227
weals, 122
weed walks, 256-257
  burdock, 91-94
  chickweed, 116-118
  dandelion, 136-140
  nettle, 168-170
  oatstraw, 198-199
  seaweed, 218-221
  violet, 241-242
weight, 123-124, 172, 178, 227-228
wens, 283
whooping cough, 99, 103, 121, 178, 245, 246, 247
windburn, 149
wines, 151, 178
wintergreen *(Gaultheria procumbens)*, 269
Wise Woman tradition, 1, 2-3, 5-45
  death, 12-13, 21-22
  healers, 33-34
  healing, 20, 32-33
  health, 12
  holographic understanding, 18-20
  men in, 40-41
  nourishment, 13-14, 18-19, 35-38
  pharmacy, 255, 256, 263, 268
  references, 42-44
  rules, 33
  simples, 38-39, 263
  spirals of transformation, 74-75, 79-81
  symbol, 11
  uniqueness, 9, 27-28
witch doctors, 40-41
woman-hating, 52
wormers, 174, 177
wounds, 205, 245
  infected, 96, 102, 122
  open, 97

Yarrow *(Achillea millefolium)*, 263
yeast overgrowth, intestinal, 121, 227, 265
yellow dock *(Rumex crispus)*, 108

Zinc, 96, 120, 143, 172, 216
  RDA, 284
Zingiber officinale, 38

Recipe Index

Alaria Minestrone, 233
Anne's Marinated Hijiki, 233
Aunt Violet's "Chicken" Soup, 252
Bacon, Chickweed, & Tomato Sandwich, 127
Beverages, 151, 152, 154, 189, 215, 229, 248
Biodynamic Fertilizer, 250
Bladderwrack Tea, 229
Breads, 208, 209, 230
Burdock 'n' Brown Rice, 105
Burdock Stalk Marinade, 107
Burdock Vinegar Poultice, 103
Carrot/Onion/Hijiki, 230
"Chicken-Fried" Burdock Stalks, 105
Chickweed Eye Lotion, 125
Chickweed Pesto, 126
Chickweed Poultice, 124
Chickweed Tabouli, 126
Cooked Chickweed Greens, 125
Cosmetic Preparations, 125, 182, 183, 207, 248
Creamy Violet Soup, 251
Dandelion Apéritif, 152
Dandelion Blossom Soup, 154
Dandelion Bud Breakfast, 155
Dandelion Coffee, 154
Dandelion Dip, 157
Dandelion Egg Noodles, 153
Dandelion Wine à la Laughing Rock, 151
Dandy Autumn Dish, 159
Dandy Pumpkin Soup, 156
Doctor Dandelion's Homebrew, 152
Dulse Cold Cure, 215
Fast Flower Fritters, 155
The Fast Root, 106
Festival Oatcakes, 209
First Blush Greens, 252
Garden Preparations, 103, 184, 228, 250
Grain dishes, 105, 126, 153
Green and Purple Salad, 229
Green Goddess Plant Food, 184
Herbal Compost Activator, 184
Herbed Burdock, 107
Hijiki Caponata, 231
Homemade Litmus Test, 250
Hot Stuff Dandelion, 160
Japanese Sweet and Sour Gobo, 106
Love of the Earth, 159
Mild Curried Chickweed, 127
Mother Earth/Mother Ocean Soup, 229
Nettle Beer, 189
Nettle Face Saver, 183
Nettle Goat Cheese Casserole, 187
Nettle Hair Lotion, 182
Nettle Hair Rescue, 183
Nettle Juice, 182
Nettle Porridge/Pudding, 188
Nettle Rennet, 183
Nettle Sesame Salt, 185
Nettle Soufflé, 186
Nettles Plain or Nettles Fancy, 188
Not Fishy Chowder, 231
Oat Tonic, 207
Oatcakes, 209
Oatstraw Hair Rinse, 207
Oriental Dandelion Soup, 158
Parsnips Love Burdock, 103
Plant Food Feast, 228
Rare and Common Soup, 232
Rich Russian Nettle Tonic, 185
Rosemary's Violet Moon Dreams Brew, 248
Salads, 107, 125, 126, 153, 229, 248, 251
Sesame Nettle Salt, 185
Sesame Seaweed Cornbread, 230
Shitake-Nettle-Tofu Quiche, 187
Sister Spinster's All-Purpose Insecticide, 184
Skin Soother, 207
Soups, 108, 154, 156, 158, 159, 186, 229, 231, 232, 233, 251, 252
Spring Song Soup, 186
Spring Tonic Soup, 108
Standard Greens, 157
Stinging Nettle Hair Tonic, 182
Stir-Fry Dandelion Roots, 156
Summer Flush Supper, 108
Sweet Aunt Vi, 249
Think Spring Salad, 125
Very Fancy (but easy) Dandelion Salad, 153
Vietnamese Healing Soup, 232
Violet Complexion Lotion, 248
Violet Syrup, 249
Violet Vinegar, 248
Violet Vision Salad, 251
Wild Oatmeal Bread, 208
Wild Oats 'n' Breakfast, 208
Worthy Winter Soup, 158